The Ambulance

The Ambulance

A History

RYAN CORBETT BELL

McFarland & Company, Inc., Publishers
Jefferson, North Carolina, and London

The present work is a reprint of the illustrated case bound edition of The Ambulance: A History, *first published in 2009 by McFarland.*

LIBRARY OF CONGRESS CATALOGUING-IN-PUBLICATION DATA

Bell, Ryan Corbett, 1967–
The ambulance : a history / Ryan Corbett Bell.
p.   cm.
Includes bibliographical references and index.

ISBN 978-0-7864-7301-4
softcover : acid free papers ∞

1. Ambulances—History. 2. Ambulance service—History.
3. Emergency medical technicians—History. I. Title.
[DNLM: 1. Ambulances—history. 2. Emergency Medical Services—history. 3. Emergency Medical Technicians—history. WX 215 B425a 2008]
RA995.B45   2012   362.18'8—dc22   2008033939

BRITISH LIBRARY CATALOGUING DATA ARE AVAILABLE

© 2009 Ryan Corbett Bell. All rights reserved

No part of this book may be reproduced or transmitted in any form or by any means, electronic or mechanical, including photocopying or recording, or by any information storage and retrieval system, without permission in writing from the publisher.

On the cover (from top, left to right): 19th century sketch, gathering up the ailing and the dead (C. Gastognola, in Landini's "Istoria della misericordia," 1843); Life Saving Corps, R.N.C. lifeguard training (courtesy "To the Rescue Museum," Roanoke, Virginia); police call boxes were telegraph stations; 18th century "street chair" (J.L.G. Ferris, c. 1930. Library of Congress Prints and Photographs Division, LC-USZC4-9906); cigarette premium; Bellevue ambulance surgeon (courtesy the National Library of Medicine); 20th century use of pneumatic tires (photograph by William Shipler, Utah State Historical Society); Plymouth ambulance, 1943 (University of Washington, Special Collections, C. Kinsey 2855); Gernster Field aero-ambulance (courtesy National Library of Medicine); "squad" rig suitable for transporting medical and rescue equipment; Paramedic motorcycle; ambulance at hospital emergency entrance (both © 2008 Shutterstock); medevac helicopter (courtesy Kenn Kiser); modern ambulance © 2008 Shutterstock

Manufactured in the United States of America

McFarland & Company, Inc., Publishers
Box 611, Jefferson, North Carolina 28640
www.mcfarlandpub.com

To my grandparents,
Seth, Curly, Evana, and Thelma,
and to my parents,
Karen and Jesse

Acknowledgments

This book could not have been written without the efforts of the librarians and archivists who preserve our common history. I am indebted to all who gave so generously of their professional time in the course of my research, but would like to take a brief space to mention those whose services were particularly kind.

The genesis of this book was a paper submitted to the Rochester (New York) Academy of Medicine in pursuit of a generous prize underwritten by the Kluge family, an award that financed a research trip to Cincinnati that not only introduced me to five-way chili and White Castle sliders, but which was successful enough to convince me that there was enough new material in old archives to warrant a book. At the start, my historical sleuthing was mostly accomplished in the Rochester General Hospital's museum and archives, curated by local historian emeritus Phil Maples. His generosity of spirit and time, and his ability to conjure up interesting photographs and documents from the vaults, kept the project alive. (A trip up the winding staircase to an attic bursting with banker's boxes of documents, racks of ancient uniforms, and doll-sized dioramas from forgotten fund-raising fairs was also a welcome reprieve after another thirty-hour shift on OB/GYN or Internal Medicine.)

Stephanie Brown Clarke, of the University of Rochester Medical Humanities Department, was generous with advice that helped shape the first draft of this manuscript. Thanks are also due to the ebullient Lisa Lazar at the Heinz Regional History Center in Pittsburgh, and to Phil Hallen and Mike Margerum, two pioneers of the ambulance who added immeasurably not only to the historical record but to the readability of the final book. I also wish to thank Kevin Reynolds for graciously sharing both his collection of Emergency Service Unit photographs and his knowledge of the service. Also notable for their efforts on my behalf are Christina Forte at the Santa Barbara Library, who helped trace the final days of the 19th century ambulance hero Edward Dalton, and Frank Hines of the Belmar (New Jersey) Rescue Squad, whose resources were instrumental in laying to rest an enduring mystery surrounding the earliest days of the volunteer rescue squad in the United States.

Lastly, I thank my wife, Brooke, for her tolerance of the time spent on the book. No one has ever been luckier in their choice of a partner than I, and it gives me great pleasure to commit my gratitude to the page. Finally, to all those not mentioned but who contributed to the completion and publication of this book, my sincerest thanks. May you all be as fortunate in the pursuit of your own dreams.

Table of Contents

Acknowledgments vi
Preface 1

1 • Prelude to the Ambulance 3
2 • Debut of the Ambulance 11
3 • The Modern Ambulance Appears 18
4 • Developments During the Civil War 30
5 • "Let Us No Longer Add Murder to Maiming": The Civilian Ambulance in America 49
6 • Badge and Bandages: Police Surgeons and Patrol Ambulances 80
7 • The Ambulance Surgeons 104
8 • First Aides: Early Ambulance Attendants and Emergency Hospitals 126
9 • From Horses to Horsepower 146

Between pages 176 and 177 are 8 color plates containing 12 images

10 • Siren Call: The Lure of Speed 177
11 • Specialty Squads and Disaster Cars 190
12 • The 1950s: Losing the Battle 227
13 • The 1960s: Changing Tactics 243
14 • An Incomplete Revolution: 1970 to 2000 302
15 • The Ambulance in the 21st Century 332

Appendix I. In Search of the Origins of the Misericordia 341
Appendix II. Barber Surgeons 345
Appendix III. Dalton: A Life of Service 347
Appendix IV. Shock of Life: The Portable Defibrillator 349
Chapter Notes 355
Bibliography 371
Index 379

Preface

There is no comprehensive history of the safety movement; someday it will be written and we shall find it a romance of high adventure. It will tell a story of desperate struggles against enormous odds, against nature's relentless forces, against the perils of scientific discovery, against the little understood working of change, and, sad to say, against ignorance of life saving methods so often improperly applied. Wars come and go in the world's history, but the war against accidents must go on forever.
—Julian Stanley Wise, ambulance pioneer, April 1938 [*First Aider,* Vol. 2, 4:6]

Seven decades after Wise wrote the above words, the comprehensive history of emergency medicine is yet to be written, and each passing year makes the prospective task more daunting, the material to be canvassed more expansive, and the likelihood that one chronicle could contain it all more remote. The aim of the present book is simpler, to take the most exciting element of emergency medicine—the ambulance itself—and tell the story of its origin and evolution, an epic with its own "high adventure" and "desperate struggles." While several photographic atlases of the ambulance have been published over the years, instead of another lush taxonomy for car enthusiasts (tracing the evolution of roof-lines and tail-fins like an automotive Darwin), *The Ambulance: A History* is a centuries-long look at the development of the ambulance's function, as well as its form. Naturally a subject so thoroughly associated with speed and drama deserves more than a dull compilation of dates and august names, so *The Ambulance* makes extensive use of source material to re-create, not simply recite, the critical moments in ambulance history, stretching from the dusty byways of Byzantium to our own asphalt boulevards.

My particular interest in ambulance history was sparked in medical school, when I idly wondered when interns had stopped "riding the bus" as part of their hospital training. Originally the question reflected nothing more profound than an opportunity to think about something other than biochemistry for an hour or two, but a quick turn through the card catalogue and a few minutes creeping among the stacks revealed a staggering paucity of source material on ambulance history—odd, considering the ambulance is without question one of medicine's more romantic and dramatic interventions and so presumably had a correspondingly interesting story behind it.

In fact, when I looked for the origins of the ambulance, the only work on the general history of the ambulance, aside from a few photo books, was 1978's *Ambulance!* by Katherine Traver Barkely. While *Ambulance!* remains an excellent introduction to the topic, it is stronger on description than background, and my purpose in writing this volume was to explain, not merely describe, ambulance evolution through its political, economic, and social influences, and to introduce topics omitted from previous work: for example, the critical role played by police ambulances in the development of our first emergency medical services, a concise history of the ambulance intern, an explanation of why the emergency ambulance was perfected in the United States in the late 1860s, instead of the more promising venues of Europe (where modern ambulance service had been created nearly a century earlier), new material on the role played by women in ambulance development, and a fresh look at the first paramedic services. In telling these stories every effort has been made to rely on primary sources, and the extensive endnotes will, ideally, become a set of coordinates from which other scholars will launch their own investigations—expanding and elaborating the work started here.

Of course, it was impossible to include everything that could be found, known, or plausibly inferred. (Not that I didn't try.) The threshold limitation was confining this history of the ambulance to the civilian world, referring to the battlefield only when necessary to understand developments on the boulevard: for those with an interest in military ambulances, I recommend John Haller's *Farmcarts to Fords: A History of the Military Ambulance, 1790–1925* (Southern Illinois Press, 1992), and Miller Stewart's *Moving the Wounded* (Old Army Press, 1979). Secondly, while an attempt has been made to give notice to significant developments overseas, the bulk of the material concerns the United States and Great Britain, two countries that inarguably dominated the earliest years of the civilian ambulance. Only the most dramatic and influential developments of a more global scope could be included, but absence of notice should not be equated with absence of action, although the present work is sufficient to describe the general outlines of early ambulance history.

Lastly, although the early history of the ambulance was long overdue for a thorough excavation and reconstruction, developments from the late 1960s forward have been much discussed in the literature, and this book should be considered a sort of unofficial adjunct to several previous works concerning themselves with the last thirty years or so of ambulance history. Without doubt, the definitive examination of the emergency services in the 1970s remains James Page's *The Paramedics* (Backdraft Publications, 1979). An emergency responder himself, Page's insider account of emergency service development between 1969 and 1978 is vivid, richly sourced, and invaluable. Here, a much less ambitious survey of this critical period is given, one sufficient to communicate the scope of the changes remaking ambulance history during these important years, but which aims to complement Page's history rather than replace it. Another excellent look at this era is Mickey Eisenberg's *Life in the Balance* (Oxford University Press, 1997), which provides a close-up of several influential paramedic services in the late 1960s and early 1970s while also pulling back to examine the larger forces that helped, and often hindered, their development. Carl Post's *Omaha Orange* (Jones and Bartlett, 2002) is a fast-paced account of the legislative and political history that has transformed ambulance services since 1964, augmenting its overarching survey with a road-level look at what it has meant for the practicing emergency medical technician. Finally, for those who will be satisfied with nothing less than a definitive account of each bill, regulation, and policy argument that has roiled the field in the last thirty years, there is the magisterial *Prehospital Systems and Oversight,* edited by Alexander Kuehl (Kendall Hunt, 2002). Published under the auspices of the National Association of EMS Physicians, it is a definitive and beautifully researched look at recent EMS practice and history. The present work can only touch briefly on what has been so ably done by others, but I hope *The Ambulance: A History* will not only satisfy curiosity about how the ambulance came into existence and why it followed the course it has, but will provide a context in which to appreciate the contributions of generations of men and women who dedicated their lives to the rescue of others in the hour of greatest need. Hopefully when more is understood about the challenges of the past we will be more generous in helping our emergency first responders meet the challenges of today.

· 1 ·

Prelude to the Ambulance

For the ancient Greeks the healing arts were embodied by Asclepius, son of Apollo and the apotheosis of that god's association with medicine. While revered and honored with numerous temples across Greece, Asclepius represented the somewhat chilly and impersonal abstraction of the very idea of medicine itself, and his cult was soon embellished with a more approachable junior league of minor deities who could personalize the concrete and practical aspects of the healing arts. Most illustrious were his daughters (including Panacea, goddess of cures, Hygeia, representing the state of good health, and Iaso, goddess of recuperation), assisted by a lesser constellation of sons associated with surgery. In this pantheon of names the portmanteau of medicine was unpacked and its diverse elements honored according to their utility. (Hygeia was widely revered, for example, in keeping with the idea that the best medicine was the one that prevented disease, while her unlucky brother, the surgeon Machaon, was killed off during the siege of Troy, a fate he likely shared with many of his patients in the days before antibiotics and aseptic surgical technique.)

Among all the children of Asclepius, however, there was no deity associated with the transportation of the ill, no demigod whose special charge was the ambulance (although Asclepius' first teacher, a centaur named Chiron, would have been an obvious choice). Which isn't to say that the injured and ill were simply being left where they fell, of course. Certainly from the earliest times human beings were inventing more or less elaborate versions of the stretcher, whether borne by men or towed by beasts of burden, and when wheeled carts and chariots appeared they were soon serving as impromptu ambulances to convoy the casualties of ancient life. A true ambulance, however, is more than a vehicle carrying the ill in some semblance of comfort: it is a specialized vehicle with a particular destination—namely, a hospital or its like—and incorporates in its design haste in dispatch and speed in delivery. In this way, the ambulance, like Asclepius, is actually a vessel for a host of medical ideas, ideas that must be individually realized in order to understand the nature of its intervention. Without hygiene, pharmacy, surgery, and recuperation there is no healing art, and equally it was the absence of three critical qualities coexisting together—a vehicle intended to transfer a patient, associated with a receiving place of care, and designed to move with all available speed—that sifted the stretchers, palanquins, and hammock carts of ancient history from the few antecedents clearly presaging the rocketing emergency room on wheels represented by the modern ambulance.

Under this definition of an ambulance, a vehicle specifically created to rapidly transfer a patient from the place of their injury to a dedicated point of care, the ambulance is not so old after all. Indeed, the first prototype likely appeared in the 6th century, when the Byzantine Emperor Mauricius deployed a system to convoy wounded soldiers from the battle-lines directly to the surgeon's tent. While the practice may have predated him, in Mauricius' *Ars Militaris* (circa 590 C.E.) he left the first surviving description of how a squad of horsemen was assigned to each troop of infantry, the riders pacing the action two hundred feet behind the skirmish

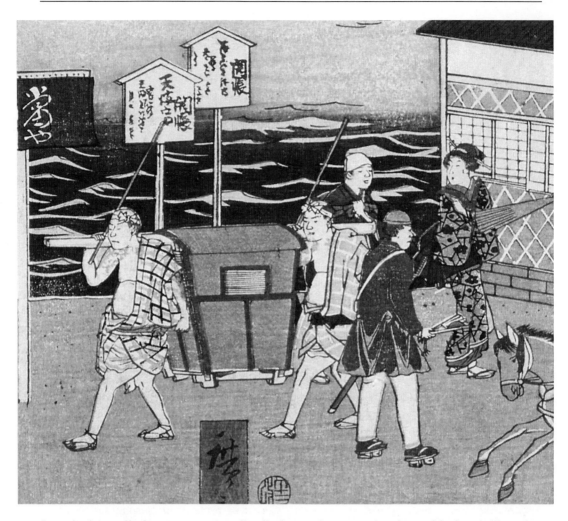

In antiquity, medical centers were usually pilgrimage sites attracting those with chronic illness but well enough to travel. The suddenly injured were carried home in impromptu "ambulances" like this Japanese version of the sedan-chair (Hiroshige Utagawa, 1870. Chadbourne Collection of Japanese Prints, no. 46, Library of Congress Prints and Photographs Division).

line. Wounded soldiers finding their way back through the chaos of battle found a rider with two iron stirrups hanging over the horse's left flank, one at each end of the saddle.[1] These scalae let the injured climb up for a swift gallop back to the medical tents, where the hard riding *deputati* received one gold coin for each man salvaged from the altar of Mars.[2] While devices such as travois, stretchers, and various carts had been used for centuries all over the world to haul the sick and injured, these Byzantine "horse ambulances" formally united the three ideas essential to a true emergency service: rescue immediately following injury, use of specially designed "vehicles," and direct transfer to a place of care.

From this humble beginning came—nothing. Mauricius' scheme was kept on the rolls for an emperor or three after him, but without elaboration within, or imitation without, the Empire, and in time it simply disappeared. For the rest of the world, the stretcher and the common cart sufficed to bring the wounded and sick to whatever refuge stood to receive them, be it their own bed, a caliphate hospital in 8th century Baghdad offering cool sherbet along with its prescriptions, or a European monastery with an abundant herb garden. In fact, Mauricius was six

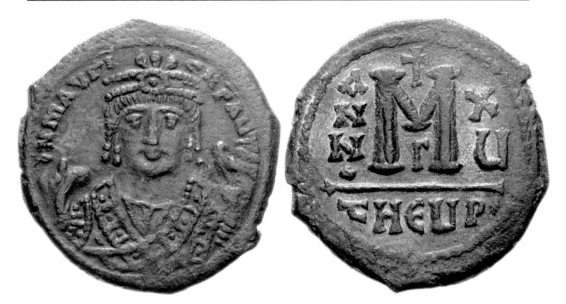

Mauricius, memorialized on a coin minted during his reign, sought to reassert the primacy of the Roman Empire over a fractious Europe and Middle East. His "horse ambulance" reflected an interest in preserving his military capital for the inevitable next campaign.

hundred years in his tomb before a humble Italian laborer raised his eyes to the example set by the emperor and founded the Brothers of Mercy, the world's first civilian ambulance service. The story begins in 13th century Florence, an autonomous city-state where poverty and sectarian strife united to create a charity that has endured for seven hundred years.

Mitte nobis, Domine...

> *We go forth, Lord, with charity, humility, and courage.*
> —Traditional prayer of the Brothers of Mercy

Within the walls of a medieval city a somber peal sounds in the night, and a train of men emerge from a rounded arch near the bell-tower, silent men clad in scarlet cloaks and the cloth mask of the *penitente*: leading the procession are two figures shouldering a crimson stretcher shaped like a deep-sided casket held aloft on long poles. Without a word the group strides along the greasy cobblestones, the folds of their long robes almost brushing the ground. Summoned by the tolling of the iron bell they will go to the bedside of some victim of fever, or perhaps of violence, load the victim into the basket-stretcher and carry him or her to a charity hospital. If they are too late, and the victim has died, they will offer to deliver the body to a chapel for a funeral mass and, if need be, will remove the remains to a pauper's graveyard for interment at their own expense. The hands that reach out to lift the body will be thick and calloused, for under their robes they are not clerics, but laborers, men who hire their backs to carry the thick bolts of wool cloth that make their city rich. This is Florence, Italy, in the middle of the 13th century, and the men who carry the stretcher are *facchine*, porters, and their office is the living embodiment of the oldest ambulance service in the world.

This slightly macabre fraternity evolved from the strange mélange of charity and brutality characterizing pre-modern Italy. Sharing a language but little else, the medieval inhabitants of the Italian peninsula formed a region but not a nation. The landscape was sectioned into tiny, disputatious city-states, each municipality further subdivided into factions of family, professional guild, religion, and allegiance to either Pope or Holy Roman Emperor. It was an age of heretics and war, of famine, pestilence, and civil unrest. It was, in short, the perfect environment for an ambulance service to make its appearance. The organization that assumed the role was the Compagnia della Misericordia, later known as the Confraternity della Misericordia or "The Brothers of Mercy." It is assumed to have taken shape in 1240, but from what rough stuff it was fashioned, by whom, or even precisely when, is a subject of debate. Anyone seeking the definitive history of the origin of the Misericordia soon finds that the trail stops cold at the banks of the Arno River, whose unruly waters flooded Florence (and the Misericordia's archives) five times between 1269 and 1288, repeated inundations that destroyed the company's oldest documents and obliterated the written history of its earliest days. Ignorance is rich soil for speculation, of course, and this fertile effluvium was left in quantity by the retreating floods. A number of competing stories have survived to explain the origin of the Misericordia, and if none are substantial enough to rout all doubters, by far the most popular tradition is the one recounted in Placido Landini's *Istoria della venerabile arciconfraternita di santa maria del misericordia*, first published in 1779.[3]

More gossip than hard-nosed historian, Landini's history skewed towards the recent past and flattering biographies of the bold-face names of his own day, so it isn't until Chapter 10 that he almost reluctantly turns to the origin of his title subject, after warning readers that "*the exact time when the venerable organization of Santa Maria Misericordia started, as well as the custom of bestowing it, cannot be found.*"[4] Despite his own misgivings, he proceeds to reveal an origin that came to him by a fantastically circuitous route. It originally appeared in a lost book written in Gothic script by Francesco Ghislieri (he provides no date, but Italian Gothic script was only used between the late 1200s and the early 1500s, when it gave way to more modern typography). Ghislieri's history was then translated in 1605 by Father Lorenzo Fici, and it was this version (itself now presumed lost) which found its way into the hands of Antonio Magliabechi, an avid bibliophile who poured his meager resources into collect-

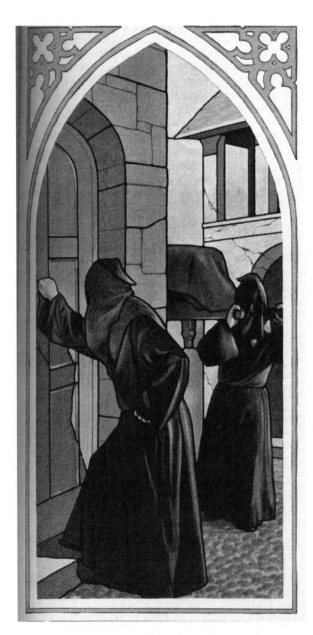

"**Dark Angels**": The Brothers of Mercy offering aid (*The Modern Hospital*, December 1923).

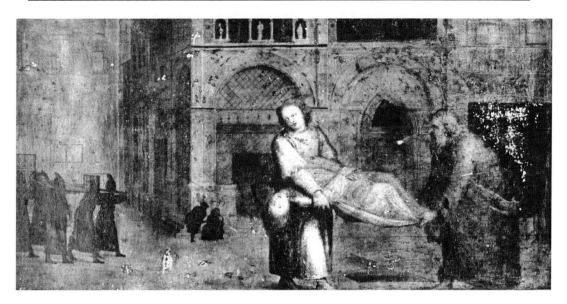

The Brothers of Mercy with their traditional shoulder-borne litter in a 1515 altar piece by Ghirlandaio. The building in the center was their oratory, where the bodies of the poor received the funeral rite before internment in a pauper's cemetery maintained by the brethren.

ing some 30,000 books and thousands of manuscripts, a collection that became a public library after his death in 1714. One of his early librarians set down a paraphrase of the 1605 translation, and, at last, it is this second generation summary that Landini quotes in his own book. The story has been broadly accepted as fact ever since, in part owing to its presumed antiquity and in part owing to its alluring narrative, and it dates the origin of the Misericordia to 1240 and the efforts of a casual laborer named Pietro Borsi.

At the time Florentine wealth was based on the wool trade, drawing buyers from all over Europe to annual fairs where enormous quantities of material were sold and vast fortunes realized by the city's merchants. Even absent the great fair days there was ample work for the city's *facchini*, or porters, lugging the wool and fabric from market to dye shop, from dye shop to merchant, from merchant to buyer, and so on through the long days and wearying years. As the work was tiring and offered no prospect for wealth or advancement, it is not surprising the porters were famous for indulging themselves with the company of good friends and bad wine, usually loitering with an abundance of both in the Piazzas of San Giovani or Santa Maria del Fiore while between jobs. On a cold night in 1240, during one of the annual fairs, several scores of them were crowded into a sort of cellar serving as a canteen, warming their outsides with a pleasant fire and their insides with wine. Among them was an old porter named Pietro di Luca Borsi who, being rather more devout than the local standard, was irritated by the frequent oaths uttered by his fellows. He suggested that each time a man blasphemed he should put a coin in a small box, by way of repentance. Surprisingly, this idea was accepted with good will by his rowdy compatriots, but the fine must have been too lenient for soon the little box was overflowing. Borsi then made another suggestion, that the money be used to finance a stretcher service whereby the city would be divided into six sections and volunteers would go out and collect the destitute sick and those injured in the street or during their work, carrying them home or to the hospital of their choice. It was Borsi's idea that this office be done for a small fee, but his fellows decided it would be better for their souls were it done gratis, and so from this humble beginning the Misericordia ambulance service saw its origin.[5] (The scheme was not so far-fetched as it may sound to a contemporary cynic, as such lay charities were actively encouraged by the church, which saw them as worthy displays of piety; were heartily endorsed by city officials, who saw in them an opportunity to have important civic functions performed at no cost to themselves; and were useful to the participants, who used the organization as an excuse to socialize and could depend on it as a sort of mutual aid society in the event of their own need.)

In keeping with a general practice of Italian charitable groups at the time, the porters went out disguised with the fabric mask and concealing robes of the penitent, the disguise guaranteeing that their charitable actions would not be contaminated by the sin of pride. At first their garments were a rich vermillion, as was the coffin-like litter that they carried. At some early date they decided that a somber black was more suited to their purpose, especially as they often were carrying away the impoverished dead to be buried in a pauper's cemetery maintained by the brotherhood.[6] The litter was borne on the shoulders of two brethren, and at intervals they would change places with those following in the van—not only to decrease their own fatigue, but also to allow the merit of their work to be shared by all. As individuals they maintained strict anonymity, but their guild was known and their work quickly earned the porters the respect of their fellow citizens: it was a respect they were jealous of, and initially the porters did not admit outsiders into the ranks of the Misericordia, apparently leading to the appearance of at least one other lay group performing a similar function.[7] In October 1423, the original Misericordia reportedly reached a rapprochement with their rival, and the two organizations affiliated themselves into a newly reorganized Compagnia della Misericordia; it is probable that the existence of early parallel groups has led to much of the mystery surrounding the origins of the service.[8] (The parochial bias persisted for centuries, and even in the 1800s, long after they had accepted volunteers from beyond the ranks of the porters, they still excluded members of the "vile arts" like butchers, fishmongers, sausage makers, servants in livery, cobblers, and coachmen.)[9]

Eventually the Company became known as the Confraternity de Misericordia (still later it became an Archconfraternity when it was given a grant to sponsor franchises in other towns), and while the group operated with variable fortunes for its first one hundred years or so, by the 15th century their work was widely acclaimed and increasing patronage financed equip-

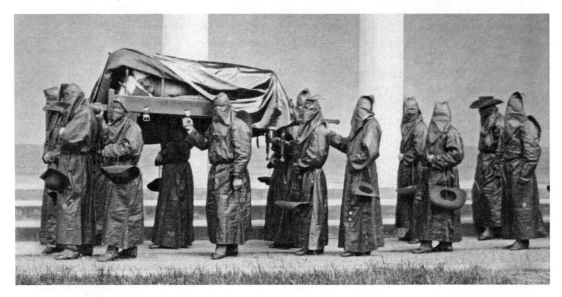

In this 19th century photograph the Brothers of Mercy pose in costumes identical to those worn by their 13th century predecessors.

ment upgrades like sedan chairs and ever more opulent shoulder borne litters. (From a relatively early date they had also expanded their charitable work to the restoration of lost children and the care of orphans, an office facilitated by putting their wards on display inside a grilled porch where passers-by might claim them.) They acquired a substantial property to conduct their meetings and store their equipment, and received ample bequests of money and property in recompense for their work during plagues in the 1300s. By 1425 they were sufficiently prosperous to attract the avaricious eye of Coismo Medici, political puppet-master of the Florentine city-state, who at the time was prominently affiliated with another medical charity, the ancient Bigallo Hospital. The Bigallo's finances were in disarray and its coffers virtually empty, so Medici schemed to rehabilitate his pet charity with a forced marriage between the Bigallo and the wealthy Misericordia. Once the societies were united Coismo promptly set about plundering the corporate dowry the porters had brought with them, raiding this endowment to erect statues of the Bigallo's patron saints over the entrance to the Misericordia's oratory: the funds were also appropriated to stage elaborate feast days honoring the Bigallo's Saints Lucy and Peter the Martyr, leaving the Misericordia to cater its own St. Tobit with the crumbs that remained.[10] In time, the demoralized porters began to drift away, and the work of the Misericordia was left undone. By 1475 the Misericordia was only a name, but that year a dead man was picked up off the street by a passerby and carried to the door of the old oratory

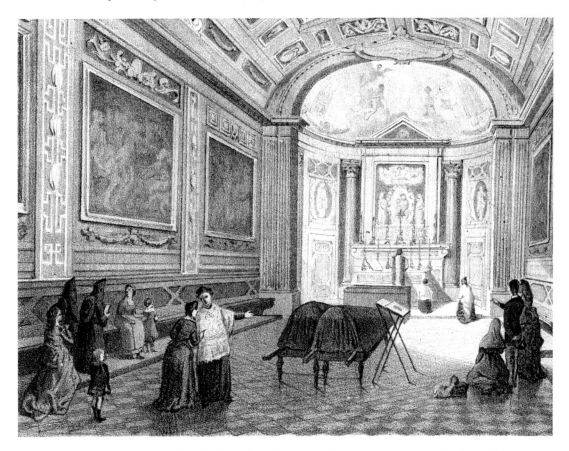

In the 19th century the once humble Misericordia was wealthy enough to support a beautiful oratorio for religious services, such as this mass for the dead. Of note, their costume remained a somber cassock surmounted by a peaked hood, with a broad-brimmed black hat (G. Castagnola, in Landini's "Istoria della Misericordia," 1843).

and left there as a cold rebuke to the ancient, nearly defunct, charity.[11] In shame the porters regrouped, set up housekeeping away from the Bigallo and soon obtained their independence by municipal decree. Never again would the Misericordia be absent from the streets of Florence, and as the centuries passed the company's antiquity and merit gave it a cachet that would have been inconceivable to the humble class of men inaugurating it, until by the 19th century even the nobility were listed among its members, shouldering the sick in anonymous silence with brethren of every stripe and station. Members were summoned by the tolling of a great bell to a meeting hall standing in the shadow of the Duomo Cathedral—one peal for the common case of illness or injury, two for a serious accident, while a triplet of sonorous notes proclaimed a death and that the litter was needed as a hearse, not an ambulance.[12]

In time the Brothers of Mercy, like the gondoliers of Venice, became a working tourist attraction whose antique pageantry and romantic history embellished, but did not replace, their genuine purpose. Eerie in their black cowls, moving silently through the streets, the Brothers were eagerly memorialized by generations of visitors in letters home, perhaps most illustriously by Alexander Dumas in 1842. His richly descriptive account preserves the conservatism of the order's traditions, nearly unchanged after six hundred years:

> The seat of the brotherhood is in the place del Duomo. Each brother has ... a box enclosing a black robe like that of the penitents, with openings only for the eyes and mouth, in order that his good actions may have the further merit of being performed in secret ... he puts on his black robe and a broad hat, takes the taper in his hand, and goes forth where the voice of misery has called him.... And when these brothers of mercy have quitted the house, the children whose father they have carried out, or the wife whose husband they have borne away, have but to look around them, and always, on some worm-eaten piece of furniture, there will be found a pious alms, deposited by an unknown hand [from *Souvenirs de Voyage en Italie*, quoted in *Blackwood's Edinburgh Magazine*, May 1843].

In after-years their equipage was modernized to horse wagons and, inevitably, the motorcar, although even into the automotive age members wore masks and monks' robes on duty. Finally, The Brothers of Mercy had inspired domestic imitators as far back as the 14th century, and today a network of Misericordia ambulance groups exists throughout Italy, honoring the foresight and piety of men humble in station but great in compassion. Still, pious and useful as he was, a medieval Florentine in a monk's cowl and carrying a wicker basket was not a true ambulance—but this idea was destined to resurface in more recognizable form some two hundred years later, during the titanic contest between the royalty of Spain and the Moors of Al Andalus, when the ancient relationship between war and medical evacuation took its defining turn, and the promise of the Byzantine *scalae* was finally redeemed when Spanish armies debuted the first vehicular ambulance service.

· 2 ·

Debut of the Ambulance

In the twilight of the Middle Ages, Spain witnessed the critical moment when the certain proximity of a receiving hospital, the inevitability of mass casualties in war, and a commitment to improved care inspired, under the auspices of Queen Isabella, the first true ambulances, albeit crude in construction and use. The inability of early military surgeons to actually *do* much to save their patients quickly dampened enthusiasm for ambulances, but their perceived effect on morale ensured that the mercy wagons were never completely unknown, however illusory their benefit appeared to objective observers. Meanwhile, away from the battlefields only the Brothers of Mercy and their Italian franchisees provided organized medical transportation, a monopoly lasting into the 17th century before yielding to ambulance services organized by city governments elsewhere in Europe. This stagnant interlude ended as it began, with war and its carnage inspiring the best in humanity to ameliorate the worst when Napoleonic surgeon Dominique Larrey matched his genius for healing against his generation's appetite for war, in the process organizing the first recognizably modern ambulance service.

Crude Medicine and Simple Wagons

In the 15th century the Spanish kingdoms of Aragon and Castile, united by the marriage between Ferdinand and Isabella, resolved to expel the last Islamic kingdoms from southern Iberia and cleave the fringe of minarets clinging to the hem of Catholic Spain. The battles were destined to drag on for years as the Moors tenaciously defended their adopted land, having little appetite for a return to the scrubby desert of North Africa after several happy centuries in Al Andalus. As her armies slowly hacked their way to the Mediterranean, Queen Isabella displayed a tender regard for the welfare of her *reconquistadores*, an interest taking tangible form with the introduction of *ambulancias*: not vehicles, but tent hospitals that could be struck and carted to whatever piece of land was being wrested from the Moors next (this tender regard did not extend to her Jewish subjects, whom she expelled, or to religious free thinkers, whom she put to torture under the Inquisition). Then, sometime around 1476, Isabella authorized the construction of special bedded wagons, each covered by an awning, to carry wounded soldiers to the shaded sanctuary of the fluttering *ambulancia* tents. Whether these wagons did double duty trucking the tents and medical equipment or were specialized vehicles traveling in the midst of the great hospital trains is not clear. In any event, their design and integration with a hospital service made them the first true ambulances and, creaking and groaning, they entered the historical record during the siege of Otrera in 1477.[1] When the Moorish citadel at Malaga fell a decade later an enormous tide of these wagons rolled into the city to collect their burden of human—or at least *Catholic* human—suffering.[2]

This idea inaugurated by the Spanish monarchs found its way into other European armies, and after a battle bedded wagons were often sent forward to collect those hurt too badly to walk. In time these *fourgons* (French for "wagon") grew to monstrous size, being drawn by as many as forty horses, and they were configured more for the convenience of the driver (fewer trips) than for the comfort of the men piled in back.[3] What is most notable about developments after Isabella dispatched the first ambulance wagons is how feeble were any efforts to improve them, despite the sanguinary excesses of the next three hundred years: for one example out of many, the opposing sides had plenty of time during the Thirty Years War (1618–48) to come up with something more elaborate than hammering benches into a wagon and stacking up the wounded when the battle was over, but no innovation appeared. Each passing century saw only the inconsistent deployment of these crude, seemingly immutable ambulance wagons. *Fourgons* were the objects of such indifference partly because an ambulance service is justifiable only when an available medical mind can reliably translate speedy attention into an improved outcome, and the outcome of a military leech's prompt attention was rarely improvement. Those injured soldiers surviving cautery with boiling oil or amputation without septic technique were delivered into the unwashed hands of a regimental apothecary and his *Dreckapotheke*, or "filth pharmacy."[4] The alchemist's chemotherapy offered there included such specifics as dog fat, scorpion oil, and mummy dust, as well as the odd potentially useful herbal like camphor and opium.[5] In such a world the absence of universal military ambulance services appears less an oversight and more a recognition of the futility of pre-modern medicine, when the creaking arrival of the ambulance offered nothing better than a jolting ride on bloodstained boards to the surgeon's tent, where the odds of survival were no better than the battlefield.

Seventeenth Century: Urban Ambulances Appear

By the early 1600s the example of the Brothers of Mercy had yet to percolate beyond the Italian states, and across Europe those suddenly stricken were carried home by whatever means was most convenient—likely a wheelbarrow or a sedan chair, depending on one's station in life. (Home was by far the likeliest disposition, as hospitals had mostly been reduced to drafty hives where, with perhaps a weekly visit from a charitable physician or surgeon, the impoverished were warehoused to recover or die as their constitutions

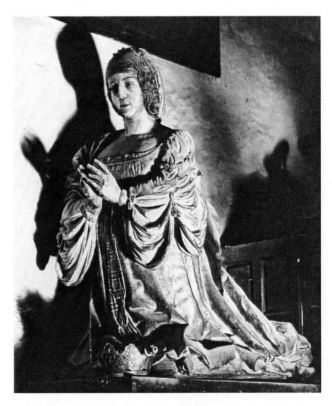

Queen Isabella I (1451–1504) is credited with the first true ambulance service, deployed during the reconquest of Spain. The last Islamic kingdom to fall was Grenada, where this statue of Isabella was commissioned to commemorate the victory (J. Laurent, photographer [circa 1870], The Library of Congress, Prints and Photographs Division, LC-USZ62-108697).

allowed.) This deinstitutionalized approach to medical care was epitomized by the earliest first aid manual published in English, Stephen Brandwell's 1633 edition of *Helps for Suddain Accidents Endangering Life, by Which Those that Live Farre from Physitians or Chirugions May Happily Preserve the Life of a Poore Friend or Neighbour, Till Such a Man May Be Had to Perfect the Cure.*[6] With the bulk of the population having its cures perfected at home by a visiting "physitian or chirugion" there was little incentive for anyone to invest in ambulance wagons to bring the injured to a hospital. In fact, prior to the 19th century hospitals did not consider it part of their mission to dedicate scarce resources for the routine transfer of the sick and injured. Even in Florence the municipally imposed alliance in 1425 between the Brothers of Mercy and the charity operating the Bigallo Hospital was crippled by the hospitallers refusal to sully their hands with the menial labor of carrying in the sick.

It was harder to ignore the needs of a patient already admitted, however, and so it is logical that the earliest report of a hospital concerning itself with patient transport involved *discharges* rather than arrivals. While the practice is likely much older, a trustees' report from 1644 shows London charity hospitals like Bridewell, Saint Bartholomew, and Saint Thomas providing "Money and other necessities" to speed the discharged homeward, often at some distance.[7] That the "naked and miserable poore" (as the hospital auditors dubbed their charges) were being given cab fare to their hovels was owed to the idea that hospitals had a responsibility to ensure patients left in a manner calculated to preserve their new-found health, and the practice of hiring transportation for the discharged persisted well into the 18th century.[8] Only in extraordinary circumstances was this concept enlarged to include a similar, if temporary, duty to patients *seeking* aid: during an outbreak of bubonic plague in 1665 the municipality of London hired sedan chairs to carry victims to a hospital or home, an action designed to limit the spread of the disease by isolating the infected as quickly as possible.[9]

A way of Sweating described by Mathiolus. There is alfo another excellent courfe to be taken (befides all thefe) by thofe of abilitie, and that is; Take a found horfe, open his belly aliue, take out all his entrayles quickly, and put the poyfoned partie naked into it, all faue his head, while the body of the horfe retaines his naturall heate: and there let him fweat well.

Stephen Brandwell's 1633 first aid guide included dubious advice about sweating out toxins by stuffing the patient inside a disemboweled horse. It would be another two hundred years before horses were routinely used to save lives in a more conventional way—by drawing ambulances to the nearest hospital.

While a brief airing-out was the only thing separating a sedan chair used as an ambulance from one used as a taxi, this ad hoc scheme stands as Great Britain's first attempt at an organized ambulance service.

Eighteenth Century: Innovative Administration, Stagnant Execution

This inauspicious beginning set the stage for the 18th century, when the civilian ambulance finally assumed a measure of importance in the history of medicine. Indeed, in 1703 the first example of a full-time *hospital based* transport service appeared in the Electorate of Saxony, a small state wedged between Poland and the Austrian-Hungarian Empire. It was here, in Leipzig, that the earliest documentation of hospital based stretcher-bearers is found.[10] Similarly, the Royal Infirmary in Edinburgh began using sedan chairs (also called street chairs) in the late 18th century: while comparing unfavorably to the comfort of recumbent travel in a Leipzig stretcher, the sedan chair likewise allowed a person to be carried straight into the hospital without the trauma of being loaded in and out of a vehicle. As an Edinburgh physician noted in 1788:

> The Great Stair [leading upstairs to the operating theater], being spacious and of easy ascent, admits of Street Chairs in which patients are brought to the Hospital with fractures, dislocations, or dangerous wounds ... without difficulty.[11]

The era of sedan chairs coincided with the splintering of Britain's Barber and Surgeon Guild into separate entities in 1745, after which surgeons distanced themselves from their

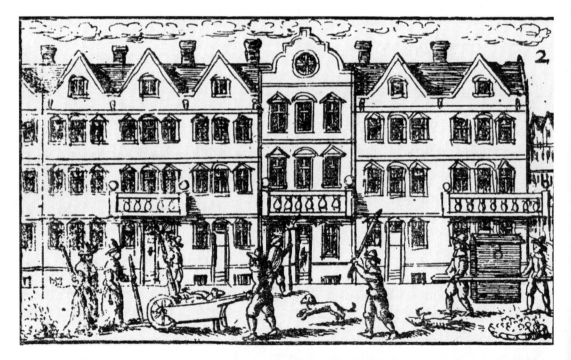

Published in London during an epidemic in 1665 this broadside included a sketch of a sedan chair being used as a plague ambulance, while in the foreground a wheelbarrow carts away the dead (John Dunstall, 1665).

embarrassing tonsorial relations, and improved their professional standing, by becoming more involved in hospital administration.[12] One of their first goals was getting more accident cases admitted to infirmaries, since consolidating their patients under a single roof not only spared the bone-smith the drudgery of calling on patients across the city, but in teaching hospitals each misadventure was another object to lecture over. That a good ambulance service might further these ends, and benefit the public, was first grasped by the Middlesex Hospital Board in 1777 when it debuted England's original hospital ambulance service: a "chair and horse" purchased to transfer the injured "in case of accidents," according to its October minutes.[13] (Located in northwest London, Middlesex Hospital was a teaching hospital serving a rapidly growing business district whose main thoroughfare was so notoriously crowded and dangerous that, if properly harvested, it could be counted on to continually replenish the curriculum with trauma cases.) This vehicle was most likely a wheeled sedan chair drawn by a horse in shafts, an equine rickshaw whose hybrid nature was a way-station between sedan chairs and the carriages soon replacing them as the preferred means of both public transit and impromptu ambulance work.

However they arrived, at the hospital the patient would have been unloaded and carried into the hospital's receiving room. Throughout the 18th century these reception wards were almost as crude as the makeshift ambulances serving them, usually being staffed by apprentice surgeons called "duty dressers." Often working alone, dressers were authorized to perform simple out-patient procedures like draining an abscess or amputating a finger. More serious matters, such as strangulated hernia or fractures, were admitted to the hospital at their discretion, upon which the surgeon would be summoned.[14] In time this direct admission of accident

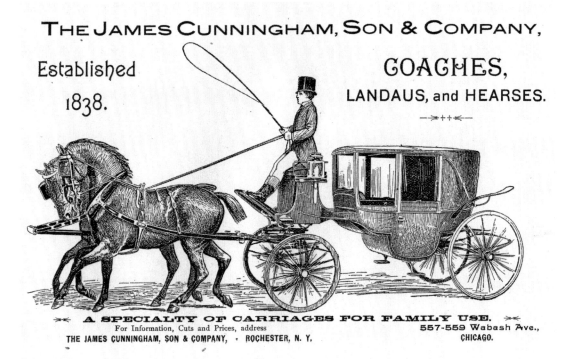

With wooden wheels and stiff springs, 19th century cabs were ill suited to transfer trauma cases, and when used for infectious cases they exposed subsequent passengers to contagion. (In 1909 Cunningham would introduce the first mass-produced automotive ambulance.)

cases to the hospital motivated improvement in both services: after all, a poorly managed casualty office would nullify the efforts of the best ambulance team and vice versa, and the integration of the two operations, though decades in coming, proved essential to the reimagining of the ambulance as a *medical* service rather than merely a delivery vehicle. Meanwhile, as hospitals made incremental investments in the delivery of the mangled and maimed to their receiving rooms, a second transportation question involving a different class of patients was becoming increasingly difficult to ignore: as the Industrial Revolution led to a rapid overgrowth of cities and towns the ensuing crowding and poor sanitation contributed to the "golden age of fever." Since the fevered ill risked contaminating whatever they touched, hauling them about in public conveyances like sedan chairs ignited a debate over whether hospitals should be required, or at least encouraged, to assume the costs of dedicated ambulance services. One of the first institutions to take responsibility for such a sanitary transportation service was the Manchester Board of Health. In May 1796 the Board opened a quarantine hospital "for the prevention of infectious fevers," and the third regulation for admission stated:

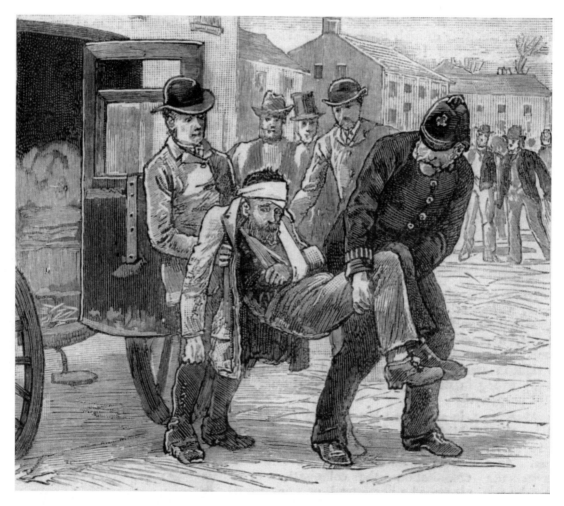

Transport by cab was often agonizing for patients with traumatic injuries, but the decentralized nature of medical and public services made it difficult to finance and maintain the sort of universal ambulance services that would spare patients these tortures (*The Graphic*, November 27, 1886).

That such patients, as the physicians shall deem peculiar objects of recommendation, either on account of their extreme poverty, or of the close and crowded state of their habitations, shall be conveyed in a sedan chair (provided with a movable washing lining) and kept for the sole purpose, and distinguished by proper marks, to the House of Recovery.[15]

With its washable lining this dedicated vehicle was as sanitary as current technology allowed, but institutional inertia, cost concerns, and even debate over the truth of the germ theory of disease meant that it inspired few imitators, and for decades longer the traveler shared public transport with small pox and typhoid victims, to the detriment of both classes. Indeed, the next evolution in ambulance service didn't separate the healthy from the sick—it just gave them a marginally more comfortable ride in which to pick up germs. It happened when the sedan chair, that workhouse of hospitals for centuries, finally give way to the coach in the early 19th century. Although the discarded carriages of royalty and gentry had been available for public hire since at least the 1600s, sedan chairs had predominated, being cheaper and more suitable for narrow, medieval streets. Increasing wealth, larger cities with greater distances and, crucially, lighter and smaller hackney coaches (typified by the French cabriolet reaching London in 1820) spelled the doom of the sedan chair by the early 1800s. Meanwhile, despite the influence of surgeons in some hospitals and the efforts of a few contagious disease enthusiasts, ambulance services remained rare as infirmaries trusted the ingenuity of their patients to arrange transportation. Where it did exist, the ambulance remained a common carrier drafted into hospital service, never an extension of the hospital or a means of delivering care. Whether it was a hack hired in the street or a second-hand cab purchased by the hospital itself to collect injury cases or bring in scheduled admissions too poor to hire their own transportation, such vehicles, like the sedan chairs before them, had been designed to transfer healthy individuals through city streets or along the country roads, and when adopted by the hospitals for invalid transfer little or no alteration was made to retrofit them for their new role, with predictable results. In the words of one 19th century surgeon, "Who ... accustomed to visit hospitals, has not seen patients with fractured limbs actually hopping out of cabs, to avoid handling ... or has not seen the floor of the conveyance deluged with the blood of the unfortunate sufferer?"[16] Ultimately, it would take a brilliant innovation by a Napoleonic surgeon to finally open the way for the modern ambulance.

• 3 •

The Modern Ambulance Appears

Dominique-Jean Larrey, the Frenchman who gave the world the ambulance as we know it today, was a slight man with a powerful mind and not only great physical bravery, amply demonstrated under fire during the Napoleonic Wars, but also the much rarer quality of moral courage: he was willing to court professional condemnation when he thought he was right, not least when he willingly wagered his reputation on an untried scheme to provide first aid on the battlefield. He was also vain, intrigued endlessly for social position, and, like many geniuses, had no patience for foolish little minds who failed to swiftly acknowledge his superiority: however, unlike many men and women even more endowed by nature than he, his worst qualities never prevented his better ones from accomplishing their ends.

Born in 1766 to a French surgeon, Larrey was practicing medicine in Paris when Robespierre jerked France out from under the slippered feet of the *ancien régime*. An adventurer who came to Paris after a turn as ship's surgeon aboard a North Atlantic schooner, Larrey embraced the revolutionary cause with ardor and by 1792 proudly wore the tunic of a military surgeon in the Grand Army of the Republic. Unfortunately, the soldiers fighting to create a modern Europe were, medically, not appreciably better off than their martial ancestors had been in the days of Ferdinand and Isabella: Larrey summarized this stagnant state of affairs in his memoirs while writing about the fall of Spire in 1792:

> The military regulations required that [field hospitals] should always be one league distant from the Army. The wounded were left on the field, until after the engagement, and were then collected at a convenient spot, to which the [field hospitals] speeded as soon as possible; but the number of wagons interposed between them and the Army, and many other difficulties so retarded their progress that they never arrived in less than twenty-four or thirty-six hours, so that most of the wounded died for want of assistance.[1]

While some units made an effort to detail men (often members of the regimental band) to stretcher duty, their scant numbers, poor discipline, and inadequate training rendered them of only marginal benefit. Overall, Larrey confronted a system designed to bring the hospital to the man, rather than the man to the hospital, with inevitable delay.

Ultimately, it was the aftermath of a comparatively trivial battle outside a minor Belgian town that triggered Larrey's monumental creation. In 1792 Limbourg, popularly known as the birthplace of odoriferous Limburger cheese, hosted a skirmish between the Prussians and Napoleon's Army of the Rhine. The French came out the worst for it, and, as only a fraction of their injured had been carried to the rear in the actual fighting, during the retreat under cover of darkness a great number of casualties were left on the battleground, abandoned to the night and the enemy. Deeply affected by the fate of his wounded men, Larrey cast about for a means for preventing such medical debacles. In considering the logistics of the problem his attention was caught by one of the French army's recent innovations—the placing of its field guns onto

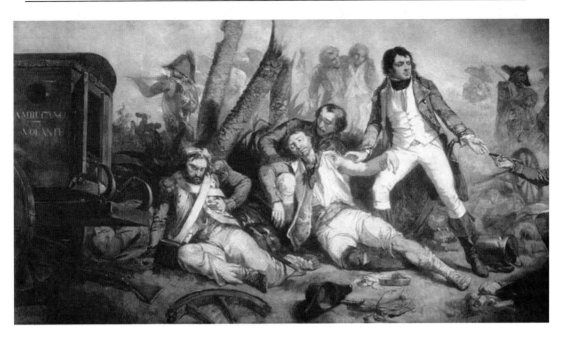

Dominique Larrey, famous for treating the wounded under fire, is shown next to one of his innovative "flying ambulances" (Charles Louis Muller, "Larrey opérant sur le champ de Bataille," c. 1860).

light, comparatively mobile carriages to create "flying artillery."¹ One invention inspired another in Larrey's active brain and, as recounted in his memoirs,

> This misfortune induced me to propose to the general, and to the commissary general ... the plan of an ambulance, calculated to follow the advance guard in the same manner as the flying artillery ... and I was authorized to construct a carriage, which I called the flying ambulance.²

Larrey lost no time organizing his pre-existing field hospitals, called *hopital ambulant*, around the new *escouades volant*. These "flying squads'" sent surgeons and attendants sallying onto the battlefield in light transport wagons to provide first-aid for the wounded before bringing them back to the *hopital ambulants* for definitive treatment. The tripartite combination of specialty vehicles for patient transport, medically trained attendants accompanying the patient to a hospital, and the goal of immediate response to an injury made this scheme the first recognizably modern ambulance service.

Larrey's Invention

Larrey actually developed two distinct transport carriages: two wheeled models for use on level terrain and four wheeled versions for uneven and mountainous ground. As Larrey described them:

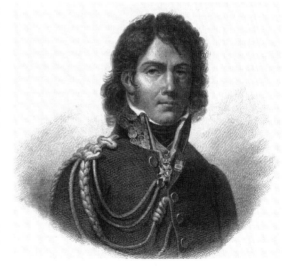

Portrait of Dominque Larrey in the uniform of a surgeon of the Army of the Republic, circa 1795.

The frame ... resembled an elongated cube, curved on the top: it had two small windows on each side, a folding door opened before and behind. The floor of the body was movable; and on it were placed a hair mattress, and a bolster of the same, covered with leather. This floor moved easily on the sides of the body by means of four small rollers; on the sides were four iron handles through which the sashes of the soldiers were passed, while putting the wounded on the sliding floor. These sashes served instead of litters for carrying the wounded; [and the men] were dressed on these floors when the weather did not permit them to be dressed on the ground.[3]

(The uniform sashes that Larrey mentions were made of heavy red wool, and when these wide bands were unwound they could be used as simple stretchers.)

Designed to carry two men lying flat, both styles of the carriage had padded wainscoting on the interior for the comfort of the men being jostled within and featured wall panels that opened outwards, permitting the wounded to be loaded from the side. Larrey also noted, with his French eye for beauty, that his Reubenesque ambulances "united solidity with lightness and elegance."[4] Supplementing the ambulance carriages were heavy wagons, drawn by four horses to the ambulances' two, which transported the bulk of the medical equipment and staff, as well as carrying forage for the horses. Each large wagon also secreted, in their undercarriage, a flat wheelbarrow for moving equipment or wounded men short distances. Surgeon-officers accompanied the carriages, carrying modified cartridge boxes stuffed with instruments, medicine, and other accouterments of first aid.[5] Where officers of the line carried large caliber cavalry pistols in saddle holsters, the surgeons carried courier bags stuffed with field dressings — and, in keeping with the "elegance" of the ambulances they attended, the flaps of the bags were trimmed in lace.[6]

Larrey's carriages first saw action when the French abandoned the mountain fortress of

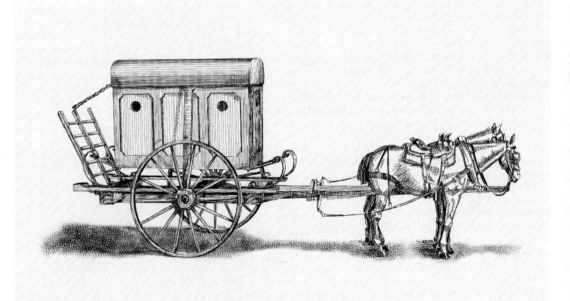

Larrey's flying ambulance. The four wheeled type provided more stability and comfort than the lighter, two-wheeled version, which tended to sway sickeningly over all but the smoothest roads (Alexander Savin, ISD Group).

Koenigstein in 1792, carrying their wounded in the new ambulances during an escape over craggy roads above the Elbe. By 1793 the ambulance had been adopted by the entire Army of the Rhine, although they were not integrated into the whole of Napoleon's forces until 1797. By then in its maturity, Larrey's hopital ambulant was a considerable force divided into divisions, each commanded by a chief surgeon overseeing sixteen carriages, twelve ambulances, four supply wagons, and sixty-four troops, including fourteen junior surgeons and thirty-seven infirmiers, acting as orderlies and nurses.[7] There were other, competing schemes, most notably Baron Percy's "wurst'" wagons, elongated caskets that were meant to be straddled by their crews as if riding a saw-horse. Unlike Larrey's plan, these wagons were intended to deliver surgeons and their equipment to the battlefield, but not necessarily to carry casualties away: it was assumed that the wounded would be brought back in stretchers, although the lightly injured could of course ride back with the surgeons if space allowed. Ultimately it was Larrey's design, which permitted not only delivery of medical care but retrieval of the seriously hurt, which prevailed and became the French standard.

By the early 1800s the French Army was fielding the most sophisticated emergency medical service yet devised, and Larrey was the object of the richly deserved adoration of the soldiers whom he served. Napoleon would bequeath 100,000 francs to Baron Larrey, declaring in his will that the surgeon was "the worthiest man I ever met," and the story is told that, amidst the carnage of Waterloo, Wellington directed his cannon-fire away from Larrey and his men as they recovered the wounded. Looking across the gently undulating field, where the French ambulances struggled to keep pace with the butchery in a fog of cannon and rifle smoke, Wellington pointed to the surgeon with his sword and remarked to his lieutenants: "I salute the

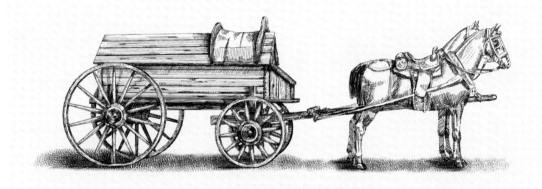

Baron Percy's wurst-wagon: While second to Larrey in ambulance design, he was a brilliant teacher and the author of influential textbooks on military medicine. His funerary monument proclaimed him "the father of military surgeons" (Alexander Savin, ISD Group).

courage and devotion of an age that is no longer ours."[8] Wellington's compliments aside, the ambulance made little progress across the Channel in the ensuing decades, due in no small part to the reluctance of the Iron Duke himself: when his medical officers asked for more ambulance wagons Wellington demurred, estimating that delays occasioned by their presence on the roads would cost more lives than they would save. His miscalculation influenced British ambulance investment for decades to come, culminating in a shocking medical collapse in the Crimea that profoundly influenced ambulance development on the battlefield and, by extension, the boulevard.

Crimean Lessons

When the Crimean War broke out in 1853 the British War Office felt the exigencies of battle could easily be met by the time-honored expedient of sending up stretchers carried by drummer boys and regimental musicians. Backing them up were a score of two-wheeled ambulance carts and an equal number of larger, four-wheeled ambulance wagons, all staffed by grizzled old pensioners.[9] In the event, the smaller carts were so unstable over the broken ground and rough roads as to be useless, and a *Times* correspondent reported that ambulance drivers discovered "not only are surgeons not to be had, but there are no dressers or nurses to attend on the sick during the intervals between [their] visits."[10] Surrounded by death and pestilence, their efforts made futile by the absence of any coherent medical service, the ambulance drivers abandoned themselves to the soporific of liquor, guzzling the "medicinal'" brandy laid in for the patients as quickly as it arrived.[11] In the Bulgarian port city of Varna a commanding officer took stock of the besotted ambulance corps and wrote their epitaph in clipped military style: "Cholera increasing.... The old pensioners sent out with the ambulance wagons are dropping off fast. I expect they will all be buried at Varna. Worn out before coming here, they get drunk when they can and die like dogs."[12]

The French, for their part, maintained the essentials of Larrey's ambulance scheme, including "flying ambulances'" deployed under fire carrying a pair of surgeons and two *infirmiers*,

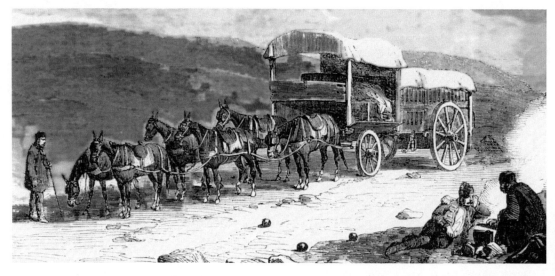

A British ambulance carriage awaits the wounded near Sevastopol in 1855. Its large frame and poor springs made it clumsy to handle and jolting to ride in (*The Illustrated London News*, June 2, 1855).

backed up behind the lines by heavier carriages ready to receive transfers and equipped with an officer, five surgeons, twelve nurses, and enough material for 1,000 dressings.[13] The difference between the nations was pointedly described in December 1854 by a *Times* war correspondent who noted "while our soldiers were creeping about with haybands round their feet and in great-coats that scarce held together" the French not only had warm clothes that fit but also "a sufficiency of wagons and ambulances, and a great abundance of mules in good condition."[14] Indeed, the reporter confessed that the British were reduced to begging the loan of French mules to carry in their own sick and wounded, as the Empire's horses were so weak and sick that it took, allegedly, forty to haul a single cannon. (It should be noted that the disastrous absence of sanitation that turned hospitals into charnel houses afflicted the French as well as the British, and despite superior ambulance services the mortality rate for France's wounded was no better than that of her allies.) The failure of the British to appropriately handle their wounded and convalescent became a scandal notorious throughout the world—or at least that portion of the world that read newspapers, which were thick with dispatches from the front detailing the misery of the Crimean campaign. In America, newspapers followed the war closely, and the deficiencies of the British medical service attracted keen interest in Washington. Indeed, a certain Major (later General) McClellan was on the 1855 "Commission to the Crimea" dispatched by the United States to observe the ruinous campaign first-hand, and one of their reports specifically addressed the want of ambulance services.[15] Later, General McClellan was the first commander to provide well-organized ambulance services in the Union armies, and it is probable his action sprang in part from his recollection of the suffering attributable to their absence from the British forces in the Crimean campaign.

Urban Ambulances of the Early 19th Century

Meanwhile, in the *civilian* world the concept of the ambulance had yet to seize the imagination of office holder, hospital executive, or the common citizen, although the coverage of the Crimean medical crisis did put the idea of the ambulance in front of every news reader for the better part of two years. Prior to 1865 no organized emergency ambulance service existed in any municipality in the United States (although infectious disease hospitals frequently used hand-carts and occasionally even carriages to drag in their charges), while European hospitals still depended on public conveyances, the independent efforts of charitable individuals like the Brothers of Mercy in Italy, or hospital porters carrying heavy, long-poled stretchers whose stout frames resembled coffee-tables, complete with stubby legs.[16] (Nor is there any evidence that the rest of the planet, from Cairo to Peking, from Buenos Aires to Muscat, was any further ahead.) Notably, Britain's experience with ambulance services predated by many years that of the United States, and yet the United Kingdom long felt the want of uniform, systematic services such as would be found in New York City and other American municipalities by the 1870s. London, in particular, was rich in hospitals, capital, and sheer need, and even in the 18th century individual infirmaries like the Middlesex Hospital had experimented with enhanced ambulance services which, had they been duplicated and maintained, would have made London the unquestioned leader in civilian emergency medical service. Why, then, did the great city, and the United Kingdom as a whole, end up a poor second to her initially inept rival, the United States? The answer lies in the complex web of jurisdictions that once separated the greatest metropolis in the western world into a smattering of principalities resembling the feuding duchies of pre-unification Germany more than a modern city. (This infirmity bedeviled other British cities as well, and so the analysis of the one will help illuminate the many.)

The story begins with the religious houses that ran the hospitals serving the poor in Great

Britain throughout the Middle Ages, just as they did in continental Europe. In 1534, however, Henry VIII took control of the Catholic Church in England and by 1540 the greater part of the country's monasteries, friaries, and nunneries had been suppressed. This paved the way for his daughter, Elizabeth I, to make public health and care of indigents the responsibility of individual parishes, rather than the obligation of local chapters of nationally organized religious institutions. The resulting decentralized system meant that the unequal distribution of talent among humanity would ensure that nothing more than chance determined whether a particular community's medical care was better than average, worse, or in the broad middle. Looking at London in particular, occasionally an institution, like the Middlesex Hospital in 1796, trotted out an innovative vehicle to bring in the sick, but despite such occasional advances *The Lancet* ruefully observed in 1856 that "the vastness of the metropolis and the incoherence of its government precludes it from taking advantage of the teachings of experience."[17] For the majority of Londoners, therefore, from the 18th century onward the fastest way to move the sick or injured was in a hastily hired public conveyance, if one could afford it, or in a wheelbarrow or carried on a plank if one could not.

The first British reform effort with implications for ambulance development, The Poor Law Act of 1831, actually perpetuated this ancient evil by creating thirty autonomous Boards of Guardians to oversee London charitable services, ensuring that no single body had the authority or resources to establish city-wide ambulance services or enforce uniform standards—had anyone even been inclined to do so. In the event, each of these tiny sovereigns displayed varying degrees of initiative when it came to the health of those within their sphere, and collectively their efforts at patient transport failed to assume an organization worthy of their responsibilities. As in centuries past hired conveyances continued to handle the majority of the sick, despite the generosity of a few newly created Boards who purchased the odd carriage to transport the destitute ill directly to a workhouse hospital. Then, a year after the Poor Law took effect, a health catastrophe challenged Britain's inadequate ambulance services when the reign of King Cholera forced the hand of reformers, prompting concerted efforts to end the substitution of public cabs for a modern ambulance service.

After evolving on the sub-continent, Asiatic cholera was introduced to the United Kingdom in 1831 through the vector of infected crew members from Russian ships. The scale of death visited by the new epidemic was shocking, with some 50,000 fatalities in the first year.[18] Still, Great Britain

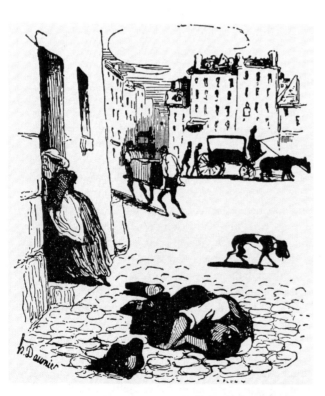

Something of the horror of cholera is given by this sketch of the French 1832 epidemic, as porters carry a victim off in an enclosed "sanitary" stretcher and a hearse rumbles along. Cholera quickly became a critical spur for improved ambulance services in England and, much later, in the United States (Daumier, circa 1832).

was no stranger to epidemic disease—small pox and scarlet fever had been afflicting the population for centuries—but cholera's virulence (the dehydration from waves of diarrhea and painful vomiting could be fatal within twenty-four hours of onset) and a loathsomeness undiluted by familiarity combined to shock the public out of the fatalism accompanying domestic breeds of pestilence. Realizing that curbing an outbreak required isolating the sick as swiftly as possible, city officials began resurrecting the ambulance from obscurity. As early as 1832 Manchester used public funds to purchase a special van to deliver victims of its first cholera epidemic to the hospital: unfortunately, the vehicle so resembled a hearse that many patients were in mortal terror of it, families were loath to summon it, and the dread it excited was presumed detrimental to the health of the sick.[19] Despite its inauspicious beginning, the fever ambulance proved its worth by providing greater comfort for those transported and limiting the spread of contagion by reducing the number of infectious who reached the hospital in a public cab. Other infirmaries slowly, but far from universally, adopted the idea of Manchester's fever van (if not its macabre shape), and by 1847 London's Kensington, Islington, and Whitechapel workhouses all owned coaches servicing their associated charity hospitals.[20] Overall, the authorities' dilatory response angered many physicians, and by 1856 *The Lancet* was using its editorial page to advocate universal ambulance service:

> It is therefore a point of urgent necessity, for the sake of the public as well as the sick, that each workhouse should be provided with an ambulance, in which a patient can be conveyed in the horizontal position. Some parishes, such as Shoreditch and others, are already in possession of vehicles of their own. We trust that the vestries will immediately turn their attention to this alteration ["Street Cabs and Contagious Diseases," April 12, 1856].[21]

The Lancet editorial coincided with the City of London (an autonomous square-mile district in the center of the metropolis) ordering its own Poor Law Guardians to provide ambulances designed to transport infectious patients in a recumbent position, after one too many sufferers stuffed upright into the rigid seat of a cab arrived at the hospital gate "dead in the arms of the attendant supporting him."[22] Unfortunately, this flurry of editorials and public activ-

This 1832 poster warned residents of a London neighborhood about the symptoms of cholera, a message made superfluous by the disease's rampant spread. Its remorseless vomiting and diarrhea could kill its victims within twelve hours of onset, and resulting interest in public health laid an early foundation for improved ambulance services in the United Kingdom.

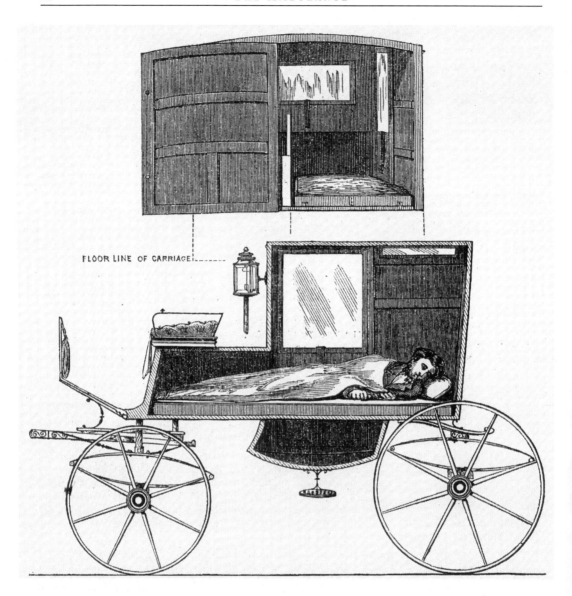

The innovative, and discreet, ambulance devised by London's Hospital Carriage Committee was likely the first civilian vehicle in Europe to meet the criteria for a wholly modern ambulance service, with its specialty design, affiliation with a hospital, and provision of medical care en route (*The Illustrated London News*, February 24, 1867).

ity did not signal a wholesale commitment to comprehensive ambulance services—indeed, it was emblematic of this general failure to sustain public investment that seven years after the City of London had ordered its Poor Law Guardians to acquire their ambulances the municipal commissioners still had no idea whether they had even been built, or, if they had, what had become of them.[23]

By 1864, fully thirty years after cholera brought systematic ambulance services before the public eye, a band of London physicians gave up on the capital's atomized parishes, Poor Law Unions, and the assorted panjandrums overseeing a slew of public and private hospitals, and set out soliciting subscriptions for a London Hospital Carriage Fund to deliver a universal alternative to packing the infectious into public cabs—which one donor called "perambulating fever nests" in good Victorian style.[24] The need was acute, as in 1865 a poll of municipal hospitals revealed that only one percent of infectious disease cases arrived by ambulance, with better than 90 percent coming by hack.[25] Reformers received a modest boost a year later when the Sanitary Act of 1866 ordered vestries to construct suitable ambulances for contagious cases and made it an indictable offense for any cab transporting an infectious person to hire out again until it had been disinfected. Unfortunately, the Act proved more aspirational than directional, and it fell to the private Carriage Fund to advance the ambulance cause. In 1866 the Fund canvassed its members and assembled sufficient funds to hire the craftsmen of John Woodall and Son to manufacture an ambulance, whose innovative design made it the most advanced "invalid carriage"' in Europe.[26]

Bearing in mind the dismal reception given earlier fever vans resembling hearses, this vehicle was deliberately camouflaged as an ordinary private brougham. The back opened on hidden hinges, permitting the patient to be loaded while lying flat, while the introduction of the bed into the carriage was smoothed with rollers built into the floor of the cab (a scheme first employed by Larrey's ambulance). Although not clearly seen here, a side door opened into a small space for an attendant to ride with the patient. Fearful that porous, textured materials like cotton, leather, or linen would offer rich soil for germ laden effluvia, the interior of the ambulance was fitted entirely in close-grained wood enameled with a thick coat of paint, and the mattress and pillow were fashioned out of vulcanized India-rubber. Taken as a whole, this carriage likely represented the first civilian ambulance in Europe to incorporate all the principles associated with a modern ambulance service: a vehicle constructed on scientific principles for the convenience of the ill, configured to permit medical attendance en route, and whose operation was integrated with a hospital.

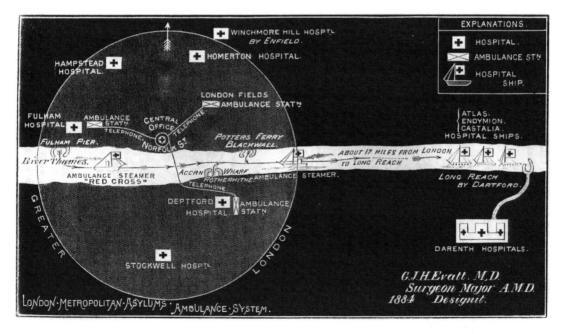

By 1884 London's ambulance system was designed to remove infectious paupers to an isolation hospital. First, a physician contacted the District Receiving Officer, who telegraphed the Central Asylums Board. The board telephoned the ambulance station and a nurse and wagon went out within three minutes (G. J. H. Evatt, *Ambulance Organization, Equipment and Transport* [London: William Clowes and Sons, 1884]).

At the not inconsiderable cost of £100 apiece the Carriage Fund bought six of the vehicles, with the first two being given to the London Fever Hospital (one for small-pox and the other for fever). The gift was conditioned on the hospital providing a suitable stable on the grounds, which was done, and the ambulances were available for anyone to use—anyone, that is, who could afford to pay for the necessary hire of the horse. The other four carriages were donated to the London, St. George's, St. Mary's, and Middlesex Hospitals on similar terms.[27] After this initial success London's hospital carriage movement languished until late 1881 when the ambulance reformers were invigorated by the timely intervention of the American physician Dr. Benjamin Howard. Originally from England, Dr. Howard returned with fresh ideas and some unkind comparisons to recent successes in New York, and his enthusiastic support helped rekindle interest in a uniform, organized ambulance service for the metropolis.[28] While the ultimate scheme depended on staging the apparatus at many city police stations, neither it, nor slightly later efforts by the charitable St. John Ambulance Association to assemble an Invalid Transport Corps, succeeded in providing the truly universal and comprehensive ambulance service that reformers had long hoped for, one that covered the entire city with a guarantee of medical attention en route to the hospital. On the other hand, even as Dr. Howard and his allies in the Hospital Carriage Committee struggled to bring truly universal ambulance service to London, governmental changes were finally being entertained that would, by the end of the century, finally see their dreams realized.

Since ambulance reformers had continually ran afoul of the decentralized nature of city governments, realizing their ambition depended on a complete legislative restructuring of British municipalities into more coherent administrative units. The first step towards this goal had actually taken place when the Metropolitan Asylums Board was created in 1867, centralizing some of the powers strewn among individual parishes and their aggregated Poor Law

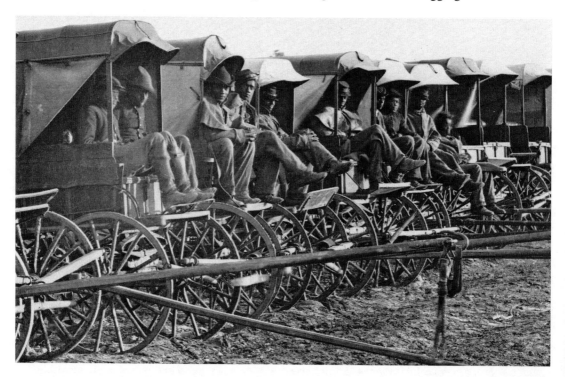

Union ambulance crews at City Point, Virginia, July 1863 (The Library of Congress, Prints and Photographs Division, LC B811-2585).

Unions, but only in 1879 was the London Asylums Board finally granted the city-wide legal authority to operate ambulances for the conveyance of patients with infectious diseases. The board was swift to act upon its new writ, and by 1884 its ambulance stations were servicing a constellation of fever ships moored on the Thames and shore-based isolation hospitals. (While a dramatic improvement over the necessity of sitting upright in a carriage or being toted along in a wheelbarrow, this innovative system represented a commitment only to the transfer of infectious cases, not emergency work, and so represented a distinct departure from nearly contemporaneous developments in the United States where, as we will see, ambulance services were built around accident and urgent medical cases.)

In the end, the reality of city-wide ambulance wagons providing universal services to all those in need of medical attention, not just the contagious, debuted not in Europe but in the New World. The Civil War became the proving ground for this uniquely American invention, and the development of a modern civil emergency medical service was one of the dearly purchased fruits of that horrendous carnage. The way would be long, and there would be many false steps, but when Lee proffered his sword at Appomattox Court House the outlines of civilian ambulance service, from emergency dispatch via alarm bells to the shape and size of the wagons, had been seen and tried on American streets. The modern civilian ambulance service would be the result.

• 4 •

Developments During the Civil War

> THE AMBULANCE SONG
> Let the broad column of men advance!
> We follow behind with the Ambulance.
> * * *
> Through rattling bullets and clashing steel,
> We steadily guide the leaping wheel.
>
> Writhing in agony they lie,
> Cursing the Ambulance, praying to die.
>
> While some in a dreamy deathlike trance,
> Bleed life away through the Ambulance...
> —Anonymous, *Vanity Fair*, November 30, 1861.

The 19th century was a bellicose age whose innumerable battles brought predictable casualties at well defined places, and most European armies had well-organized medical units poised to execute prompt medical attention and removal. The convenience that came with destroying large numbers of soldiers in a well-defined area was missing from the cities of the day, where illness and injury were widely scattered, unpredictable, and, generally, under no single entity's jurisdiction or responsibility. Civic emergency medical care was thus haphazard and largely left to individual initiative, as it had been for thousands of years. Still, the ambulance, born in a war to unify Spain, was destined to achieve maturity in a war to reunite the United States, a conflict unwittingly setting the stage for the defining revolution in ambulance history—its permanent adoption by the civilian world.

America, without even the meager tradition of civil ambulance services flickering in some European states, seemed an unlikely place for the ambulance to complete its transition from the battlefield to the boulevard, especially considering the dismal state of American military ambulances at the beginning of the 19th century, lagging far behind that of any major European power save, perhaps, woeful England. Despite incompetence, inertia, and malfeasance, great strides were made during the Civil War in ambulance technology and deployment, improvements laying an intellectual and organizational foundation for the debut of the truly modern, and peculiarly American, civil ambulance service.

Prelude

At the outbreak of the Civil War no unified ambulance corps existed in either the Union or Confederate armies, an omission that was less oversight than official policy. Indeed, American military planners had been cutting corners on medical evacuation since the Revolution, when the medical corps waited until after the battle to collect the wounded in "wheel-barrows

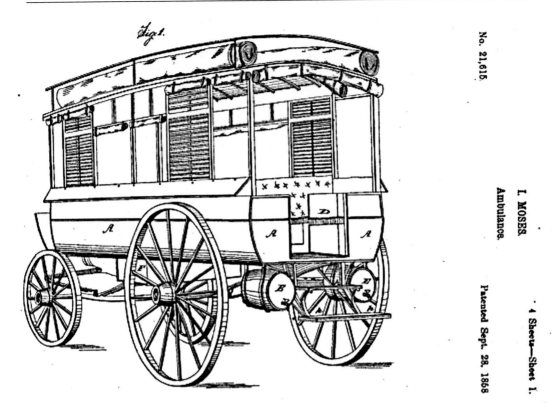

Though it received a cold reception in Congress, Dr. Moses' ambulance design appears to have deserved a better fate. It featured seating for up to 18 persons, fold-down beds, hooks to suspend hammocks for comfortable travel over rough ground (an innovation sorely missed in subsequent army ambulances), and Venetian blinds (U.S. Patent Office, No. 21,615).

and other convenient biers" according to Dr. John Morgan, the Continental Army's Physician in Chief.[1] By the 19th century even the wheelbarrows and convenient biers were gone from the Medical Department, as all ambulance material had been transferred to the Quartermaster Corps. Unfortunately, quartermasters proved to be more interested in soap and hardtack than ambulances, and placing medical officers in one command and their ambulances in another hampered relief efforts. Whether it was the War of 1812 or the Seminole War of the 1830s, the wounded were often removed in springless "hospital wagons" whose stiff, lurching ride evoked pitiful "cries and shrieks" from the injured soldiers inside.[2] In the 1840s many western units lacked even the hospital wagon, and the wounded might find themselves dragged to safety in an improvised buffalo hide travois.[3] As these contraptions demonstrated, transporting the wounded continued to be a scattershot affair absent a central, organized ambulance service on the French model. Still, American genius was not entirely wanting during these years, as in 1858 an ex-assistant surgeon in the United States Army named Israel Moses submitted an original ambulance design to Congress for adoption by the military. Despite its apparent superiority to the wagons then in use, it vanished into undeserved obscurity after receiving an adverse report from a sub-committee in the House of Representatives.[4] A year later, in 1859, the army revised its supply table and took the step of assigning an assortment of experimental ambulances to various units, but the vehicles proved unsatisfactory and the staffing and equipment inadequate.[5] So it was that in 1860, on the eve of the greatest conflict ever waged on the North American continent, the United States military ambulance service amounted to a handful of supply wagons under the control of the Quartermaster Corps, a few sketches at the patent offices, and a small supply of surgeons under the direction of superior officers who believed the rebellion would be over and done within a few months.

Of Avalanches and Agitators

While the war officially began with the bombardment of Fort Sumter on April 12, 1861, appeals for an organized, self-sufficient ambulance corps under unified command had begun appearing with increased urgency earlier that year, suggestions sent to Washington by field commanders and private citizens alike. All of them were turned aside by Secretary of War Stanton and General-in-Chief Halleck, who agreed that an ambulance corps would impede the progress of troop and supply trains, would be prohibitively expensive, would clutter the battlefield with non-combatants sowing panic and getting in the way, and, in any event, the war would be over so quickly that there wasn't enough time to organize such a project anyway.[6] Despite the nonchalance of the top command, this virtual absence of army ambulance services caused severe misgivings in many astute physicians and other lay observers once war began. A veteran war correspondent for the London *Times* passed a prophetic judgment on the havoc these feeble medical preparations would have on the warring sides, writing in July 1861 that

> The medical department is better in the Northern than the Southern armies, but even here there is not an ambulance, a cacolet, a mule litter.... Little do they, North or South, know what war must cost in money, in life, in misery. Already they are suffering, but [this] is but a tithe of a tithe of what is to come.[7]

Similarly, in May 1861 the *New York Times* had noted the city's Fifty-fifth French regiment of Zouaves was, like many other units, going to the front without a single ambulance to collect its inevitable casualties: in the disgusted words of a local physician "even hog-drivers [have] a wagon going behind the drove to pick up the fat and overdriven, and we pay less attention to our patriotic men than to swine."[8]

The first general to act as if he valued his men at least as much as fat and overdriven swine was General George McClellan. As mentioned earlier, McClellan had been sent as an observer to the Crimea, and it is probable that the medical debacle he saw there informed his support for an ambulance corps in the Army of the Potomac. On August 2, 1862, McClellan issued "General Orders No. 147," forming a basic ambulance corps within his Medical Department. Under the capable administration of Medical Director Jonathan Letterman, it depended on two-wheel and

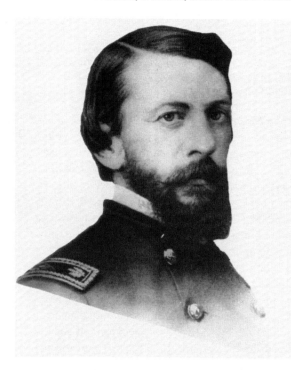

Jonathan Letterman, medical director for the Army of the Potomac during the Civil War, was responsible for organizing, training, and managing America's first ambulance service (courtesy the National Library of Medicine).

4 • Developments During the Civil War

four-wheel ambulances, along with supply carts. Individual regiments received a pair of two-wheeled ambulances and a single four-wheeled model, each staffed with two attendants and a driver. The smaller ambulances were for the actual battlefield, while the larger convoyed the most seriously injured from the field hospitals to positions in the rear, from which they could be transferred to more elaborate facilities. (In March 1863, Major-General Grant of the Union's Army of the Tennessee issued General Order 22, organizing dedicated ambulance crews but leaving the ambulances under joint control of the quartermaster and the medical director.) Merciful intentions aside, a handful of ambulances per regiment was too meager a complement when the reality of modern weaponry collided with men trained in the tactics of the previous century: no force of six ambulances could harvest the crimson windfall of several hundred men charging with bayonets against massed artillery and rifled minnie balls. (This paucity of ambulances was likely attributable to the meager stock on hand: in the summer of 1861 the quartermasters had been putting out contracts for divisions of ten thousand men, requesting supplies in proportionate abundance—ten thousand tin mess kits to be delivered, ten thousand rucksacks, twenty thousand shirts—but for ten thousand men under arms they asked their contractors to provide a mere forty ambulances, of two- and four-wheeled sizes, assorted.)[9] Poor sanitation and bad food accomplished what lead and steel could not, and it is estimated that, on average, each combatant in the war was either sick or wounded a total of six times during the conflict, placing an enormous strain on the ambulance services.[10]

The presence of an undersized but comprehensive ambulance service was still an improvement over the previous system, which had consisted of doling out stretchers to members of the regimental band, drilling them for an hour a day (with Sundays off), and then expecting pic-

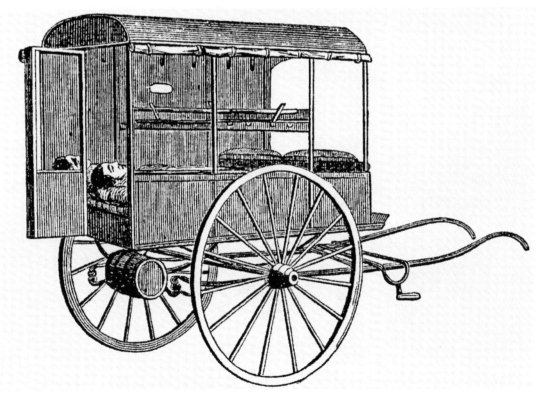

The two-wheeled ambulance was reviled by those lucky enough to survive the trip; all too often the jolting, rocking ride seemed purposely designed to complete the work of an enemy bullet.

colo players to trot into a hail of grapeshot to collect the wounded.[11] Organizational merits aside, it was not for nothing that soldiers called the ambulances "avalanches" and "gut-busters." As one anonymous "gentleman of Massachusetts, alike a scholar and a soldier" explained in *The North American Review*, in 1864:

> We believe that no man who has once ridden in the two-wheeled ambulance would willingly get into one again, even if he were well. As for the four-wheeled ambulance, it is within our personal knowledge that a soldier in our army, ill, but unwounded, lying at full length on the fore and aft seat or bed with which it is fitted, had to hold on with both hands to keep from falling to the floor ... [think] what it must be to ride over corduroy [log] roads when ill or wounded, in a vehicle which, when running on an earth road, both hands are needed to keep the passenger from falling.[12]

To be fair, some blamed the rough roads and the resulting necessity of stiff, heavy springs for the miserable ride, but most felt the ambulance was not all it could be, although its absence was felt even more acutely than its deficiencies—barely. Coming in a variety of models, however, some were unquestionably of better make and design than others. A vehicle with at least one well-considered design element was captured by the Confederates at the first Battle of Bull Run and described in considerable detail by the editors of the *Macon Daily Telegraph*, who noted that the sturdy wagon was fifty inches wide and subdivided into two somewhat cramped interior compartments. While they, at least, were impressed by its four steel springs mounted on flexible hickory shafts, plus additional springs installed under the stretchers, what they most admired was the Yankee ingenuity that went into the contrivance of the stretcher bed, which not only was mounted on rollers to facilitate its smooth transfer in and out of the wagon, but which featured a "small trap door in the centre of the bed, worked by means of a spring and a bolt, [that] offers a convenience to the sufferer that can be easily appreciated," particularly in an era when dysentery was one of the most common causes of military invalidism.[13]

Sanitary stretcher beds aside, the common military ambulance was a tough ride, but the physical limitations of the vehicles were not the only difficulty presented. Whereas Baron Larrey had staffed his vehicles with junior surgeons, the Union Army relied on privates as attendants and drivers, or it simply hired teamsters to handle the horses and took such physicians

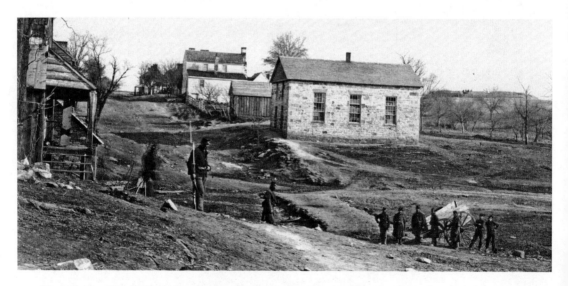

The trip described by the two doctors ended at this Centerville church, used as a hospital for evacuated soldiers. A photograph shows the church as it appeared a year earlier, following the first Battle of Bull Run. The building is in the center, to the right of the sentry (Barnard and Gibson, 1862: Library of Congress, Prints and Photograph Division, LC-B811-0302).

as were available to render aid. Two such medical volunteers were Drs. Charles Stedman and Henry Ingersoll Bowditch, and in 1862 they recorded these impressions of the men handling the Union ambulances after the defeat at Second Manassas (a.k.a. "The Second Battle of Bull Run" north of the Mason-Dixon line).

> DR. STEDMAN: Beyond all example, the driver of the ambulance, in which it was my lot to ride, was the most vulgar, ignorant, and profane man I ever came in contact with... One or two other drivers, who came under my notice, behaved themselves with becoming humanity and gentleness in their assistance of the sufferers; though as a body these drivers were such as would disgrace, it may be, any menials ever sent out to the sick and wounded.
>
> DR. BOWDITCH: I soon perceived that the drivers were men of the lowest character, evidently taken from the vilest purlieus of Washington...

These two volunteer physicians were en route to a church in Centreville, where the Union wounded had been taken after the fight. Shockingly, the battle had been over for five full days before this relief convoy set out to deliver much needed medical supplies and collect the seriously wounded for transport back to Washington, D.C. En route, the physicians had ample time to observe the lack of medical training among the teamsters hired by the Quartermaster Corps. At one point, Dr. Bowditch's section of the relief force stopped to pillage an orchard in Virginia, and, furious at the delay, Dr. Bowditch remonstrated with the men:

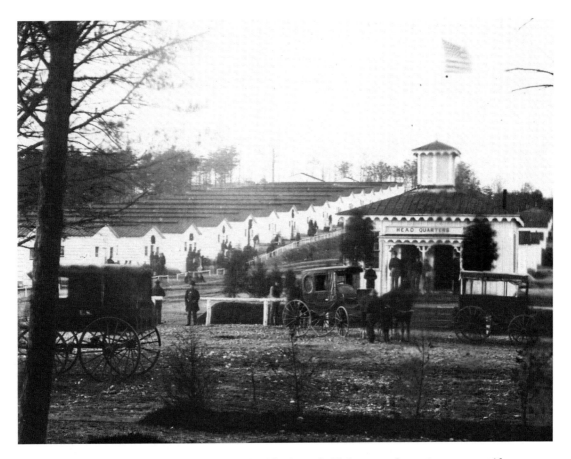

Two different styles of ambulance are seen in this view of a Union convalescent camp near Alexandria, Virginia, around 1864 (a private carriage is seen at center). (Andrew J. Russell, photographer. Library of Congress, Prints and Photographs Division, Lot 4336, No. 60.)

In vain I urged the inhumanity of leaving our starving, suffering soldiers, in order to fill our own greedy stomachs. I appealed to one of the three leaders who rode on horseback ... [h]e only smiled a smile of ineffable contempt, and munched his stolen apple with perfect *nonchalance*.[16]

When an irate farmer hurled a rock at the departing ambulance, the irrepressible Dr. Bowditch dryly remarked to the driver that "hereafter I should know why our ambulances were fired on by the enemy. The only answer I obtained was an oath."[17] Not even the actual presence of the wounded, suffering men could chasten the drivers—indeed, on the return trip Dr. Bowditch's ambulance driver was stuporously drunk, toppling backwards to make a mattress of a wounded soldier lying behind him. The physician was forced to take the reins and "drove most of the night with one hand, while with the other I supported the snoring drunkard."[18] As he propped the inebriate upright, a simpler solution occurred to Dr. Bowditch, who later wrote "I should not have cared if [the driver] had fallen forward and been crushed by the wheels. I doubt whether I should have stretched out a hand to prevent death coming summarily to such a traitor to his country and to humanity."[19]

Not a man to sit at home and wring his hands over the folly of it all, Dr. Bowditch fired off a letter to the surgeon general detailing the deficiencies he had seen. In his reply the sur-

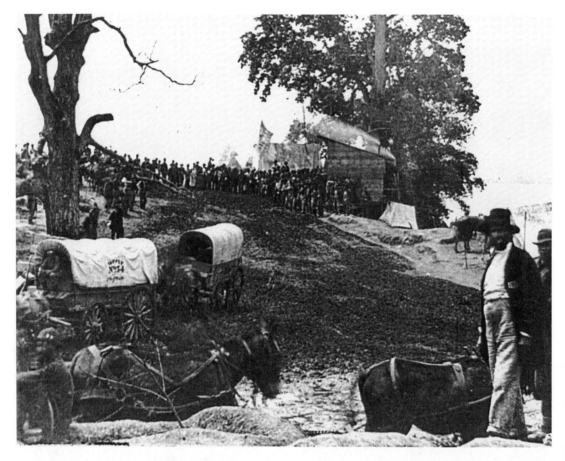

A United States Sanitary Commission camp at Belle Plain, Virginia, May 1864, with supply wagons of the kind used as impromptu ambulances. While the Union dithered over the need for comprehensive ambulance services, the privately organized Sanitary Commission provided medical necessities for the underserved troops, including medical evacuation (Library of Congress Prints and Photographs Division, Civil War Photograph Collection, Lot 4180-A).

geon general confessed he had no influence as ambulances belonged to the quartermasters (in all Union armies save McClellan's Army of the Potomac). The letter confessed that the surgeon general, had, "months since, foretold to the Secretary of War the horrors that would occur with such a set of wretches as usually were found in a body of ambulance drivers—that he had vainly endeavored to obtain some system, but there was none now."[20] Sensible to the justice of Bowditch's rebuke, the surgeon general lost no time in accumulating details of the medical catastrophe at Bull Run and using them to bludgeon opposition to a unified ambulance service under a medical department endowed with sufficient resources and given the power to allot them as needed. A letter that he sent a week after the battle is worth reprinting:

SURGEON-GENERAL'S OFFICE
September 7, 1862.
HON. EDWIN M. STANTON,
Secretary of War.

SIR: I have the honor to ask your attention to the frightful state of disorder existing in the arrangement for removing the wounded from the field of battle. The scarcity of ambulances, the want of organization, the drunkenness and incompetency of the drivers, the total absence of ambulance attendants are now working their legitimate results—results which I feel I have no right to keep from the knowledge of the department. The whole system should be under the charge of the Medical Department. An ambulance corps should be organized and set in instant operation...

Up to this date [fully a week after the battle] six hundred wounded still remain on the battlefield, in consequence of an insufficiency of ambulances and the want of a proper system for regulating their removal in the Army of Virginia. Many have died torments which might have been avoided. I ask, sir, that you will give me your aid in this matter; that you will interpose to prevent a recurrence of such consequences as have followed the recent battle—consequences which will inevitably ensue on the next important engagement if nothing is done to obviate them.

I am, sir, very respectfully, your obedient servant,
WILLIAM A. HAMMOND,
Surgeon-General.

The letter was returned to the surgeon general with a note from General Halleck, general in chief of the Union Armies: ambulances would remain under the jurisdiction of the Quartermaster Corps, and any effort to consolidate the ambulances or to standardize their staffing was denied.[21] While this decision seems almost incomprehensible, a bitter Gideon Welles, secretary of the navy, noted in his diary that the response was of a piece with the career of General Halleck, a man who habitually avoided responsibility and "originates nothing, anticipates nothing ... plans nothing, suggests nothing, is good for nothing."[22]

Dr. Bowditch did not abandon his cause after receiving the dispirited reply of the surgeon general: Fate had chosen Dr. Bowditch as its champion of the ambulance and was not squeamish about the goad used to drive him forward. In November 1861 his oldest son, Nathaniel, had left an apprenticeship with a prominent Cambridge physician and accepted a commission as a 2nd lieutenant with the First Massachusetts Calvary. Sixteen months later Dr. Bowditch received a terse telegram from his son's regiment: "Potomac Creek, March 18, 1863: Nat shot in jaw. Wound in abdomen. Dangerous. Come at once."[23] Immediately the father decamped from Washington, where he had been lobbying for ambulance services, and hastened to the Maryland hospital where his son was being tended. He arrived too late.

Later, he learned the circumstances of the mortal wounding, how the lieutenant had been in the vanguard of a cavalry charge at Kelly's Ford, Virginia, only to be cut down, horse and rider alike. The battle swirled on, the Union colors briefly triumphed and then were withdrawn in the face of Confederate reinforcements, and in the aftermath the desperately wounded young officer "had been left in torture on the battlefield by the side of his dead steed."[24] Two surgeons came upon him but, lacking any means to remove him, rode on. Ultimately a Rhode

Island trooper happened by, and, dismounting, hoisted him into the saddle and led him to the hospital tents in what must have been an agonizing trip for a wounded man jostled along as if he were a pair of insensible panniers. He died less than twenty-four hours later.

His father could never know whether his son might have lived had he been quickly carried to a surgeon's tent in a suitable conveyance, but already concerned with the improvement of the army ambulance service on the broadest humanitarian grounds, Dr. Bowditch suddenly had a consuming, personal reason to pursue his crusade. Shortly before his son's death the House had passed a bill authorizing creation of a central ambulance corps, a bill pigeonholed by the ponderous machinations of the Senate. It was against this backdrop that Dr. Bowditch wrote, published at his own expense, and widely distributed a profoundly influential pamphlet entitled:

A BRIEF PLEA
FOR
AN AMBULANCE SYSTEM
FOR THE
ARMY OF THE UNITED STATES
AS DRAWN FROM THE EXTRA SUFFERINGS OF THE LATE
LIEUTENANT BOWDITCH AND A WOUNDED COMRADE
BY
HENRY I. BOWDITCH, M.D.
PROFESSOR OF CLINICAL MEDICINE IN HARVARD COLLEGE
BOSTON: TICKNOR AND FIELDS, 1863

Realizing that most European armies had already adopted some version of Larrey's system and implemented it by central fiat, an outraged Dr. Bowditch drew on his past experiences at Centreville and elsewhere when asked what the Union did for its soldiers:

> It provides a carriage, which a perfectly healthy man would find exceedingly uncomfortable to drive in, even for a few miles, and one driver, sometimes not the most humane.... *The Senate and Government of this free people, decline to do for its volunteer soldiery, what every despot of Europe carefully looks after, with reference to his conscripts and hirelings!* [25]

(The want of adequate ambulances would, after the Crimean and Civil Wars, finally become a topic of general concern: one commentator writing in 1867 estimated that as many as 40 percent of those who had "perished on the field of battle in recent wars—many from thirst, hunger, or cold" might have been saved had there been sufficient means to "remove them without delay to places where their wants could have been attended to in safety."[26])

Ambulance Ballads and Pamphleteers

Dr. Bowditch was not alone in his pursuit of better ambulance services, and magazine articles on the subject were widely reprinted as pamphlets and distributed in churches, on street corners, and at meetings of reform minded citizens. Nineteenth century periodicals were also partial to verse that, in the tradition of the broadsheet ballad, commented on social and political issues. The following excerpted stanzas invoke the suffering of men who literally waited days for an ambulance to appear, often dying of thirst, of wounds, or exposure, and ends with a rebuke to the political inertia perpetuating this misery.

> HURRAH, boys! It's almost over now!
> Hark,—nothing but scattering shots.
> Now they'll have picked up the hurt in the rear,

4 • Developments During the Civil War

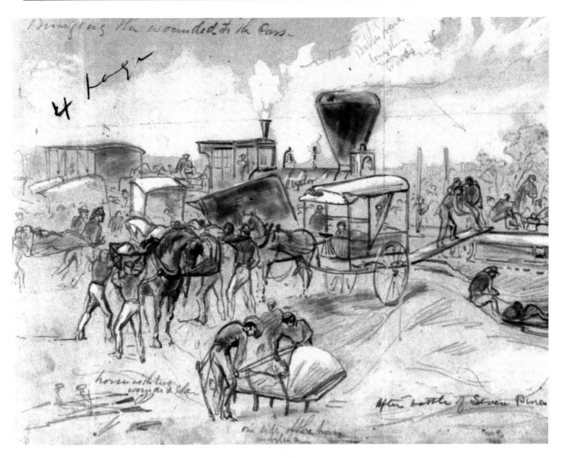

In this sketch made on June 3, 1862, after the Battle of Seven Pines, all modes of transporting the wounded are represented—simple stretcher bearers, an injured man carried by fellow soldiers, a "bonnet" stretcher with a retractable hood, pannier-style stretchers on a horse, and both two- and four-wheeled ambulance wagons. (Drawing by Arthur Lumley. Library of Congress Prints and Photographs Division, LC-USZ62-83035.)

        And make for these foremost spots.
   If my leg and arm weren't both broken,—bad luck!
      I'd manage to walk or roll
To see them coming, and give three cheers,
      There from that nearest knoll.
      Where can the ambulance be?
* * *
Of course they'll bring casks full of water, Jim?
      What's that you're eating? 'Grass'?
Put some in my mouth,—I can't move my hand,—
      It will help the time to pass.
Beasts live on it: couldn't a man, then,—think?—
      If he had to,—a day more,—two?
They'll find us soon. We must give them time.
      They're few, with much to do.
      Where can the ambulance be?
* * *
I think my soul is striking its tent;
      For like fire that's almost out
It seems now here and then elsewhere—

> Flickers and flies about.
> Just now 'twas up in the Congress Hall;
> And it heard them speak and say,
> They'd put the bill for an Ambulance Corps
> Off to another day!
> Where can the ambulance be?
> [E. Forton, "The Forsaken Soldier," *The Monthly Religious Magazine* 30, No. 2 (August 1863): 69].

Amidst the welter of articles, poems, and letters circulated around this issue, Bowditch's pamphlet was probably the most widely disseminated and oft cited, until, in March 1864, his efforts and those of like-minded reformers were finally rewarded when Congress established a uniform ambulance service for all the Union armies. The pattern was almost identical to that set out by General McClellan in 1862 (except for giving regiments of at least five hundred men three of the two-wheeled ambulances rather than a miserly pair) and, at last, it took authority for the service from the quartermasters and gave it to the surgeon general. As before, surgeons did not accompany the ambulance on its forays to collect the wounded but rather received them at impromptu surgeries set as close to the line of battle as practicable. Congress's belated directive came at a time when the military, influenced by the efforts of the private Sanitary Commission, was finally progressing with its experiments to convert the "avalanche" from an infernal machine apparently designed to tumble its occupants to death into something more humane. By the end of the war the two-wheeled ambulance was virtually extinct owing to its instability on bad roads and a tendency to rock so much as to sicken the well and doom the ill, while several versions of the four-wheeled ambulance were deployed, each supposedly improving on the last. Most were little more than spring-wagons such as might be used to haul any commodity, be it men or bags of peas, and the sheer numbers of casualties meant springless supply wagons were frequently commandeered to ferry the wounded: contemporary accounts describe how these were fitted for the purpose by strewing their floorboards with brush and hay, a measure probably appreciated more for the thought than the result.[27]

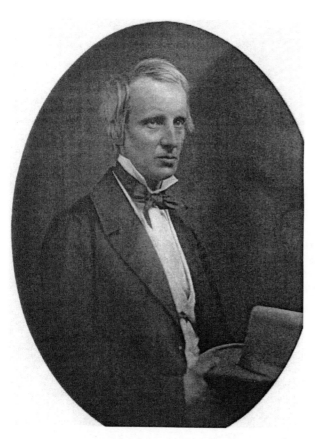

Dr. Bowditch was a passionate abolitionist and an ardent supporter of the Union. Along with his passion came unorthodox methods, as when he discovered a "bounty jumper" during an enlistment physical and deftly inscribed the letter "D" (for deserter) in the flesh of the man's arm using a wand of silver nitrate. The scoundrel sued for battery and was awarded one thousand dollars in damages, to the shame and disgust of Dr. Bowditch (Vincent Bowditch, ed., *Life and Correspondence of Henry Ingersoll Bowditch,* **Vol. 2 [Cambridge: Riverside Press, 1902], 37).**

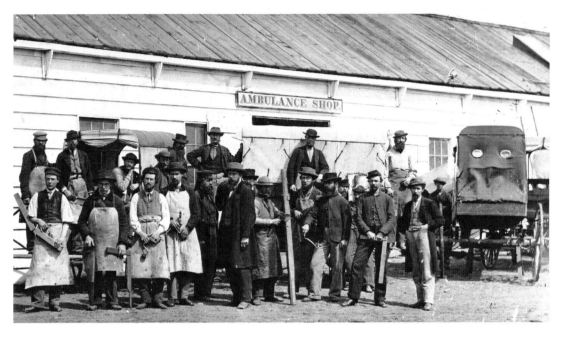

Workmen take a break from fabricating new ambulances outside of Washington, D.C., in April 1865 (Library of Congress, Prints and Photographs Division, LC-B817-7834).

Southern Ambulances

Confederate forces struggled to organize their own comprehensive ambulance service during the war, at first limited by the same medical myopia afflicting the northern armies and then further hamstrung by insufficient funds and materials. With the support and encouragement of Dr. Samuel Preston Moore, Surgeon General of the Confederate Army, individual commanders were nonetheless able to create efficient units with the dwindling resources available to them.[28] (Notable among the Confederate surgeons was Dr. Samuel Stout of the Army of Tennessee, who became particularly renowned for his superbly organized mobile field hospitals, relying in part on well-trained ambulance squads.)[29] Originally these services "enjoyed" the use of the same spring wagons being roundly cursed by their northern kinsmen, but soon, as the Confederate economy was plowed under like a stubble field, the medical corps had no choice but to replace its lost ambulances with improvisations, like ordinary mule wagons roofed with bowed wands of white oak draped with cotton-duck cloth.[30] Occasionally these rough vehicles were supplemented by captured Union ambulances, which, as the war progressed, had become slightly more comfortable than their ancestors of only a few years earlier: predictably, these prizes were almost invariably requisitioned by headquarters, putting the field regiments back into the mule wagons.[31] For example, when Confederate forces captured an ambulance belonging to General Silas Casey at the Battle of Seven Pines, the prize was given to J.S. Dorsey Cullen, Surgeon General to the First Corps, Army of Northern Virginia: a Georgia paper reported that rather than being assigned to the field, Cullen was enjoying the personal use of the ambulance wrested from the supplies of an "Abolition General."[32] Finally, just as the civilian Sanitary Commission gathered up the medical loose ends of the Grand Army of the Republic, so the Confederacy turned to the Richmond Ambulance Committee, a privately organized force of volunteers providing significant ambulance relief work, perhaps most notably at Gettysburg.[33]

From Battlefield to Boulevard

The initial, and wholly unintended, step in converting the ambulance from military to civilian use was the simple exposure of the American people to the existence and practical operation of ambulances, vehicles which had the virtue of novelty to anyone who had not borne arms or had occasion to visit a London fever hospital recently. This gentle introduction was accomplished in print, mostly in service to the crusade to establish a general ambulance corps, but also in reality, as military hospitals, inundated by the undreamed scale of casualties, shunted convalescent troops into civilian infirmaries across the country (while in 1859 the entire United States Army stood at around 15,000 men, in 1862 at least 10,000 Union soldiers alone were killed or wounded in twelve hours at Antietam).[34] Transferring wounded soldiers from depots and wharves to private hospitals required ambulances, and the vehicles became common sights in the scores of northern cities whose infirmaries eagerly sought contracts to care for the wounded.[35] (Boarding these soldiers was a profitable bit of patriotism for hospitals: for example, at a time when the city paid $1.25 a week for charity patients, Rochester City Hospital in New York received $5.50 a week from the U.S. Treasury for each soldier it cared for.)[36] Philadelphia was a particularly important hub for transports carrying ill and injured troops and saw a steady flow of hospital trains and boats arriving from the southern battlefields. When the official ambulance contractors proved incapable of keeping pace, the city fire stations raised their own ambulance squads, and in November 1862 the various firehouse ambulance teams united to assume complete responsibility for the transport of wounded soldiers entering the city.[37] This newly formed "Rescue 1 Squad" was called to action when the fire bell in Old Independence Hall rang fifteen times, with various firehouses getting the location of the arriving train or boat from the nearest police telegraph office. Notably, this was the first time in history that an ambulance service was connected to electronic dispatch.

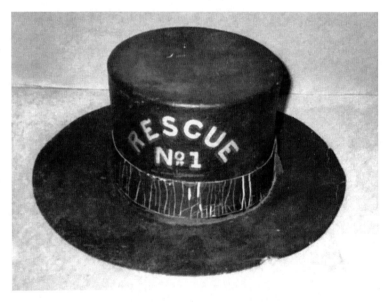

A relic of America's first civilian ambulance service, this special "parade hat" was worn by a member of the Philadelphia Fire Department's ambulance crew. The squad removed thousands of wounded and ill soldiers from the flood of troop trains and hospital ships that periodically inundated this important transportation hub.

The sheer number of firefighting companies in the largest cities led to keen rivalries between them, not only in the race to reach a blaze first, but to show up with apparatus whose magnificent ornamental flourishes would shame rivals and astound the onlooker. The Philadelphia fire company ambulances did not deviate from this tradition, and if anything the added spur of patriotic zeal pushed them into new heights of Technicolor extravagance. A model unveiled by the Washington Steam Fire Engine Company will illustrate the point: this ambulance was painted a radiant white, with every

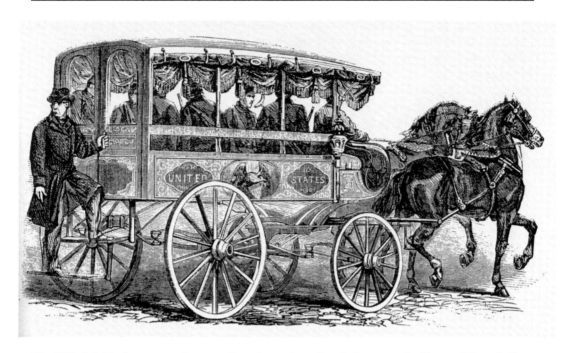

The Philadelphia fire companies contributed a variety of ambulances to the Rescue 1 Squad. Here is an omnibus pattern, suitable for the least severely wounded (F. Schell, in *Frank Leslie's Illustrated Newspaper*, May 27, 1865).

edge and border illuminated in heavy gilt; two silver lamps cast a spotlight on the driver's seat; on the splash board below the teamster's box was a large portrait of "Fame" holding a medallion, all set on a rich, blue background; and every flat surface facing the public eye was similarly adorned with allegorical paintings depicting scenes from the life of President Washington and various American historical vignettes, making this ambulance not only practical for those within, but an education for those without.[38] In the Philadelphia Fire Museum a lithograph from the period shows one of the Washington Steam Company's rivals, a tiny rolling cathedral illuminated by miter-shaped windows and tattooed all over with ovals and cameos featuring portraits and city views.[39]

After the war there was some confusion about what to do with these opulent vehicles. By July 1865 there are news reports of some of them being used for emergency work, taking injured Philadelphians to local hospitals and carrying away casualties from fire scenes, while other companies volunteered to load the cheerfully painted ambulances with children from local orphanages, like the Northern Home for Friendless Children, and whisk them off on outings to parks and festivals.[40] By 1866 several of the firefighting companies had settled into providing emergency ambulance service for their neighborhoods, although some squads, like the Globe Steam Fire Engine Company in 1868, were happy to sell their ambulances at fifty cents on the dollar to whoever wanted them.[41] By 1870 the volunteer companies, loosely affiliated under a Chief Engineer, were only in possession of four ambulances, down from at least twenty-six during the war years.[42] This gradual disappearance of the Philadelphia ambulances demonstrates how civilian exposure to ambulance operations was, in itself, insufficient to ensure the creation of robust civilian ambulance services. Far more influential was a uniquely American phenomenon: the veteran effect.

During the Civil War every soldier was exposed to the wide-scale use of military ambulances, so by sheer statistical chance a portion of the men surviving the experience were gifted with the imagination and energy to translate what they had seen into civilian applications, and America's abhorrence of standing armies made sure that they had the chance to do so. Unlike Europe, where deterrence of closely packed, hostile neighbors required large forces in perpetual readiness, America's military depended on turning shopkeepers into officers in times of war and officers back into shopkeepers in times of peace (this anticipation of radical downsizing certainly applied to the medical corps: in 1861 it was reported that after the war Union ambulances were expected to be sold off to farmers for around $30 apiece).[43] The inevitable diuresis of officers and men after Appomattox meant the genii of the civilian ambulance revolution would likely be veterans importing their knowledge of military ambulances onto the "quasi-battlefield" of modern metropolitan life, in Dr. Benjamin Howard's apt phrase.[44] Again and again we will see how groundbreaking ambulance operations were created by discharged military men with significant exposure to ambulance operations during their service, men who in Europe would likely have spent their active careers under arms. This liberality with demobilization was the signal factor ensuring that America, with its trivial and recent history of ambulance service, became the leader in civilian ambulance development after the Civil War, as opposed to a European state whose military ambulance tradition was decades, even centuries, older. Though the creation of modern municipal ambulance services depended on ex-soldiers carrying the wisdom of grape-shot into the vineyards of civil life, the campaign still had to begin somewhere. In the event, the campaign opened on *several* fronts independently, an inevitable reaction to that unique combination of expertise, access, and innovation present throughout the United States as the war wound down.

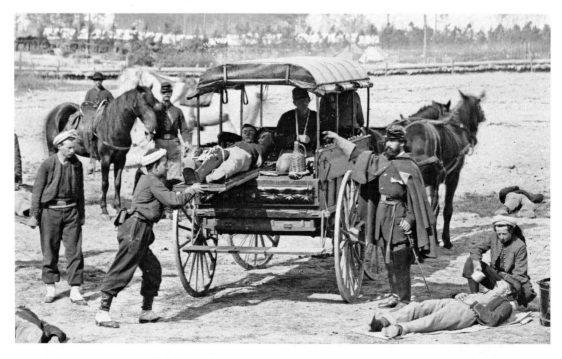

Members of a Union Zouave regiment pose with a Howard ambulance wagon during a drill at Brandy Station, Virginia. The comfortable bed was easily unloaded—unfortunately, many officers found the couch so comfortable that the privates on stretcher duty had to haul them away, bed and all, rendering the ambulance useless (Edward Munson, "Transportation of Federal Sick and Wounded," in *Prisons and Hospitals*, Vol. 7 of *Photographic History of the Civil War*, ed. Holland Thompson [New York: Review of Reviews Co., 1911], 305). (Library of Congress, Prints and Photographs Division, LC B8171-7285.)

Ambulance Ambassador

This "veteran effect" was also slated to have a dramatic impact in Great Britain, almost wholly due to the influence of one man, an expatriate Englishman turned Union Regimental Surgeon named Benjamin Howard. His influence on the struggling British emergency services movement was pivotal, and the story of how he was able to translate his war-time experience on the shot-swept meadows of Antietam and Gettysburg to the "modern battleground" of urban London and Liverpool is one of the most intriguing, and inspiring, in the history of the ambulance.

His long and varied career, described by one friend as "more meteor-like than planetary," flashed into existence in 1836, at Chesham, England.[45] While showing tremendous promise at school, he was both of modest birth and orphaned at early age and, determined to get a university education, he struck out at the age of seventeen for what he hoped would be the more egalitarian opportunities offered in the United States.[46] In America he supported himself by working in the manual trades, mostly as a paper hanger, before graduating from the New York College of Physicians and Surgeons in 1858.[47] After briefly flirting with the idea of becoming a medical missionary, his flickering curiosity lighted on the subject of slavery, the nation's all-consuming debate at that time.[48] Fascinated by the persistence of this wretched practice in a country whose vaunted equality of opportunity had given him a life undreamed of in England, he elected to comprehend by action, moving to Missouri and taking work as a clerk in a slave market. Whatever theoretical misgivings about slavery that had been smoldering in his mind were ignited into visceral hatred by his first-hand experience of the horror and brutality of the "peculiar institution," including the casual depravity of the local gentry who could wander in at will to take advantage of female slaves awaiting sale.[49] He lost no time in making contact with local abolitionists and was put to work as a conductor on the "Underground Railroad" while still clerking at the slave-house, a perilous masquerade that was quickly caught out: only a hurried warning from a friend allowed him to escape from Missouri with his life.[50] These experiences made him a militant abolitionist, and when the Civil War began in the spring of 1861 he enlisted as an assistant U.S. volunteer surgeon, serving until December 28, 1864, when he resigned for reasons of ill health.[51]

It was during the war that his inter-

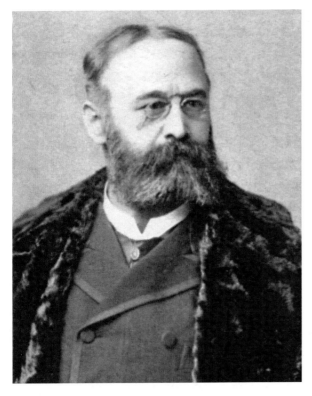

In addition to his other talents and interests, Dr. Howard enjoyed demonstrating his skill at handwriting analysis. A friend observed that merely by examining a specimen from a complete stranger he could divine, with uncanny accuracy, "peculiarities of body habit and mental action known only to intimate acquaintances" (*The Literary World* 33, no. 8 [August 1, 1902], 117).

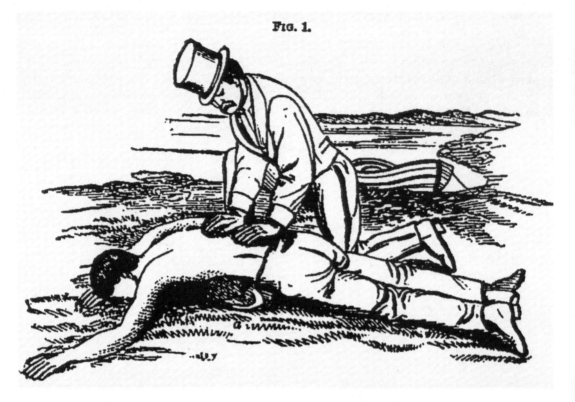

Dr. Howard's efforts to perfect means of artificial respiration were widely disseminated and reflected the same reformatory zeal informing his crusade for improved ambulance service in England (Scientific American, 21:9 [August 28, 1869]).

est in emergency transport was awakened, although he had always been a determined innovator, and an ambulance he designed while in uniform was favorably noticed at the Paris World's Fair in 1867.[52] Nonetheless, after the conflict he banked the fires of his reformatory zeal around the object of preserving the nearly drowned and asphyxiated, going on to develop new maneuvers for rescuers to pump the water out of victims' lungs and pump the air back in and helping create the New York Life Saving Society in 1873.[53] Shortly after becoming the society's corresponding secretary he went abroad in hopes of strengthening his health, and while visiting Paris he attempted to interest the civil authorities in an ambulance service, to little avail: traveling to London in 1878 he pressed his ambulance ideas to an equally cool reception.[54] When he returned to Great Britain for a lecture tour in 1881 he found England's ambulance services no better and his own enthusiasm no less. While tramping the hustings he chanced to pass a long train ride explaining his ambulance theories to the captive audience sharing his compartment. His patient listener was James Crossman, a vice-chairman of the London Hospital who, coincidentally, had been active in the Hospital Carriage Society of the late 1860s, only to see his efforts stymied by the admixture of custom, precedent, and pettifoggery that routinely thwarted efforts to dislodge the status quo in England (and elsewhere). Mr. Crossman was sufficiently impressed by the impromptu exposition that he invited the opinionated American to bring his views, and his ambulance designs, down to London for an airing.[55]

Howard seized the opportunity with the zest of a missionary discovering a lost tribe in the Amazon. Night after night he lectured, exhorted, and cajoled groups of British physicians. He was quoted in *The Lancet*, mentioned in the *Times*, and allied himself with that small cadre of Londoners who had been advocating for a municipal ambulance service since the Hospital Carriage Society had been formed in 1864. In September of 1881 he and his allies successfully persuaded the staff of the London Hospital to expand their ambulance service to include accident removal as well as transporting the infectious, and on December 20, 1881, the infirmary took possession of a Howard Ambulance Wagon, built by Mr. J.V. Burt of Gray's Inn Road and financed by Howard's former traveling companion, James Crossman.[56] From the beginning Dr. Howard stressed that realizing the full benefit of the ambulance required some way of summoning them immediately via telegraph or telephone, but even at this late date only the London Hospital in the East End, St. Bartholomew's near Fleet Street, and Guy's Hospital south of the Thames were accessible electronically, through a complicated relay system that involved sending a summons over the police telegraph to some station that had a telephone connection with the hospital.[57] By 1882 this cumbersome state of affairs was partially circumvented by placing ambulances at various police stations throughout the city, greatly expediting their dispatch.

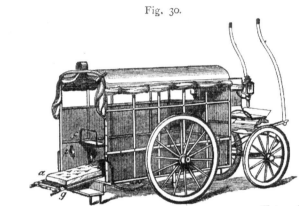

Fig. 30.

DR. HOWARD'S AMBULANCE SICK-TRANSPORT WAGGON. (External view.)

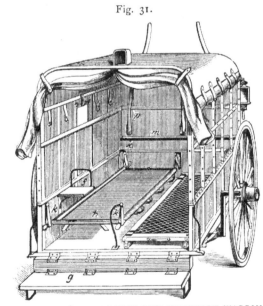

Fig. 31.

DR. HOWARD'S AMBULANCE SICK-TRANSPORT WAGGON.

The attraction of the Howard system was soon felt far beyond the capital. Liverpool's Northern Hospital installed one of Howard's ambulances in 1881 after a well-to-do American visitor miscarried on a trans–Atlantic steamer. Prostrate from her illness when she arrived in port, she was appalled to learn that her options for traveling to the hospital were to be carried through the streets on a stretcher, to be slipped inside a dusty fever van (which city authorities did offer to specially disinfect for the occasion), or consent to being toted on the police hand-ambulance, a rolling platform like a costermonger cart

Howard's Ambulance Wagon, introduced to England in 1881. Despite weighing six hundred pounds, its balance allowed a *Lancet* editor to pull it using his little finger. Howard boasted his ambulance could transfer trauma cases "from the most distant country seat in Scotland to the farthest Italian villa in safety, comfort, and seclusion" (B. Howard, "Hospital," 174; *Times*, "Hospital Ambulance," December 21, 1881).

which was usually employed to haul inebriates off the public stage.[58] Such devices had been considered good enough for the average Liverpudlian, sober or otherwise, but the scorn expressed by the wealthy American for the shabby state of Liverpool's emergency services awoke the hospital staff to the poverty of their condition, and within eighteen months a surgeon and a Howard ambulance were on twenty-four hour standby for the benefit of wealthy tourists and humble ratepayers alike.[59] By the 1890s craftsmen all over Britain were busy manufacturing ambulances of local design, but without the dedication and professional reputation of Benjamin Howard it is likely that modern ambulance services in the United Kingdom would have been even further delayed. (After successfully introducing his ambulance to England, Dr. Howard continued to teach and write on medical topics and developed an interest in penology, becoming the first English speaker to visit the fearsome prison island of Sakhalin during his tours of Siberian detention camps between 1886 and 1896.[60] On June 21, 1900, he succumbed to cancer after a brief illness, while staying at the home of a physician friend at Elberon, New Jersey.)[61]

Meanwhile, how the American public came to grips with the civilian ambulance, and the impact it would have on the world, will be the topic of the next chapter, where we encounter the first wave of prototypically American ambulances: specifically built for their task, intimately associated with hospitals, and, in contrast to the contemporaneous London fever vans seen earlier, envisioned as principally responding to trauma calls. Quickly enough the mission of the civilian ambulance services expanded from sudden injuries to general medical provider of first resort—and its attempts to keep pace have continued to shape its evolution down to the present day.

• 5 •

"Let Us No Longer Add Murder to Maiming": The Civilian Ambulance in America

LET US NO LONGER ADD MURDER TO MAIMING
Wanted, Ambulances for the Injured

[T]here are every day in our very midst human beings whose sufferings are as intense as those of the victims of the Inquisition [because] the variety of conveyances used in the transportation of patients to the hospital is as great as the variety of injured received: carriages, boards, wagons of all descriptions, none fitted for the purpose; [and] often a simple fracture of the bone, which would be well in a few weeks, is in this transportation converted into a compound fracture, the end of the bone tearing through the skin [and] producing an injury which requires months to heal, and which often necessitates amputation, or is even the occasion of death.
—Editorial, *Brooklyn Daily Eagle,* November 18, 1871.

Despite hitting the trifecta of emergency medicine—a vehicle designed solely to transfer the wounded, staffed by skilled medical attendants, and conceived with speed in mind—Larrey's "flying ambulance" was not welcome on the boulevard. By the mid–19th century the *ambulant volant* had followed French soldiers from Austerlitz to Sevastopol, but Parisian streets remained a medical no man's land; and while Great Britain boasted a clutch of specialty ambulances in its cities and towns, this tiny complement functioned mostly as elaborate sneeze-guards to dart the infectious into the nearest pest house. Meanwhile, from every vantage America had fallen far behind its European rivals by 1863: in the midst of civil war the two sides struggled to field enough ambulances to clear battlefields a week after the last shots had been fired, while the only civilian ambulances in the country were rude wagons and hearses used by smallpox and fever hospitals. So how was it that by 1871 the penny press of Brooklyn could claim emergency ambulance services to be the birthright of every bricklayer born on the banks of Gowanus Canal? The answer was presaged, but not delivered, in 1865, when a municipal hospital in Cincinnati, Ohio, became the first American infirmary with a general ambulance service: obscure in its day and overshadowed by imitators in more famous hospitals, the Cincinnati experiment nonetheless introduced ideas that shaped the first decades of American ambulance services.

Asclepius Comes to Porkopolis—The Cincinnati Ambulance

In my next [letter] I hope to send you a full account of the beautiful and hospitable city of Cincinnati—its swine and its wine.... All Cincinnati is redolent of swine. Swine prowl the street and palaces and villas are built, and vineyards and orchards cultivated, out of the proceeds of their flesh, their bones, their lard, their bristles, and their feet ["From Washington to Cincinnati," *Illustrated London News,* Feb. 27, 1858, and "The Queen City of the West," *Illustrated London News,* March 20, 1858].

The people of Cincinnati have not only provided, probably, the best Hospital accommodations in the country for her citizens, but have made such arrangements as to enable those who are sick and unable to walk, or in case of accident, to be taken to the Hospital without delay [12th Annual Report of the Cincinnati Hospital, for the ten months ending December 31, 1872].

Cincinnati's reputation as the 19th century pork-packing capital of America was built on hogs with drawls. Separated from Kentucky by the Ohio River, the city once known as Porkopolis depended on southern pens and farms for the bacon that built its fame. When the Civil War separated Cincinnati's shambles from their traditional southern suppliers, the Queen City adroitly traded butter for guns, going from importer of southern hogs to exporter of Union military equipment—especially ambulances, which became a prominent industry.[1] By 1864 Cincinnati wainwrights were hammering out so many ambulances for the North that probably no city in the world had more ambulances per capita. Such proximity alone cannot explain why Cincinnati was the first American city to operate an exclusively civilian emergency ambulance service, however, since other towns supported ambulance manufacturers without connecting army surplus to a revolution in emergency medicine. The city's relative abundance of ambulance shops was likely a *force* in this historic decision, but it was a force acting upon a uniquely susceptible infirmary: the beleaguered Commercial Hospital of Cincinnati.

Today's University of Cincinnati Medical Center has annual revenues exceeding a billion dollars and employs more than fifteen thousand people. Although currently enjoying prestige commensurate with its wealth, it started out as the Commercial Hospital of Cincinnati, a city charity administered, somewhat haphazardly, by the Medical College of Ohio. Just *how* haphazardly was made public in 1864 when a commission of inquiry reported that the entire two-hundred-bed infirmary was staffed by a single resident physician and a pair of medical students.[2] Facing stiff competition from a host of rivals (throughout the 19th century more than twenty medical schools came and mostly went in Cincinnati), the Medical College of Ohio was often on soft footing financially, and the city subsidy for running the Commercial was a guaranteed paycheck its competitors would have been happy to cash. Shortly after the caustic report hit the mayor's desk, the faculty hired Dr. Roberts Bartholow, a prominent physician who had previously overseen military hospitals in Baltimore and Washington, D.C., infirmaries with dedicated ambulance services to deliver the wounded from nearby battlefields and transfer points.[3] Thus, by early 1865 the Commercial Hospital was surrounded by ambulance manufacturers; had a physician on staff with experience in hospital and ambulance integration; and was faced with a city council whose members were unimpressed with the quality of the hospital's administration. Whether due to this confluence of expertise, equipment, and need for social rehabilitation, or simply coincident with it, the payroll record on the opposite page appeared in the 1866 *Annual Report of the Trustees of the Commercial Hospital.*

Six hundred years after the Brothers of Mercy shouldered their first wicker basket, two centuries after Queen Isabella sent wagons to collect her wounded, and fewer than eighteen months after the American military had belatedly organized its own ambulance service, the North American debut of the hospital emergency ambulance was formally announced. The first driver, Mr. James Jackson, was no stranger to the Commercial, as he previously appeared in the handwritten payroll for 1864 as a "wagoner" at the same salary. His perch atop this historical marquee was brief, since the next annual report dropped the honorific of "ambulance driver," making Mr. Jackson a seven-dollar-a-week teamster who occasionally drove the ambulance.[4] Unfortunately, no descriptions of the Commercial Hospital's first ambulances have been found.

Geography undoubtedly conspired against the kind of elaborate emergency service that would have commanded Mr. Jackson's attention full time, since the Commercial Hospital was near the heart of town at 12th Street and Central Avenue, just over a mile from the waterfront. This location would have been conducive to passerby transferring accident cases straight to the hospital rather than waiting for a runner to secure the ambulance absent any telegraphic link to the Commercial. In fact, it wasn't until 1872 that trustees assured Cincinnati that, thanks to new telegraph wires linking the hospital with the city's station houses, "the Hospital ambulances can be summoned to any part of the city at any time, day or night."[5] An identical dispatching scheme had been pioneered by New York's ambulance service three years earlier, in 1869, and the immediacy of treatment it promised was cited by contemporary sources as crucial to that program's success. Had such a plan been in place when Cincinnati started its service in 1865 it is likely the service would have achieved greater acclaim in proportion to its greater utility.

Although the absence of telegraphic dispatch was eventually remedied, a second omission became fixed in the amber of habit: while hospital annual reports from 1865 onward include detailed lists of the duties expected of resident physicians, they are invariably silent about an obligation to accompany the ambulance on its runs. Although dispatching interns on ambulance duty was the norm by the 1870s, Cincinnati's house staff stayed indoors long after their absence had become unique among big city hospitals. In its defense, when the Commercial introduced its ambulance operation in 1865 its only models were military ambulances which, federal and Confederate alike, seldom carried surgeons. Equally significant, Cincinnati's ambulance was attached to a two-hundred-and-nine-bed hospital whose five physicians admitted two thousand four hundred and forty-one patients in 1867, a quantity that likely made it difficult for the medical staff to leave the wards.[6] Whatever its staffing deficiencies, the Commercial Hospital's ambulance was a durable one, lasting more than a century and inspiring local imi-

NAMES AND ANNUAL SALARIES OF THE EMPLOYEES OF THE COMMERCIAL HOSPITAL

No.	Name.	Rank.	Salary.
26	Bridget Lanhady	Night watchwoman	180 00
27	James A. Jackson	Driver of ambulance	360 00
28	James Carr	Man of all work	360 00

Commercial Hospital Payroll Record, for the fiscal year ending February 1866.

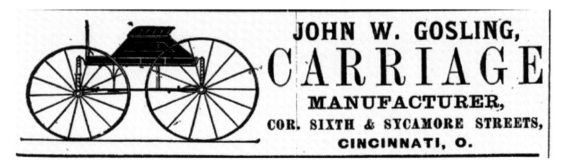

This advertisement for J.W. Gosling appeared in the 1867 Cincinnati City Directory, the same year the Commercial Hospital purchased an ambulance from the firm for $350.

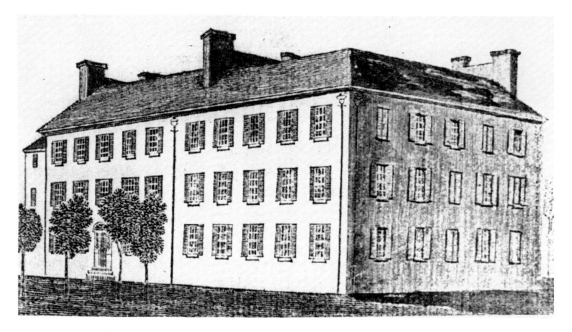

The Commercial Hospital in 1865, when its historic ambulance service debuted (courtesy the National Library of Medicine).

tators: indeed, by 1882 every hospital in Cincinnati was fielding its own ambulance, as were a few of the city police stations.[7]

As it was, by 1866 the nation had seen the birth of civilian emergency ambulance services midwifed in several cities: wounded soldiers being transferred to Philadelphia hospitals in ornate fire bureau ambulances beginning in 1863, the modest Cincinnati Commercial Hospital ambulance service in 1865, and a St. Louis municipal dispensary ambulance that was operational by 1866.[8] Together, these services represented the premiere of fire department ambulances, hospital providers, and municipal ambulance services—a triumvirate that would shape emergency medical services in the next century. Yet owing to a combination of limited press and inherent weaknesses in design, not one of these pioneers inspired nationwide imitation. Instead, if an American hospital were inclined to give any thought to patient transport it was apt to purchase a few wheeled stretchers called "hand ambulances," at best a minor improvement over public cabs and stretchers improvised from wooden planks.[9] It wasn't until 1869 that a new model of civilian ambulance service—one incorporating specialty wagons, immediate telegraphic dispatch, and expert medical attention on the scene—appeared on the national stage. Its location in America's greatest city attracted national attention, and its skilled administration guaranteed that it would merit the admiration of the world. It was the Bellevue Ambulance Service of New York City, and it changed emergency medicine forever.

Bellevue

> It has been the practice, when a person has been injured or taken sick in the public street, for the Police or passing citizens to take the patient to the nearest druggist, and after administering restoratives, convey him on a cart or other vehicle to a hospital or his home. There was always a great suffering from the rude means of conveyance and great loss of time before proper surgical aid could be obtained, resulting frequently in the loss of life [New York City's Commissioners of Charity justifying their new ambulance service, from their 1870 Annual Report].

Bellevue Hospital originated in Manhattan's "Public Workhouse and House of Correction," built in 1735 at the cost of eighty pounds sterling and fifty gallons of rum.[10] In 1736 the city fathers belatedly conceded that New York's deserving poor might fall prey to sickness as well as sloth or delinquency and with terse magnanimity put medical care within reach of the humble by stating, "We report it is our opinion that the upper room of the West End of the said House be suitably furnished for an Infirmary and for no other use whatsoever," a six-bed afterthought that was destined to become one of the world's most celebrated hospitals.[11] When yellow fever scourged the eastern states in 1794 the original infirmary was overwhelmed, and a private mansion on spacious acreage overlooking the East River, christened *Belle Vue* by an earlier owner in a happier time, was leased to receive the overflow. In 1811 construction of a proper hospital (along with a penitentiary and almshouse to replace the colonial antiques downtown) began on land adjoining this site, and the name of the old mansion became attached to the new facility forever.

By the 1860s the city had embraced this rural enclave, the almshouse and penitentiary had relocated to nearby islands in the East River, and Bellevue was an enormous teaching hospital with more than six hundred beds and its own medical school. An imposing edifice whose main building stretched two city blocks, this bulwark of brownstone and brick was separated by a dull wall from the shabby tenements nearby (built in 1853, the wall largely went up to keep friends and family from passing bottles of liquor to thirsty patients inside).[12] The street leading to its somber gate was a garbage-strewn jumble where hospital officers glumly admitted that "daily and nightly cases of severe injuries and very sick patients [are] brought in by the Police and others, on wagons and carts ... [the] poor patients trying to steady their broken and fractured limbs while being driven and shaken over the rough stones of the street."[13] Inside, Bellevue was dark with ancient wood and redolent of carbolic acid, soap, old timber, and dust.[14]

As the premiere charitable hospital for the largest city in North America, Bellevue's wards were inevitably overflowing with every species of human suffering. Whatever its effects on the patients, such overcrowding meant no teaching hospital in the country offered the variety that Bellevue could—be it raving delirium tremens cases in the alcoholic pavilion, puerperal fever sweeping through its maternity ward, the police wagons dumping out the stabbed and the beaten, or downtown factories churning out crush injuries as efficiently as watch cases and

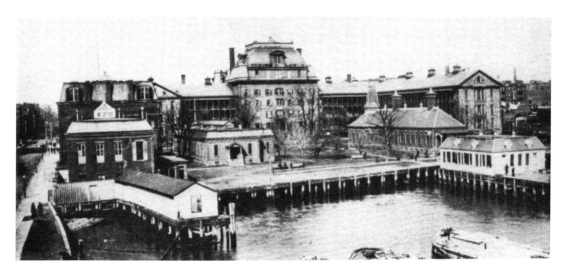

Bellevue Hospital, circa 1878, with the main building as it appeared when the ambulance service started in 1869 ("An Account of Bellevue Hospital," Carlisle, 1893).

buggy whips, all on a scale befitting the Manhattan colossus. If Bellevue was the last resort for the city's sick, its unparalleled curriculum in misery made it the first choice for the most brilliant and ambitious graduates of New York's medical schools. Internships were awarded by competitive examination and conferred a professional prestige on graduates that would follow them like a golden halo throughout their working lives.

One such rising personality was Edward Barry Dalton, a scholarly, bespectacled Harvard graduate who appeared to have directed all his vital energy into the development of his mind at the expense of the delicately proportioned body in which it traveled. Heir to a prominent medical family in Lowell, Massachusetts, Dalton graduated from New York's College of Physicians and Surgeons in 1858, and his acumen and talent earned him a place at Bellevue.[15] At that time the only ambulances in America were the occasional wagons hauling smallpox and fever cases to isolation hospitals, and Dalton himself was more interested in the ailments of the adrenal gland (having written his dissertation on Addison's disease) than on the technical merits of patient transport. Nonetheless, he was about to take a keen and deeply personal interest in ambulance operations when the Civil War pulled him from a comfortable post at the new St. Luke's Hospital (Bellevue was a fine place to train, but few interns elected to remain there permanently). After enlisting under the Union flag in 1861, Dalton served with distinction as a regimental surgeon, ultimately assuming command of the Army of the Potomac's field hospitals in 1864, a position placing him on intimate terms with ambulance organization and operations.

Resigning his commission in May 1865, Dalton returned to Manhattan. This decision coincided with a decision by the New York legislature to create a Metropolitan Sanitary District encompassing New York City, Brooklyn, and the adjoining counties, with a new Board of Health given jurisdiction for the district and broad police powers over matters of sanitation and disease prevention. In casting about for a suitable chief executive, the board received a recommendation from no less a celebrity than General Ulysses Grant, who stated that, in his view, "Dr. Edward Dalton is the best man in the United States for this place," a high opinion based on the excellent administrative work Dalton had done organizing field hospitals during the Peninsular Campaign.[16] Grant's recommendation was given the effect of an edict, and Dalton assumed the office of sanitary superintendent on March 5, 1866. As it happened, he had little time to find his footing because on May 1 a woman living in a sodden tenement, where the sewer drain filled the cellar with bilge, had been spreading the contents of a privy over her vegetable garden when she was seized by unremitting diarrhea and fever, her bodily fluids wrung from her bowels as if by some supernatural mangle.[17] She died within hours, and her pitifully desiccated remains were a bulletin any doctor could read: cholera had returned to New York. Against this ancient evil Dalton was to unleash a novel idea, one that would profoundly influence the evolution of emergency medicine and the ambulance.

In the 19th century only the terror of smallpox rivaled the dread inspired by cholera, a fearsome pestilence leaching quarts of fluid from its victims with such relentless diarrhea and vomiting that a person could sit down to breakfast in good health and yet be dead of shock and dehydration before noon. Cholera was lethal, contagious, and untouchable by the crude medicines of the day. Dalton knew that arresting its spread required immediately identifying the stricken, isolating them, and creating a sterile cordon around any possible source of infection while sanitation procedures were executed. To accomplish his task, Dalton created a rapid response team that, although forgotten in our own time, was unquestionably the first draft of the most successful ambulance service in history. Fifteen years later, in 1882, his old medical school classmate Dr. Benjamin Howard addressed an audience of London surgeons and outlined the four pillars of the successful American ambulance, by then the pattern for the world: "Although the manner of working [an ambulance service] is not in each city alike, in all cases

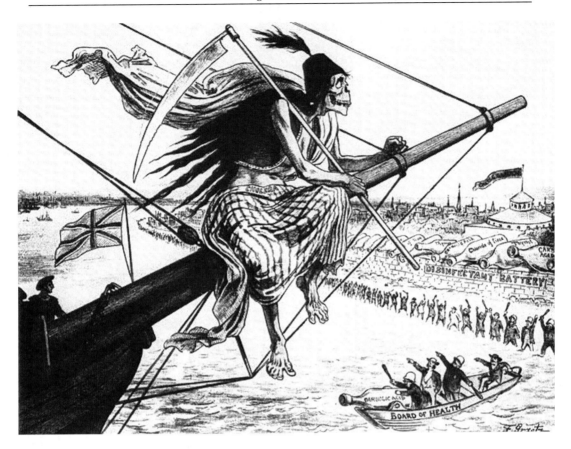

This 1883 cartoon from Puck shows cholera arriving in New York aboard a British ship. The specter wears a Turkish fez, indicative of its Asiatic origin, and is greeted by a "Disinfectant Battery" manned by members of the Manhattan Board of Health and their jurisdictional allies, the city police.

there are four invariable factors: these are the police, the hospitals, the horse ambulance carriages, and the electrical communication."[18]

Each one of these elements had its origin in Dalton's plan for a cholera interdiction force, whose success was much acclaimed by the same public health officials who would inaugurate Bellevue's ambulance service a few years later. First, under Dalton's orders all suspected cholera cases were to be immediately reported to the police. The precinct notified a sanitation inspector who visited the patient and, if cholera were confirmed, had the police telegraph the news to the Board of Health. Adjacent to the Board of Health headquarters Dalton installed a laboratory and a depot with wagons kept in constant readiness, and when a cholera report came in the wagons were dispatched with disinfectant crews (and medical attendance if required) so the residence and its surroundings could be sterilized and fumigated while contaminated bedclothes and the like were burned on the spot. If needed, those requiring hospitalization could also be transported in the wagon, although this purpose was admittedly secondary. The crews generally reached the scene and set to work within one hour of receiving a report, which was considered quite rapid for the day. The success of the program was widely acclaimed by city officials, who credited it with significantly reducing the number of cholera cases in the city, although none could yet foresee that the combination of police, a supporting infirmary, medical wagons on stand-by, and electronic dispatch would be recycled to create the world's most influential ambulance service a few years later.[19] In fact, ever since he had overseen ambulance dispatch for his field hospitals during the Peninsular Campaign, Dalton had been unwittingly gathering the experiences that would lead to an ambulance revolution: the next ingredient was going to be a murder, and it wasn't long in coming.

By April 1867 the cholera epidemic was over and Dalton's flying wagons and interdiction crews were gone. Around the 16th of that month Jackson S. Schultz, president of the New York City Board of Health, was visiting the New York Hospital—the only infirmary in the city below Houston Street. At the time Lower Manhattan was bursting with factories, train yards, and crowded docks, dangerous enterprises that kept surgeons in New York's "reception room"

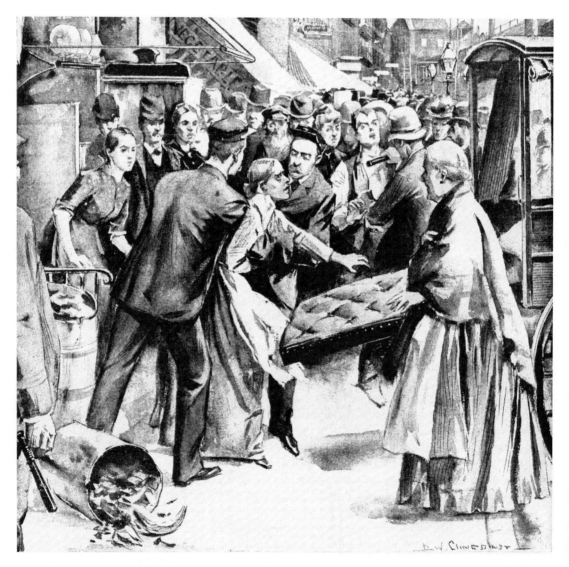

The elements Dr. Howard believed crucial to the American ambulance—the police as first responder, telegraphic dispatch, specialty wagons, and hospital support—were pioneered by Dr. Dalton's cholera interdiction squads. Here, a Bellevue ambulance pays homage to its predecessor as it removes a cholera victim under the watchful eye of the police (*Frank Leslie's Illustrated Weekly*, September 29, 1892).

active with scalpel and catgut and the orderlies busy with their mops. Schultz was touring the receiving ward with members of the Board of Health when a man was carried in from the street with a gunshot wound to the abdomen. The patient was a sailor, injured in a shipboard dispute some days before the ship made port, and when the surgeons opened his shirt they found a flaming pit of infection, the awful wound compounded by his rough cartage from the docks. Fifteen years later Shultz told an interviewer how Dalton, accompanying him as Sanitary Superintendent, told the group that Manhattan could use an ambulance service along military lines in cases like this, where an injury had been aggravated by jolting travel and ignorant care.[20]

Although one of the New York Hospital attending physicians invited Dr. Dalton to come back and expand on his ideas at a meeting of the hospital staff, it took two years, until February 23, 1869, for the governors of the New York Hospital to take Dalton's advice and adopt the following resolution: "Resolved, that the Visiting Committee be requested to procure for the use of this hospital an ambulance of the most approved construction."[21] A few months later, before the Visiting Committee had time to implement its instruction, the hospital's landlord declared his intention to terminate the lease and raze the hospital to the ground in July, in preparation for more profitable tenants. Only the satellite structure called "South House" would be spared, since its leasehold ran a few months longer than the main estate, but it too was slated for demolition, and when it was gone the New York Hospital would hold no property south of Central Park on which to rebuild its infirmary.[22] Reluctant to abandon busy neighborhoods whose factories and docks provided ample emergency cases, the governors of New York Hospital gave orders for South House to be fitted up as "a place for the treatment of surgical and other urgent cases as long as we are permitted to do so."[23] Looking to the day when this last remnant would be closed, James H. Beekman, secretary of the Hospital Committee, sought to salvage the ambulance scheme by writing to the Commissioners of Charities and Corrections in April 1869, asking them to provide "for the treatment of sudden accidents and urgent illness in the lower part of the city, and for the easy transportation by ambulance of the sick to the various Hospitals at present open."[24]

The commissioners immediately accepted the New York Hospital's suggestion and on May 1, 1869, they closed the circle by contacting Dr. Edward Dalton, who had first suggested a city ambulance service while standing beside a dying sailor at New York Hospital two years before. Noting pending legislation to fund a small reception hospital to handle emergency cases in lower Manhattan after the New York Hospital was closed, the board asked Dalton to "frame a Code of Rules suitable for the contemplated Hospital, and especially for an Ambulance system for the prompt and careful removal of the sick and wounded."[25] The board was prepared to go further, however, and expressed its intention to not only install an ambulance service in the proposed reception hospital somewhere south of Canal Street but also to create an identical service at Bellevue for the relief of "such patients as may be taken ill in the upper part of the City."

By now Dalton was no longer the sanitary superintendent, but his role as an associate physician for the municipal Lunatic Asylum meant he was still working for the Charities Commission, and this professional proximity likely made his selection as the ambulance architect more likely. What made him the obvious choice was his unique resume, including his internship at Bellevue hospital eleven years before; his experience as a surgeon and field hospital administrator in the war; and the creation in 1866 of the rapid response cholera interdiction teams, whose elements prefigured those required for an urban emergency ambulance service. Given this opportunity it is scant wonder that the brilliant young physician needed just four days to submit his complete plan. As with his cholera squads, speed was essential and once again he relied on the police department. City patrolmen were already in the habit of rendering casual first aid as required, but now their station houses would use the police telegraph to summon

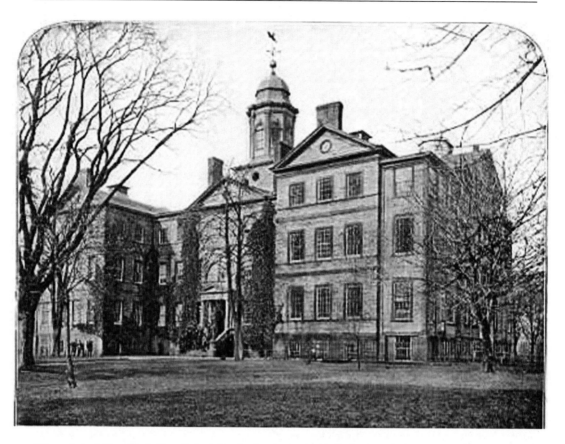

The original New York Hospital: After losing its lease in 1869 the infirmary abandoned plans to inaugurate ambulance services in south Manhattan. While Bellevue's ambulance started in June, it was a year before a satellite ambulance station served the New York's old neighborhood.

the ambulance, just as they had done with his cholera teams. Remedying a defect from his army days, the ambulances (like his cholera wagons) were staffed by surgeons, an innovation giving the nascent field of emergency medicine an ideal of medical professionalism later services struggled to maintain, and, finally, as with his cholera squads the service was built around light wagons kept on twenty-four-hour standby and supported by the full medical resources of the city government.[26]

Once submitted, Dalton's scheme moved forward with astonishing speed. The plan was formally accepted by the commissioners of charities on May 27, 1869, and by June 4 the service was answering calls from Bellevue (the reception hospital had yet to be built).[27] The first runs used house staff since the original ambulance surgeons, Drs. Duncan Lee and Robert Taylor, weren't hired until a week later.[28] While the commissioners planned to hire ambulance surgeons from graduating members of Bellevue's training program, the offer of $50 a month plus room and board proved insufficient incentive once graduates heard about the duty schedule: daily twelve-hour shifts, with the man allegedly "off-duty" taking all calls when the duty surgeon was out—a dreary program relieved by a single day off each month. Not surprisingly, it wasn't long before the Bellevue ambulance was staffed by pliable resident physicians still in training.

A hypothetical case from the first month of the ambulance service helps illustrate Dalton's plan. At this early date the reception hospital in lower Manhattan had yet to open, so four

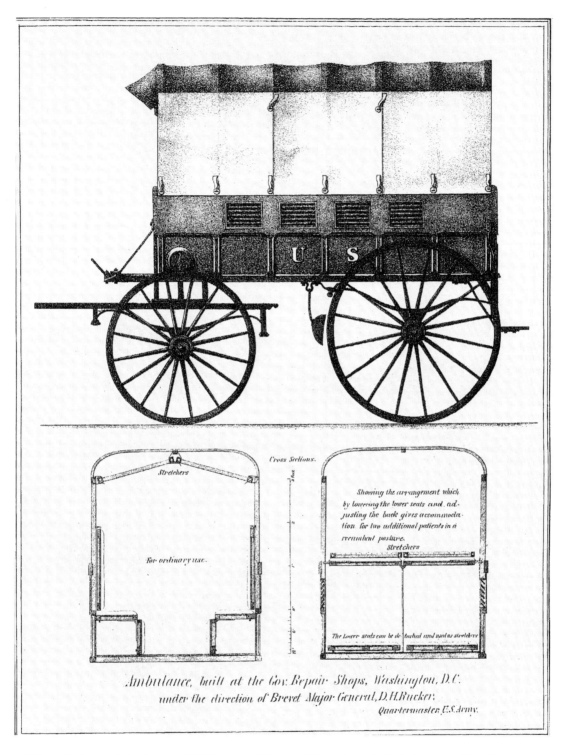

This ambulance plate, from an 1865 Surgeon's General Report, was included as a model pattern in the proposal Dalton sent to the Commissioners of Charities on May 5, 1869 (*Reports on the Extent and Nature of the Materials Available for the Preparation of a Medical and Surgical History of the Rebellion* [Philadelphia: Lippincott, 1865], plate 85).

ambulance wagons built by the Abbot-Downing Co. were stationed at Bellevue Hospital. (Light enough to be drawn by a single horse, each ambulance was seven feet long and thirty-eight inches wide, with retractable canvas side-walls and a large foot-powered gong bolted to the splashboard.) According to Police General Order No. 567, a patrolman coming across "any accident or case of sudden illness in any thoroughfare or public place" was to relay word to his precinct. Immediately men would be sent to the scene carrying one of the stretchers that, on Dalton's orders, were now kept in every station house, and the patient would be carefully carried back to the precinct.[29] Once the patient was safely indoors, the officer on duty made an educated guess as to whether the ambulance was required: if so, a telegram was flashed to the 18th Precinct, which stood nearest to Bellevue. From there it took eight minutes for a runner to cover the distance between the green lamp at the station door and the gaslight at Bellevue's gate, where he handed over a slip of paper with the address of the requesting station house.[30] (By the end of the year Bellevue was connected to the police wires directly, to the relief of footsore patrolmen.)[31]

The surgeons on ambulance duty were summoned by bell and, with one horse always in harness, the ambulance could roll out almost instantly. Arriving at the station house the invalid was carefully loaded, stretcher and all, onto the ambulance's sliding bed while one of the ambulance's litters was taken out and left by way of replacement. Unfortunately, to accommodate

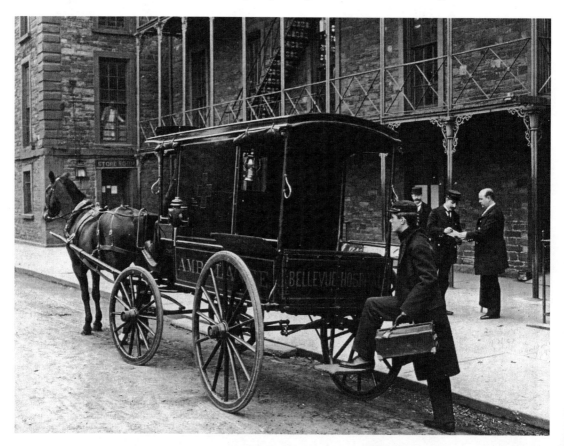

A Bellevue ambulance surgeon poses alongside the "wagon" as his driver is handed a destination slip. Originally the ambulance request would have been telegraphed to the nearest precinct and carried over by a patrolman, but by 1870 the summons could be wired to Bellevue direct (courtesy the National Library of Medicine).

its robust suspension, the cabin rode high off the pavement, forcing the attendant and surgeon to lever the bed up and into the ambulance. Still, it was better to risk lumbago in the crew than to see the injured jostled into the next world at taxpayer expense, and the inconvenience meant the ambulance was "so mounted as to produce no jolting over the roughest pavement," according to an enthusiastic reporter for the *New York Times*.[32] Of course, no 19th century wagon spring could absorb every heave and bump sent upwards by Manhattan's rough streets, and the bottom portion of the cabin was liberally padded for the comfort of the stretcher-case being tumbled on the floor, while the stout leather strap hanging over the surgeon's bench provided a handhold to keep him from being spit into the street like a watermelon seed whenever the wagon bounced out of a pothole. (To further spare the bones of patient and surgeon alike, the commissioners ordered drivers to use whenever possible roadways covered in Belgian pavement, those smooth granite blocks slowly replacing cobblestones or mud on some busy thoroughfares.)[33]

At the scene and en route the surgeons were equipped to provide proper first aid, both with their own bags and the Victorian equivalent of a portable emergency room salted away beneath the driver's bench. Inside this stout wooden box were a quart flask of brandy, two tourniquets, splints, strips of discarded blankets for padding, buckled straps for immobilizing fractured limbs, a half-dozen bandages and an equal number of sponges, and a two ounce bottle of persulphate of iron, used as an astringent to stop bleeding.[34] (After a few exciting episodes handcuffs and a straitjacket were added to secure the violently insane and "patients of a demonstrative disposition.")[35] On night runs a swaying lantern would have thrown leaping shadows around the cabin, mixing its sweet odor with the tang of sweat, the brisk perfume of freshly washed sheets, and the smell of linseed oil and varnish leaching out from the gleaming wood. Finally, responsibility for ensuring these technical marvels and their highly educated cargo made it there and back again fell to the drivers, Daniel McGuire and James Stone, who, after an unexpectedly busy summer on the job, were given a raise to $30 a month in September—a respectable wage for the day.[36]

Upon reaching Bellevue patients were unloaded and carried into a basement receiving office located adjacent to a gloomy quadrangle, an office whose door stood open around the clock, until at last the location of the key was literally forgotten.[37] Those cases deemed eligible for city care were given an iron-framed bed in an enormous ward upstairs and economically maintained on sixteen cents a day.[38] Regrettably, the mortality rate at Bellevue ranged from appreciable to shameful, so a fair number of ambulance cases wound up in the morgue next door. The unclaimed and unidentified were laid out beneath large viewing windows for inspection by passersby, but those who remained anonymous until putrefaction set in were carried down to the East River for one final journey at city expense, this time aboard the steamer *M.V. Hope*, a name at odds with a vessel that one observer described as "grim, black, [and] demoniac-looking."[39] The *Hope* ferried the unclaimed bodies to Hart's Island, where they were piled thirteen coffins deep in huge trenches, their remains guarded from body-snatchers by feral mastiffs deposited on the island for that purpose.[40]

Although Dalton's outline proved remarkably durable, a few rough edges had to be smoothed down. The original stretchers proved unnecessarily awkward and were swiftly replaced by a simpler, lighter model permitting the gravest fractures and maimings to be "transferred without infliction of unnecessary pang," according to the commissioners.[41] Finally, after constables proved too eager to call the wagon for every inebriate they tripped over on patrol, the telegraph key was initially restricted to the Police Surgeons. These private physicians, salaried by the department but keeping their own practice, proved reluctant to attend casualty cases at two in the morning simply to approve an ambulance call, so by January 1870 the scheme had been abandoned, and once more the officers themselves decided whether a groggy citizen found on

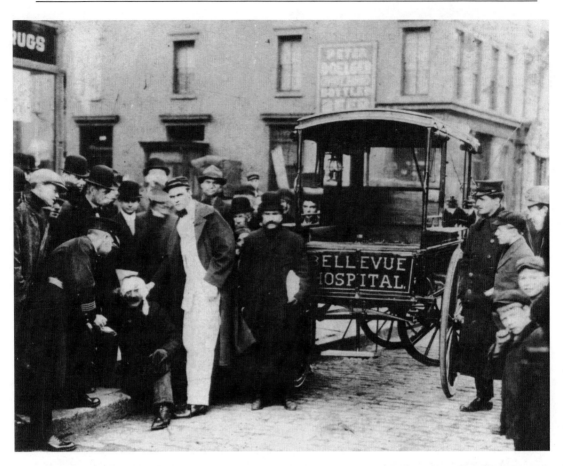

A police officer, whose precinct telegraph would have summoned the ambulance, assists a Bellevue surgeon with a patient. The ambulance driver is at the far right, in the long coat (courtesy Ehrman Medical Library, NYU Medical Center).

the sidewalk was destined for the drunk tank or the medical ward.[42] In its first six months the little service handled five hundred fifty-eight patients, at an amortized cost of just under six dollars per call.[43] Where once Bellevue had received Gotham's casualties in carriages and rough wagons, now they arrived in well-equipped ambulances staffed by skilled surgeons, and it was the proud boast of the ambulance crews that in the first eighteen months of service only four lives were lost during the swift ride to Bellevue.[44] In all, it was forgivable overstatement when the Medical Board of Bellevue Hospital noted in their annual report of 1870: "All that can be said of this organization is, that it seems perfect in all regards, and its management leaves nothing to be desired."[45] Troubled times lay ahead, but at its debut the ambulance scheme of Dr. Edward Dalton was a triumph for the city and a living monument to the many hands that, at last, had created a model civilian ambulance service. The world had waited long enough.

Crimes and Casualties: Early Ambulance Exploits

Once they took to the streets, Bellevue's ambulances were swiftly lauded in the pages of the *New York Times*, a valentine ascribed to by the entire city. And why not? In 1869 Manhat-

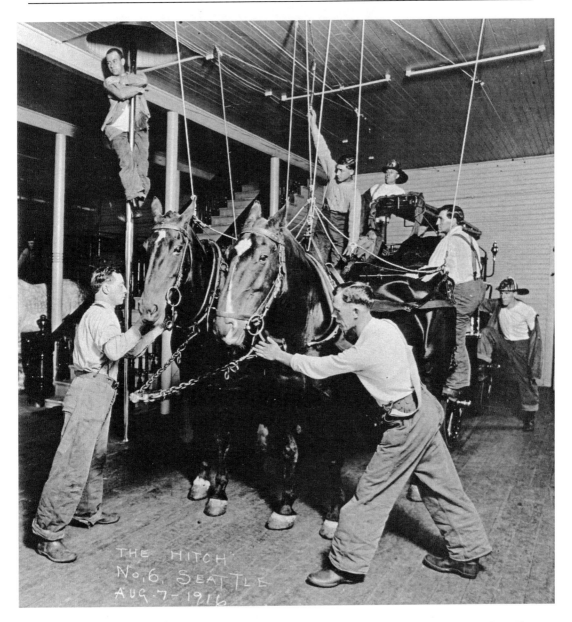

Originally designed for fire departments, the "drop harness" allowed a horse to be rigged in as little as thirty seconds. The mechanism is shown in considerable detail in this scene from the Seattle Fire Department in 1916 (courtesy the Seattle Museum of History and Industry).

tan was a polluted bedlam of violence and pestilence where endemic violent crime left victims sprawled in gutters and tenement halls, maiming and crush injuries were commonplace in the abattoirs of industry, and there was enough disease in the poisonous slums to keep the ambulance horses in Derby-winning trim. A random sampling of calls answered in its first sixteen months of service include a man hurled from a third story window by his wife; numerous attempted suicides by poison, straight razor, and hanging; victims of gas explosions and fire; and several men with cracked skulls, either from a drunken fall or a chance meeting with a blackjack.[46] Getting to these calls provided its own splash of drama to the city's gory palette of mayhem, and a visitor from Rochester, New York vividly described the appearance, and passage, of the new machine:

> Walking up Broadway, [a passerby] may suddenly have his attention arrested by an unusual agitation up the street: a bell clangs harshly, and he is startled to see omnibuses and carts and carriages pull suddenly to either side, leaving an open lane between. Down this course comes a covered four-wheeled wagon drawn by a powerful horse galloping hotly. The driver is cool and alert, and has control ... on the rear seat a uniformed young gentleman carelessly contemplates the press on either side.
> The vehicle is an ambulance summoned by telegraph from one of the large public hospitals to attend to some casualty and to carry the sufferer to a place of relief. It has the right of way over all other vehicles. It is supplied with all appliances necessary in emergencies, and the young man on the rear seat is an ambulance surgeon.[47]

The excitement and chaotic social conditions feeding the new service reached a crescendo in July 1870 when the service marked its first anniversary with a climactic role in the sanguinary Elm Park Riot. The trouble began when Protestant "Orangemen," celebrating the anniversary of the Battle of Boyne with a parade and picnic, ran afoul of a mob of Irish Catholic laborers sympathetic to the losing side of that 1690 battle between the English and a Franco-Irish army.[48] The three thousand men, women, and children attending the festivities in Elm Park were soon beset by a thousand or more Fenians, mostly drawn from the nearby work gangs laying pave-

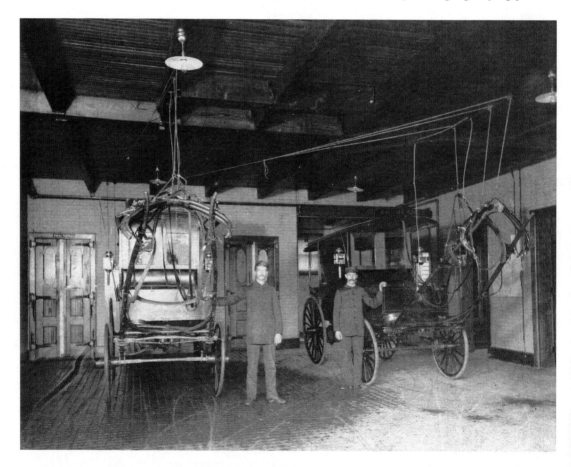

Valuing speed as much as fire crews did, ambulance squads were quick to adopt the drop harness, which was gentler than leaving the horse standing in tack. Here, a turn-of-the-century ambulance crew in Rochester, N.Y., shows off their new gear (courtesy ViaHealth Consortium Archives).

ment, excavating foundations, and putting up new buildings—occupations that put to hand a lethal assortment of improvised weapons like picks, shovels, and planks. For several hours the rabble clamored outside the fenced grounds until pistol fire from the street seemed to signal a general attack, and the mob broke through the palings of the park, scattering the picnicking families. The rioters clubbed and booted down their victims without regard for sex or age, and a general slaughter was only narrowly averted by the arrival of a hastily summoned band of sixteen police officers swinging their locust wood clubs with desperate strength as they closed with the incomparably larger mass of rioters.

Behind them the call went out to summon the entire reserve force, even as a police telegrapher hammered out an urgent wire to the Bellevue ambulance barn. At the other end a drop harness plunged from the ceiling, men with coat tails flapping scrambled aboard a gleaming black wagon, and then, with a flick of the reins, the first ambulance barreled along on the four-mile run to Elm Park. Even as the familiar wagon clattered into sight fresh casualties were being carried into the station house, so the teams swiftly loaded the most grievously injured and turned the horses around for the dash back to the East River. Thousands thronged the streets that gory day as screams and shouts echoed down the brick canyons, but the marvelously tempered horses never panicked, only pressing on, sometimes alone, sometimes with a police escort (and on at least one run a burly patrolman was stationed *inside* the ambulance to keep the four injured passengers from finishing their vendetta en route).[49] Long into the night the ambulances ran back and forth, as each hour revealed more victims hiding in cellars, alleys, and dark corners of parkland, too terrified or injured to break cover on their own.[50] Ultimately, out of untold numbers of maimed and injured, there were only eight confirmed deaths, but it was universally understood that Bellevue's swift, effective ambulance service could claim the difference between the numbered dead and the expected harvest of such violence, a tribute to Dalton's planning and the dedication of the men and steeds of the ambulance squads.

The pace of the work, even aside from rioting Irish expats, was such that five more ambulances with matching steeds were added by the end of 1870 (just in time for the inevitable sequel, the Orange Riot of 1871).[51] Matters had been made worse that year by a summer memorable for what the *New York Times* called an "unprecedented continuance of heat and solar phenomena" that saw ambulance calls increase from an average of ninety-five cases a month between January and May 1870, to more than one hundred seventy cases a month from June through August.[52] Welcome as the new wagons were, the city not only needed more ambulances, it needed more staging areas, since Bellevue's location on the eastern shore of Manhattan created long delays when the ambulance was needed in the remote reaches of the western piers or the industrial district in the extreme south. The availability of the ambulance service also meant that cases were being brought into Bellevue that in an earlier day might have traveled by cab to a closer hospital, and the mighty infirmary was in danger of inundation.

Clearly, satellites were needed for the relief not only of Bellevue's crowded reception rooms but for the patients who otherwise faced several jolting miles over rough streets.[53] Fortunately, the lower Manhattan infirmary which had been part of the original ambulance draft was in full service by July 1, 1870, with Drs. Vandewater and Marsh in attendance and an ambulance with horse in harness standing by at all hours.[54] Apparently the funds were not so generous as originally hoped (or a larger than usual percentage was skimmed off as graft), because the new city ambulance service found itself attached to a tiny infirmary tucked into City Hall Park, a location offering ambiance but little else: its unlucky ambulance driver shared an eight-by fourteen-foot apartment with an engineer, a druggist, and the orderly—accommodations only slightly more meager than those afforded the three surgeons in their single dorm, or the patients, who soon found themselves crammed five and six into rooms barely big enough for three.[55]

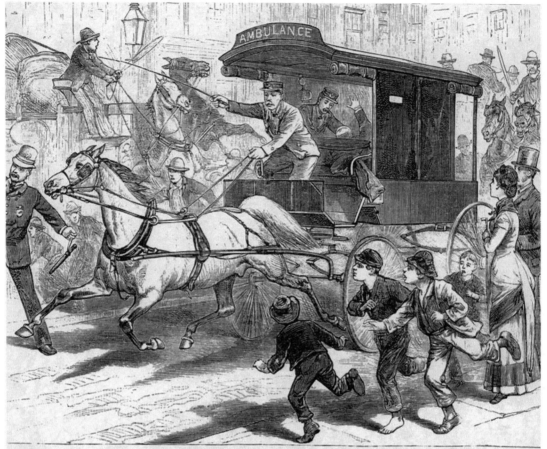

A TORRID DAY IN NEW YORK CITY.—THE AMBULANCE SERVICE OF THE PUBLIC HOSPITALS.

Note the patient flailing in the back, as well as the rearing horses at the intersection and the frightened little girl standing dangerously near the wagon's left rear wheel. By the 1890s some disgruntled New Yorkers had come to view the ambulance as a nuisance to pedestrians and other drivers (*Frank Leslie's Illustrated Newspaper*, 1881).

Whatever the limitations of the Centre Street hospital, the speed with which new wagons were added and new stations commissioned vindicated Dalton's vision and confirmed the success of his venture: within two years of its inception in June 1869, the Bellevue Ambulance Service had made the transition from innovation to institution, and the nascent field of emergency medicine found itself poised on the threshold of national acceptance.

Capital Improvements—Wealthy Donors and the Ambulance Movement

The limelight bathing the Bellevue ambulance service cast the city's private infirmaries into an unaccustomed and unwelcome shadow from which they were eager to emerge. In short order they initiated their own ambulance operations to serve the public's need for rapid emergency aid (as well as its appetite for speed and spectacle), and by 1878 New Yorkers had a plethora of ambulance services attending them. The largely undeveloped upper West Side, near Harlem, was served by the city-run 99th Street Hospital Ambulance Corps, while near the southwest corner of Central Park the Roosevelt Hospital attended the emergency needs of the swells near Columbus Circle; almost due west of Bellevue, midtown was guarded by the august New York Hospital, whose eviction from south Manhattan had precipitated the original ambulance service a decade earlier, while since 1875 the New York Hospital had operated a small emergency hospital at 160 Chambers Street, roughly midway between City Hall and the Hudson River.

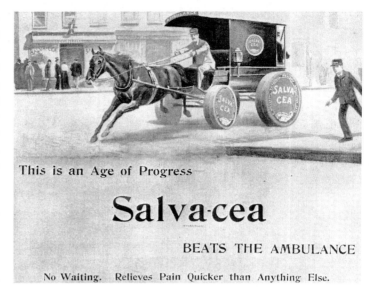

This 1895 advertisement for Salva-Cea (guaranteed to relieve burns, bruises, ulcerated teeth, and hemorrhoids, among much else) traded on the speed that was popularly associated with the ambulance service.

Unlike the ambulance services at the Bellevue, 99th Street, and Centre Street (Park) Hospitals, these new emergency services were privately funded, with each ambulance wagon, crew member, and horse financed by civic-minded plutocrats.[56] Fortunately, benefactors lived up to the prediction of medical reformer Dr. Benjamin Howard that "[a]n ambulance carriage is just the kind of thing many donors would like to give ... [and] an ambulance station is just the kind of thing that many would like to endow, its benefit being daily visible."[57] The benefit, however, was not one that the donors had any expectation of enjoying. As one contemporary commentator pointed out, "the ambulance subject is usually a person in poor circumstances. One rarely sees a well-dressed occupant being carried to the hospital by ambulance."[58]

(Indeed, absent the technological marvels of a later age, hospitals had nothing to offer that could compete with a house call at a well-appointed mansion, where at least the patient would not be sharing a ward—if not an actual bed—with fellow sufferers being treated by physicians who walked from autopsy to bedside without thought of changing their clothes or even washing their hands, since an obstinate profession resisted consensus on the germ theory until the 1880s: indeed, so far as the destination of the ambulance was concerned, it was scant exaggeration when one 19th century commentator fulminated that "it were better for a man to be placed on a dunghill or in a stable than to let him remain in a house of charity.")[59] Still, one philanthropist investing in this new project was usually all it took to precipitate an avalanche of ambulances, since others in their rarefied social orbit found it socially untenable to see their own pet hospitals publicly upstaged and dug deep into their railway dividends to buy a carriage or endow an ambulance barn. (For example, the Brooklyn Health Service enjoyed a monopoly on ambulances in 1873 until the privately operated St. Mary's Hospital acquired an ambulance in 1883. This set off a fund-raising race, with other private hospitals swiftly adding their own ambulance services: St. Catherine's in 1887, the Homeopathic and Methodist-Episcopal, both in 1888, and the privately funded Brooklyn Hospital in 1890.)

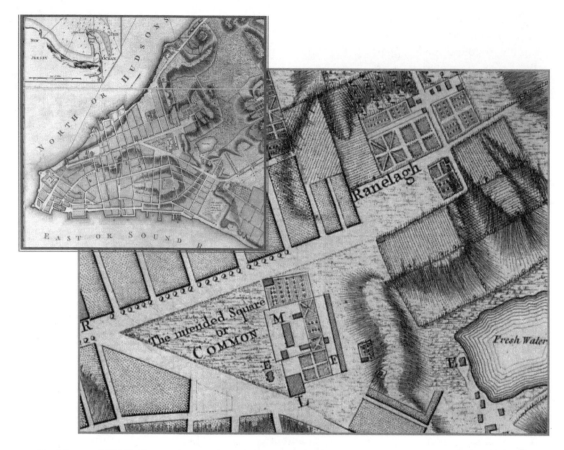

In this map "M" indicates the location of the original workhouse whose infirmary was the forerunner of Bellevue Hospital. Coincidentally, Bellevue's southern annex, the Centre Street Hospital, occupied the same location a century later (John Montresor, A plan of the city of New-York & its environs, etc. [London, 1766]). (Library of Congress, Geography and Map Division, G3804.N4 1766 .M6 Vault.)

Thanks to the efforts of socially conscious benefactors, by the end of the 1870s Manhattan's ambulance fleet was unparalleled in fame and success and unmatched in size. Engravings in the national magazines carried its image across the continent while feature articles described its operations and achievements, inspiring wealthy donors and city officials to finance their own local ambulance operations.

Institutional Ambulances and Mortuaries

Meanwhile, other agencies began to appreciate the peculiar benefits of a well-organized ambulance service: following in the carriage tracks of London's Hospital Committee, municipal Departments of Health realized that ambulances reduced transmission of contagious disease by keeping the infected from traveling to the hospital in public cabs (before 1870, for example, Brooklyn acquired separate ambulances for typhoid and small pox cases); teaching hospitals embraced the ambulance as a reliable purveyor of surgical cases, as with Massachusetts General Hospital's acquisition of an ambulance in 1878, a combination of pedagogy and charitable feeling first seen when London's Middlesex Hospital introduced its "chair and horse"

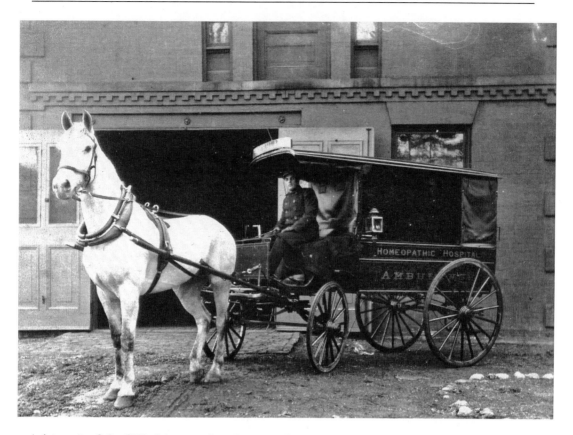

Aristocrats of the Gilded Age purchased status with investments in social capital like this ambulance from Mrs. Henry H. Perkins. Her gift to the Rochester Homeopathic Hospital included two ambulances, horses named Edward, Zip, Doctor, and Florence Nightingale, and a barn (Rochester Homeopathic Hospital, *The Hospital Leaflet*, September 10, 1895). The lace gauntlet thrown, within three years patrons of all the city's major hospitals had sponsored their own ambulance services (Teresa Lehr and Phillip Maples, *To Serve the Community: A Celebration of Rochester General Hospital 1847–1997* [Virginia Beach: Donning Company, 1997]). (Courtesy ViaHealth Consortium Archives.)

almost a century earlier to bring in surgical cases for its teaching wards; and across the country compassionate hospital managers recognized that a well-appointed ambulance saved lives that might otherwise be lost when the severely injured or ill were subjected to the rough usage of cab or cart.[60]

It is not surprising that Philadelphia, whose volunteer fire companies had started offering non-emergency ambulance service in 1863, was peculiarly susceptible to such influences. As mentioned earlier, the various fire companies had gotten information about the arrival of hospital ships and trains from the police telegraph at their closest precinct house, and it was the second city in the country to rely on a dedicated telegraph line to dispatch an ambulance—the Philadelphia Board of Health was using the wires to summon a fever ambulance from the municipal hospital by May 1870, just a few months after the Bellevue telegraph station had been completed.[61] After the volunteer firefighting companies were replaced by a paid force in 1871 their ambulances appear to have been withdrawn from the emergency service, and so in 1872 Dr. Morton of the Pennsylvania Hospital suggested to the Mayor that the police and fire telegraph wires be extended to the infirmary and a general ambulance service be installed.[62] Ultimately it wasn't until 1876 that the hospital acquired its first ambulance wagon, but in 1874

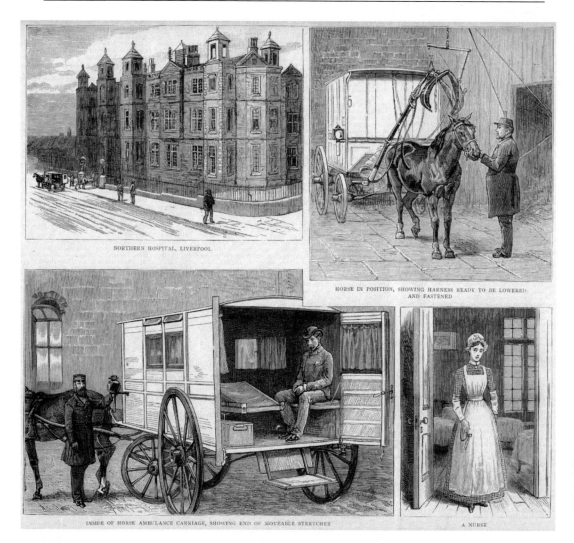

While the ambulance made slow progress on the continent, the influence of American reformers like Dr. Benjamin Howard took hold in England by the early 1880s. The Northern Hospital in Liverpool started with a Howard ambulance in 1881, but five years later replaced it with the locally designed model seen here (*The Graphic*, November 27, 1886).

the Guardians of the Poor purchased four ambulances for the Almshouse Hospital, at the suggestion of Dr. William H. Pancoast, who, in common with ambulance pioneers like Dalton and Howard, had been a surgeon in the Civil War.[63] The Almshouse infirmary was also linked to the police telegraph, not only allowing for instant dispatch anywhere in the city but which also permitted the house surgeon to get the particulars of the case before setting out and equip the ambulance according to the need of the patient. While Philadelphia was thus an early adopter of many innovative techniques, the progress of its hospitals was quickly followed by other communities as a well-developed ambulance service became a point of pride for many institutions.

Also taking note of the new technology were America's undertakers, a profession uniquely poised to capitalize on the public's new expectations for handling the sick and injured: their training in embalming gave morticians, particularly in small communities, an aura of practical medical knowledge, and hearses were ready made for ambulance work, being naturally configured for a recumbent passenger. (Indeed, it was common for 19th century towns to hire out the funeral coach during epidemics to deliver the infected to special fever hospitals.) From the funeral home's perspective converting an otherwise idle hearse into an ambulance was potentially profitable with only a modest investment in a stretcher and blankets. In addition to whatever modest fee they might charge (let alone collect), an ambulance service increased the firm's visibility and, if the patient died, a grateful family might hire the mortuary for the burial arrangements—possibly using the same hearse. In fact, the occasional funeral secured this way was often the best economic reason for mortuaries to provide ambulance services.[64] (If there was an inherent conflict of interest in operating an ambulance as a loss-leader for funerals, people were apparently too polite to have mentioned it.)

Some of the first funeral homes entering the market were in Cleveland, whose mortuaries advertised ambulance services as early as 1879.[65] By 1920 Cleveland had over one hundred funeral parlors providing the bulk of the city's ambulance service—and using embalming fluid to disinfect the vehicles after transporting infectious cases.[66] This creative use of formaldehyde aside, some of the nation's mortuary ambulances maintained high standards, providing clean bedding and comfortable stretchers in vehicles staffed by attendants trained at least in the use of tourniquets and splints and provisioned with basic medicines such as stimulants: others offered little more than a hearse with a cot.[67] Staffing was equally scatter-shot. A driver might be a former hospital orderly, or might have learned the rudiments of first aid from long service, but, as one physician observed, often ambulance drivers were hired solely on the basis of their ability to drive a horse at sufficient speed to get to the accident scene first and secure the "fare," while the attendant who rode in the back was frequently nothing more than an idler who had been "simply loafing around the barn and [who] finds delight in making runs."[68]

Aside from their technical merits, it often happened that in a particular town more than one funeral home set up an ambulance service, and the existence of competing private services operating independently of the municipal authorities made it difficult to establish a rational dispatching system, with firms taking whatever call came in regardless of whether a competitor was closer to hand. (Similarly, manufacturing firms with a high incidence of injury often contracted with specific mortuaries for ambulance services, usually choosing cheaper rates over proximity and exposing their employees to undue delay.) The impossibility of knowing when a private ambulance might arrive, and what it would look when it did, usually resulted in a large percentage of the population voting with their feet in towns where mortuary

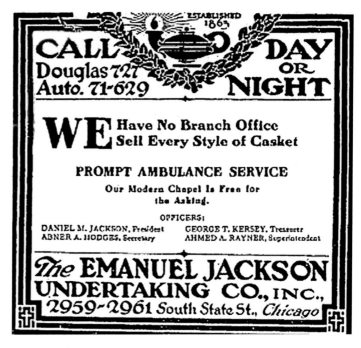

A 1914 newspaper advertisement for a Chicago mortuary with ambulance service.

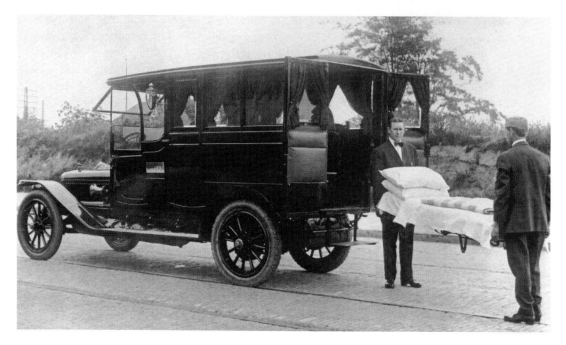

Butterworth and Sons, a mortuary and ambulance service in Seattle, around 1919 (Seattle Museum of History and Industry).

ambulances ruled the streets. For example, in 1906 Cleveland had an ambulance service strongly dominated by funeral homes and a population in excess of 430,000, yet that year just forty-two hundred accidentally injured persons arrived at city hospitals via ambulance, while many more came in buggies, wagons, and other ad hoc conveyances.[69] In the 1950s Chicago was another city whose funeral homes owned a near monopoly of the ambulance market, and by one survey only 6 percent of city accident cases arrived at the hospital in an ambulance.[70] By comparison, the Rochester, New York, ambulance system was hospital run and police dispatched, guaranteeing quick physician service in a completely modern aid car: not surprisingly, by 1932 fully one-third of patients reached the hospital in an ambulance.[71]

Still, whatever their faults the pioneering mortuary ambulance services appearing in the wake of Bellevue's grand experiment were essential in carrying the idea of the ambulance to the smallest hamlet: after all, hospitals with the resources to support transportation services were likely to be found only in cities of at least modest size, while few communities in the country were so healthy that they weren't supporting at least one undertaker. Whether it was a funeral home, a civic spirited infirmary, a great teaching hospital, or a police department putting stretchers in its patrol wagons, the ambulance was finding new homes across the nation. Behind Bellevue's barn the East River was just a muddy creek to be forded by Dalton's wagons in short order, and the boulevards they traveled soon stretched from the Battery to the Pacific: Dalton's ambulance corps now belonged to the world.

Missing in Action—The European Ambulance

Or at least the New World, since adoption of the emergency ambulance was much delayed in Europe. Assuming that the United States, by virtue of the Civil War and its aftermath, had been singularly well situated to pioneer the modern ambulance movement, the question remains why the idea was so slow to take hold on the Continent despite the free exchange of news, journals, and professional visits. While political factors, such as London's decentralized government and the relative paucity of active-aged military officers entering commercial or public life, conspired against wholesale adoption of the ambulance scheme, other factors contributed as well. One was the comparatively conservative cast to European society, an environment where novel ideas were not recommended simply by virtue of their novelty, as was arguably the case in the more bumptious United States. A second, and more flattering, explanation is that continental Europe was already experimenting with a novel approach to emergency medical aid—the Night Medical Service.

The earliest mention of the Night Medical Service was in France, when Dr. Passant proposed it as a way of reducing death and morbidity among the impoverished. His plan, proposed in 1869, called for police stations to maintain lists of physicians willing to answer night calls in exchange for a guaranteed minimum payment from the government.[72] The thought was that the poor were often unable to obtain prompt medical attention at the onset of a crisis, waiting until their condition was dire before seeking admittance at a charitable hospital—by which time their care cost the city many times the going rate for the simple house call that might have arrested their illness early in its course. Paris did not implement the program until 1875, but the scheme was adopted by Berlin by 1872 and St. Petersburg in 1874, and by 1880 it was operational in Moscow, Warsaw, Rome, Lisbon, and Algiers, as well as several smaller cities.[73]

Could the presence of such a scheme actually have reduced the incentive for an ambulance service? A comparison between the experience of New York and Paris suggests that it

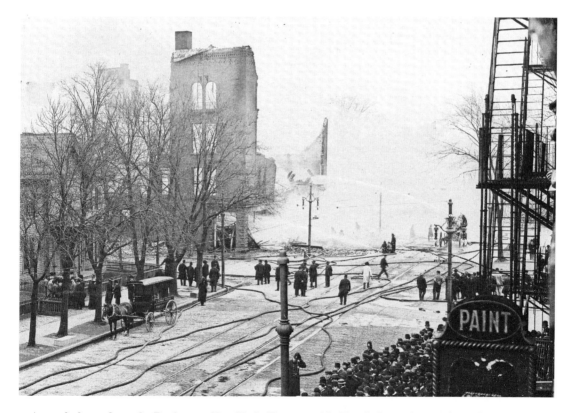

An ambulance from the Rochester, New York, Homeopathic Hospital stands guard at a fire in 1909 (from the Albert R. Stone Negative Collection, Rochester Museum & Science Center, Rochester, N.Y.).

could—while also demonstrating that the ambulance had unique benefits the European model could not duplicate. The story begins with Dr. Henri Nachtel, a Frenchman who spent the early 1880s trying to bring the New York ambulance to Paris—and the Parisian Night Medical Service to New York. In early 1880, Dr. Nachtel read a paper to the New York Academy of Medicine proposing that Manhattan adopt a Night Medical Service like the one operating in France; in 1881 he delivered an address to the French Academie de Medicine proposing a New-York-style ambulance service for Paris.[74] Of the audiences, the Americans proved the more receptive, and his proposal for a Night Medical Service swiftly caught the approving eye of the *New York Times* editorial page.[75] A bill establishing the scheme in New York City was signed by the governor in July 1880, and the first patient was seen shortly after one A.M. on September 4, Dr. O.L. Dusseldorf attending.[76] As originally proposed, those willing to participate in the service were vetted by the registrar of vital statistics to weed out incompetents; the surviving names were forwarded to the precinct nearest their homes, and after a certain hour of the night they could be summoned by constable at the request of any citizen.[77] Each house call was reimbursed at three dollars, with the city honoring the bill when the patient could not. This scheme (which was also proposed in Philadelphia at about the same time) was in every particular identical to that in effect in Paris. The only difference was that New York's Night Service operated in a city with an efficient ambulance operation, while in Paris it served a metropolis where the Count of Wimpfen could commit suicide on the Avenue Monceau and then lay sprawled on the cobblestones for two hours until a vehicle could be located to remove his remains.[78]

The difference in results was dramatic. In Paris the Night Medical Service immediately averaged more than two hundred fifty calls a month, while in New York the service made thirty-six calls a month after almost a year and half in operation.[79] Even allowing for the difference in population the Paris service was proportionately four times as busy as New York's. At its apparent peak in the 1890s, as New York's population continued to grow, the Medical Service was only averaging sixty-six calls a month, a fraction of what was expected of the Paris service.[80] While Gallic disinterest in Nachtel's efforts to deliver an American-style ambulance to Paris was considered by many New Yorkers as an example of European prejudice and conservatism, it is plausible the Night Medical Service served as a sort of safety valve for public discontent, each successful case depriving the ambulance cause of one more partisan and making the status quo incrementally more tolerable and change less imperative.[81] Meanwhile, in New York the active and efficient ambulance service won the popularity contest as measured by the volume of calls, letting the generous volunteers of the Night Service sleep through their shifts while hospital interns tended the city's ailing in the small hours.

Trampled by the Iron Horse

> In this age of rapid transit, swiftly-moving street cars, numerous railroad crossings at grade, speeding automobiles, electrically charged overhead wires, thousands of factories vibrating under the power of dangerous engines, these and countless other factors have great possibilities for injury to men, [and] demand some effort to reform [the] atrocious and haphazard way of mishandling the accidentally injured [Dr. Myron Metzenbaum, "History of the Cleveland Ambulance," 1907].

There can be no doubt that the rapid industrialization of the United States abetted the success of Dalton's scheme, a triumph assisted by the lively press of the day which publicized both the terrors of new forms of devastating injury and the thrilling rescues executed by the dashing ambulance wagons patrolling Gotham's bustling thoroughfares. For example, when Manhattan debuted its ambulance service in 1869, its neighbor across the East River, Brooklyn, was a grease-under-the-fingernails kind of town, seething with boiler shops, factories, sugar-houses, and brick yards: a place where railways punched their way through the thronging streets, bringing in raw materials, hauling away finished goods, and woe to the careless pedestrian whose foot got in the way of high-speed commerce. Limited safety measures and crowded conditions meant that a proliferation of exploding steam boilers, railway accidents, and miserable "crush" injuries on factory floors kept Brooklyn's dailies well-provisioned with grim headlines. Looking over the river towards Manhattan, the future borough watched with envy as the new ambulances brought relief and the hope of survival to the kinds of people who, in Brooklyn, were dying unattended in the backs of wagons and horse-drawn cabs clattering towards the hospital.

For two years the Bellevue ambulance was a beacon casting a shadow but no spark, until in 1871 a Brooklyn coroner's jury became the first municipal body to officially advocate duplication of the Bellevue ambulance service. No signal catastrophe moved this gathering of taxpayers to militate for medical reform, as their cue was an uncomplicated death of a sort that had become commonplace. Undoubtedly influenced by their foreman, a physician employed by the City Hospital, in plain prose they asked the political powers to give them some hope that in a month one of their own number would not be the topic of yet another coroner's jury:

> In our opinion Adam Hadden, the deceased, came to his death from excessive loss of blood, after he had been run over [on the South Side Railroad], and we believe that had he received immediate sur-

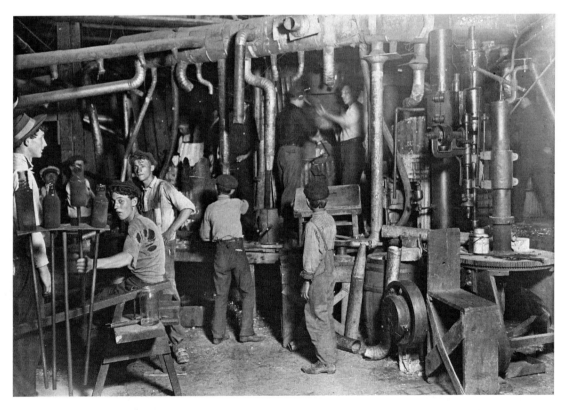

By the late 19th century 3 percent of America's industrial workforce was killed or injured each year, largely due to appalling working conditions, as in this glass factory. Unlike agricultural employment, each victim of a factory accident could literally be seen by thousands in a crowded city, multiplying the effect and contributing to demands for better emergency care. (Lewis Hines, 1908. Library of Congress Prints and Photographs Division, LC-H501-120.)

gical attention his life might have been spared, and would most earnestly call the attention of the Common Council to the urgent necessity of better means of transporting the injured, and recommend that there be immediately established ambulances ... furnished with tourniquets and all necessary appliances.[82]

Soon after the verdict was delivered a city-wide petition appeared, demanding the "establishment of an ambulance system for the speedy conveyance of injured persons to a hospital in the city," and when the ultimatum was delivered to the Brooklyn Council in January 1872, it had the weight of three thousand signatures behind it.[83] Happy to save voter's limbs (and their own jobs), the council took a break from approving paving contracts and appropriated $5,000 to purchase and equip at least five ambulances, to be outfitted with, in addition to the usual medical supplies, "necessary implements and appliances" for water rescue and resuscitation.[84] After substantial delay, the service finally started receiving patients in 1873.

Where Brooklyn led, others followed, with the surge of ambulance operations from the 1870s onward reflecting the urbanite's escalating concern for personal safety as the streets beneath their feet seemingly turned into macadam conveyor belts dragging them faster and faster into a maelstrom of steam-driven mandibles, belching smokestacks, and boulevards shaking under passing trains and phalanxes of bawling teamsters. Thus, when a Philadelphia physician wanted to expand his city's ambulance services in 1883, he had only to appeal to the frenzied city dweller's instinct for self-preservation:

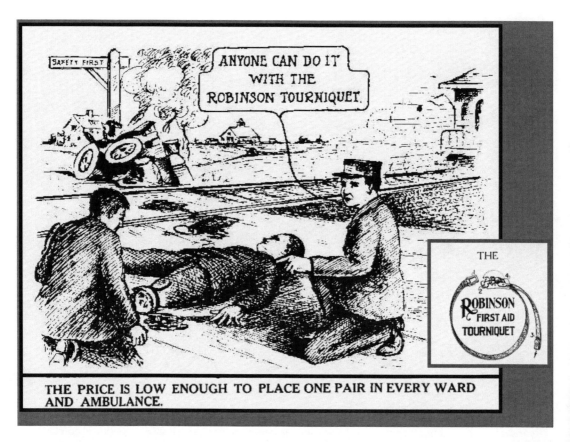

A man run over by a train illustrates a tourniquet's effectiveness when applied by an ambulance surgeon, a scenario mirroring the 1871 case that led a Brooklyn Coroner's jury to demand a municipal ambulance service.

The city of Philadelphia is urgently in need of a thorough and complete system of rendering speedy aid and comfortable transportation to those unfortunates who may be injured in her streets and busy workshops.... Any of us may fall in the street, suddenly stricken by an overpowering disease; we may be thrown from a wagon, or be struck by a running horse, or receive a blow from a chance brick or timber, or may trip over some slight obstruction, or may become the victims of a railway accident, or crushed by falling walls. Maimed, perhaps insensible, and our identity temporarily destroyed, we are all proper subjects for the kindly care of our mother city. Machinery and railway cars produce especially a form of injury known as crush, which is often of exceeding gravity and requires the most skillful attention ... [i]n the past, each sufferer has been dependent upon the hospitality of a neighboring store or office, or must lie [in the street] exposed to cold and wet.[85]

While his oration painted an unappetizing picture of a city where hapless bystanders were being crushed by falling walls and any taxpayer was apt to have a brick hurled at his head by a passing leper, his plea found its mark: within a year nineteen police stations were equipped with wheeled litters, and by 1888 ten of the city's hospitals provided ambulance services.[86]

Last Rites of Way: Ambulances and Trains

Nationally, railway accidents were an especially feared source of injury, with derailments and collisions only the most spectacular versions. Absent the modern trucking industry, rail-

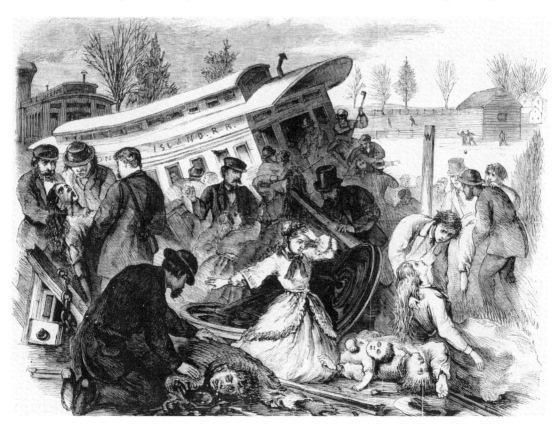

While catastrophic railway disasters seized the public's imagination, the casualties due to running track at street level through crowded cities claimed far more bloody tribute at the altar of Mammon than derailments and collisions. The number and severity of these daily injuries fueled demands for ambulance services across the country (*Frank Leslie's Illustrated Newspaper*, May 8, 1869).

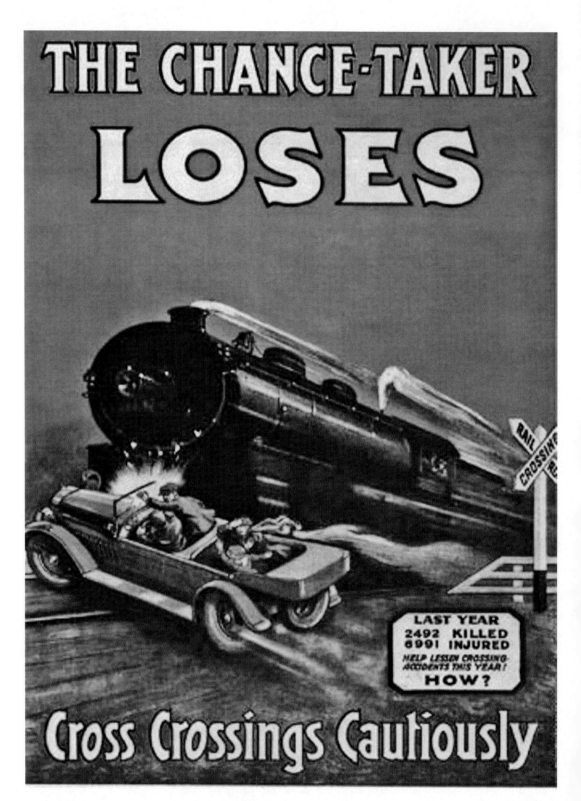

A vintage safety poster illustrating the locomotive's role in creating work for the ambulance. After a *New York Times* story in 2004 revealed steadily escalating crossing casualties and accused federal regulators of laxity in enforcing maintenance of roadway crossings, advocacy groups demanded additional oversight (courtesy Operation Lifesaver Archive).

roads ran through urban areas the way a modern expressway might, but usually without an equivalent buffer zone. The predictable results were summarized by the Rochester, New York, *The Hospital Review* in 1888:

> The many railroads that now enter our city and the extensive building operations in its different parts, while they give employment to our citizens, increase also the rate of exposure, and every few days the ambulance brings to the Hospital some wounded man who needs immediate treatment.[87]

Just as in Brooklyn, where a pedestrian killed by a train provided the literal impetus for the ultimately successful petition to establish a municipal ambulance service, so it was across the country as the increasing number of victims of the transportation revolution led to more and more demands for improved emergency medical services. In later decades it would be the escalating traffic fatalities of the automotive age that prompted wholesale ambulance reform, as we will see in a later chapter, but for now let us conclude by examining the unhappy ways in which these two inadvertent ambulance proponents intersected in the life of a particular ambulance driver. Grover Sampson was a long-time chauffeur of the Genesee Hospital ambulance in Rochester, New York and in his career he had many occasion to respond to calls involving trains, autos, and, sometimes, both. In his *Reminiscences* he recalls a collision case involving a passenger train and a delivery truck that took place in the 1930s. As he describes the scene:

> upon arrival we find that a fast train ... has hit a mayonnaise truck loaded with all kinds of bottles and cans of mayonnaise, boxes of cheese, and other items: you can judge for yourself what happened to the driver—all that was needed was a bushel basket. But would you believe it, the [truck's] engine was at least a good half mile beyond the crossover when it came to a stop, and on the bumper of that engine, as if placed there for show, were *two small jars of mayonnaise* no worse for all that had happened and a two-ton truck smashed to bits and one more life wiped out.

A happier collision is described later. In this case the ambulance arrived at a railroad crossing where a carrier loaded with automobiles had driven smack into the path of an oncoming freight. To Sampson's astonishment he found "the [truck] driver sitting holding the steering wheel—the train having taken everything off clear up to his brake and clutch pedals. Some lucky boy, I'd say, but badly frightened."[88] (Such dramatic accidents became increasingly rare during the post-war period as trains were removed to the outskirts of town and automobile accidents became the *bete noir* of the surgeon and the civic reformer. Still, even today the "Iron Horse" contributes its gory mite to the public safety debate, as new allegations arise over the safety of railway crossings.)[89]

Ultimately the American emergency ambulance service was established by a combination of successfully organized services whose reputations inspired imitators and the sheer need of a society whose rapid industrialization outpaced its ability to effectively police the safety of its citizens. By the 1880s the ambulance service was thoroughly entrenched across the country, although Dalton's original creation was destined to be reshaped by many hands. In time police departments and mortuaries supplanted hospitals as the natural purveyors of ambulance services, before giving way to newer models of care. Dalton's founding principles, however, including centralized dispatch, electronic communication, and employment of highly trained medical personnel, were accepted from 1869 onward as the benchmark for quality emergency medical transportation. Ironically, neither Dalton nor his family appeared to have thought that his ambulance scheme would be the defining achievement of his career: at the time of his death the memorial published by his brother testified that his renown would rest on his military service first and his efforts to arrest cholera second, never even mentioning the dashed-off proposal that has kept Edward Dalton's name alive a century and a half after his death.

• 6 •

Badge and Bandages: Police Surgeons and Patrol Ambulances

If you live in a rough neighborhood, go to the station by one route and return by another, with variations. You don't want to be stopped on the way ... by an ungrateful patient.
   —Advice to police surgeons responding to emergency cases, from *Police-Surgeon's Emergency Guide,* by C. Graham Grant, L.R.C.P.S., Divisional Surgeon H and Thames Division, Metropolitan Police, Surgeon Poplar Hospital (London: H.K. Lewis, 1907, 1)

While Larrey deserves his title as creator of the modern ambulance, more than a vehicle, however improved, was necessary to realize the civilian ambulance service. Cincinnati showed that an ambulance wagon operating on its own, independent of a well developed supporting organization, could only be a vague idea of emergency care, not a functioning model. Even New York's ambulance service did not succeed solely by virtue of its technical merits: it entered a city whose charters, ordinances, and professional staff had already accommodated an organized emergency medical responder system for nearly fifteen years—the original New York City Police Surgeons. Imperfect and often unpopular, they were the first civilian emergency medical responders in the United States, playing a role as overlooked as it was important in the evolution of the ambulance. In time, their work would be continued by police ambulance services, which at one time provided the bulk of emergency medical services in the United States but whose vital contributions have long since slipped into obscurity. The development and ultimate disappearance of these cardinal services forms one of the most intriguing chapters in the history of the ambulance, and their contributions were critical to the evolution of our modern emergency medical services.

Primitive Police Forces

From antiquity through the early 19th century cities and towns relied on some variation of the "Night Watch" for security. These forerunners of the police were assigned neighborhoods to patrol, usually given a box to rest and warm up in, and turned loose with no special training and no requirements other than a willingness to do the job and the ability to carry a lantern and cudgel. Rochester, New York, in 1837 was typical in its employment of a few men as a "Town Watch" who patrolled from dusk till dawn, recounting their activities in neatly ruled pocketbooks. Judging from the logs, their duties seemed principally to have involved gathering up public inebriates, whom they classified according to the following scheme: "some drunk," "drunk and sleeping," and, worst of all, the "beastly drunk." They found them in ditches, on the sidewalks, and, in one case, ensconced in a lumber-pile with a recently acquired

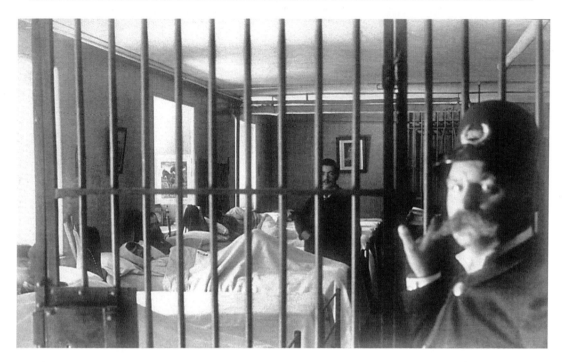

Prisoners awaiting treatment in Bellevue's "cage," circa 1890 (courtesy the Edward G. Miner Library, University of Rochester Medical Center, New York).

lady friend.[1] They also provided rude medical care, principally by taking into protective custody the wandering insane, as described in the following entries:

> August 25th, 1837: Mary Leo found in the streets going from store to store [and] put in Watch House before Police Charge of Insane (given over to her father).
> September 17th: James Mix found back of arcade at Mr. Thomas Beard's. Deranged [so] put in W. House before Police-charge of Insane (Delivered over to Poor Master).[2]

(Note that the "Watch House" was a small cell in a corner of the courthouse basement.)

The inefficiencies of such a system, amounting to little more than deputizing your neighbor to walk around the block with a flashlight looking for burglars, became glaringly obvious as the industrial revolution expanded the size of cities and magnified both want and the opportunity to assuage it by criminal means. By the 1840s crime was so prevalent, and social order so strained, that ancient prejudices against "standing armies" in the guise of large police departments yielded to a new reality of prevalent fear, and New York led the country by forming a modern police force in 1845. (Sir Robert Peel had invented the first such organization—large, specially trained, organized on military lines—for the city of London in 1824.)

Gotham's Tactical Surgeons

Ten years later, in 1855, Mayor Fernando Wood of New York announced he would hire seven "first class physicians" for a new Surgical Department of the Police. Physicians so appointed would receive $700 per year (the same salary as a policeman) and would provide medical services to members of the police department, to prisoners, and to such accident victims as were brought to the attention of the police.[3] *The New York Times* was hostile towards this innovation, probably because the municipal police force Mayor Wood was seeking to aug-

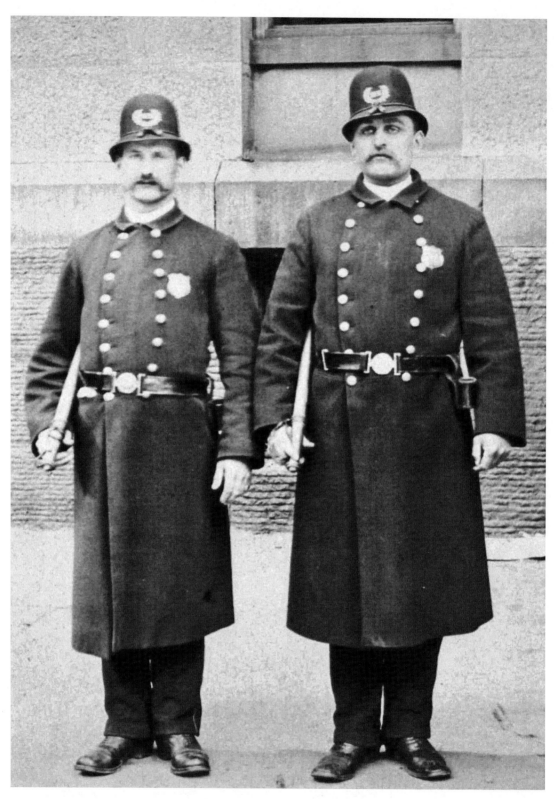

Two policemen in Rochester, New York, circa 1885. Modern police forces appeared in the U.S. in the mid–1800s, and by the 1880s "patrol ambulance" services were featured in many departments—including Rochester's (from the Collection of the Rochester Municipal Archives).

ment had become the largest organized criminal gang in the city, thanks to the aiding and abetting of the spectacularly corrupt Mayor, who profited handsomely from their well-organized extortion rackets. (The situation was so notorious that in 1856 the state legislature was forced to disband the mayor's Metropolitan Police and substitute a new Municipal Police Department answering to a superintendent appointed by the governor.) In attacking Woods' plan *The New York Times* editors pointed out that department regulations forbade police employees from accepting outside employment, and the paper was skeptical that honest physicians would "lay aside all other opportunities of business, emolument and fame, for the honor of being appointed Policemen at $700 a year!"[4] This criticism was apparently well taken, for the police surgeons were quickly permitted to continue their private practices. In addition to hiring district surgeons, Wood also decreed that station houses would be retrofitted to serve as surgical hospitals, supplementing their role as jails and administrative headquarters. Here, too, *The Times* was skeptical, expressing grave doubts that the city's small (and frequently decrepit) station houses could support even modest infirmaries absent costly improvements: "However, 'where there's a will, there's a way,'

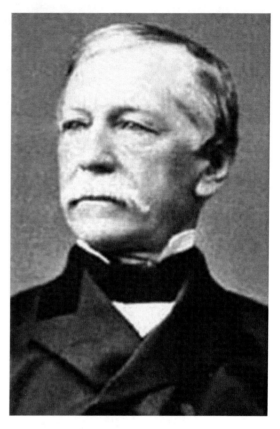

Mayor Fernando Wood: grifter, scoundrel, emergency medicine pioneer.

and if the Mayor has really set his heart on turning each of the Station-houses into a one-horse hospital with a hard-working Tammany man as its surgical supervisor, we have no doubt it will be done — and the Comptroller will be called on to pay the money."[5] The plan to install surgeries in the precinct houses was swiftly abandoned, however, and one supposes it might have suffered from the criticism of the surgeons themselves: providing such costly roosts would have made it difficult for them to justify spending their time elsewhere ... when elsewhere is where they would be seeking those emoluments, business, and fame *The Times* expected them to be pursuing. As it was, Police Surgeon General Dr. Stephen Hasbrouck (himself a politically active member of various Democratic factions and a former alderman) took charge of the assistant police surgeons on July 30, 1855, commencing work the following Wednesday.[6]

Complaints soon appeared that although the surgeons were contracted to perform certain duties, they were living down to the Tammany standard by shirking their work, and when they *did* perform their appointed jobs they were wont to submit bills for services they were salaried to perform. In order to clear up any confusion (by either the public or the surgeons), as soon as the mayor's police force had been forcibly disbanded and its grafters, extortionists, and thieves relieved of their badges, the surgeons were bodily transferred to the newly installed Metropolitan Police Department: the occasion was marked by having their several responsibilities slightly revised and then boldly published in *The New York Times* in 1857, where all might read and understand them — and remind the surgeons themselves if they happened to forget. Of interest, police surgeons were required to provide immediate medical relief to all accident victims in their district upon request from the foot patrol, as well as fulfilling numerous duties related to the public health such as inspecting meat for sale and noting the location of any animal carcasses requiring removal ... duties they were ill inclined to abandon their private practices to perform.[7] (After all, poking one's nose into the rancid meat for sale at back-alley butchers and monitoring the overflow from the neighborhood privies had little allure when compared to profitable attendance on paying patients.) Nonetheless, by the late 1850s police surgeons were functioning as *de facto* emergency first responders, willingly or not. Being on the city payroll their services were free; whether they would be summoned or not depended on the officer at the scene, and this arrangement—a physician employed by the city, dispatched by the police, and responding to emergency cases with free medical care—was an administrative simulacrum of the forthcoming ambulance service. (The absence of an ambulance vehicle in this schema is easily explained: patrol wagons only came into widespread use after the Civil War, quickly followed by police ambulances.)

Soon after the inception of the Bellevue ambulance service in the summer of 1869 the police department and its surgeons found themselves at cross-purposes with the newest addition to modern health care. Between June 4th and the 11th the Charity Commissioners alleged that the ambulance had been summoned thirty-six times by the police—and in all but seven instances the Bellevue surgeons found themselves carting off a common inebriate.[8] This was considered not only an affront to the dignity of the service but a practice certain to exhaust both the ambulance crew and their horses, rendering them all useless if a real emergency arrived. *The New York Times*, who despite the recent reforms still had few kind words for the police department, fulminated that "the ambulance system is a good one, but the Police arrangements bid fair to make it a complete muddle and inoperative for good."[9] The solution, announced June 18th, was to require a police surgeon to attend every medical case reported by a patrolman and to personally authorize an ambulance order, rather than leaving it at the discretion of the responding officer.[10] Authority over accident cases coming to the attention of the police had been vested in the police surgeons since 1855, of course, so this solution amounted to a reminder to the police surgeons that they yet retained nominal responsibility for all accident cases, even if they had lately taken to avoiding the inconvenience of night-time calls. As *The Times* noted, "For many months no Police Surgeon, except, indeed, the indefatigable Dr.

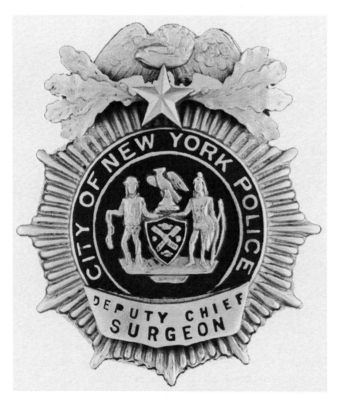

Contemporary New York Police Surgeon badge. Formed in 1855, New York's police surgeons originally provided free medical service to injured individuals who came to the attention of the police. Today, they provide medical care and training to police officers and perform fitness exams. (Copyright 2001. New York City Police Department, all rights reserved. Used with permission.)

Armstrong at the Central Office, has made it his business to respond to calls at night; their private practice affording a ready and plausible excuse for their seeming neglect...."[11] Ultimately, the deficiencies of giving hard-to-corral police surgeons veto power over ambulance calls led to the abandonment of this requirement. In its place the constables on patrol were thoroughly drilled on when (and when not) to summon an ambulance, a responsibility they learned to meet with excellent sense. Having been relieved of the duty to vet ambulance calls, some began to question what role police surgeons had left to play in the emergency services. Indeed, in 1880 the ex–Police Commissioner James Voorhis testified before the state Senate that the current force of nineteen police surgeons could be reduced to twelve, considering that the new ambulances were handling most of the casualties that had once been the exclusive responsibility of the police surgeons.[12]

In time, however, the sheer number of cases began taxing the ambulance services, and the hospitals asked the police surgeons to take on minor cases coming to the attention of the force. Indeed, by 1895 hospital representatives alleged that 60 percent of ambulance cases could have been disposed of by the district police surgeon: the police surgeons, ill inclined to resume a responsibility they had scarcely kept even *before* the ambulance, replied that they were too few for the work, and ambulances were, in any event, quicker.[13] As it was, by the turn of the century the New York police surgeons had left the streets to the ambulances, confining their pro-

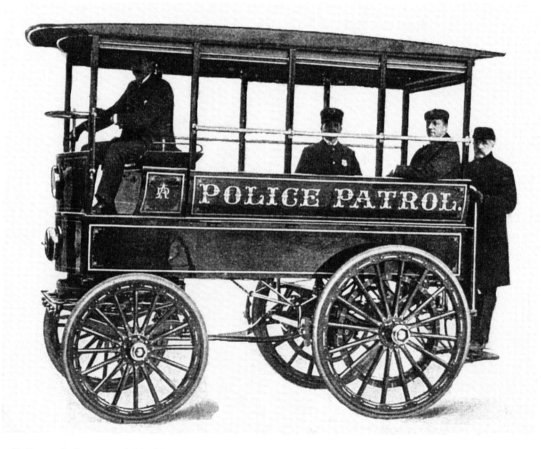

Police ambulances quickly followed the introduction of the patrol wagon in the late 19th century, and were often nothing more than a paddy-wagon with a stretcher or two. Akron, Ohio's original motorized patrol in 1900 set the stage for improved police ambulances nationwide.

fessional duties to the care of departmental employees. The First World War called them once again to the streets as emergency responders, in a final reprise of their original role. Shortly after the United States entered the War to End All Wars, New York City's police and fire surgeons, along with medical volunteers, were organized into brigades ready to respond to any massive medical emergency—like a surprise zeppelin attack by the Huns. A field dressing station was kept in the chief surgeon's office at Police Headquarters and was available for motor transport to wherever disaster struck. In addition, emergency medical bags were kept in each district station house, allowing Police Surgeons and their comrades to instantly form automobile flying-squads in the event of catastrophe.[14] (Although these impromptu ambulance services were never called into action, the idea of an NYPD emergency medical team was revived a few years after the war when the Police Emergency Squad was formed to deal with the mayhem associated with the violent years of Prohibition.) This wartime medical melodrama marked the final performance of Gotham's police surgeons in the evolution of the ambulance, after which their contributions to the emergency services were unjustly forgotten, leaving not even a footnote to mark their passing.

Police Surgeons Nationally

While New York may have pioneered the institution of the police surgeon as emergency first responder they held no monopoly on the franchise. As early as 1878 San Francisco's police surgeons supervised the ambulance service and ran the city's emergency hospitals, setting a

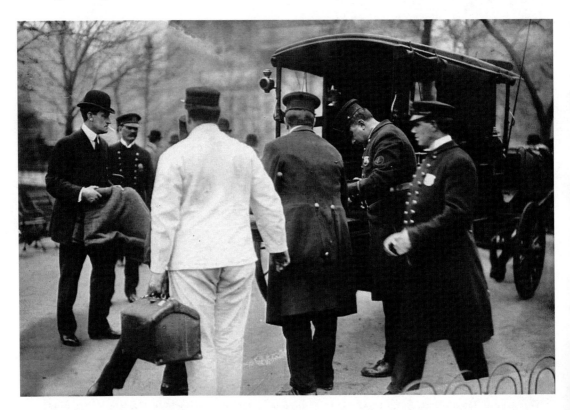

New York City police load a victim into an ambulance after a 1908 anarchist riot (George Bain Collection, Library of Congress Prints and Photographs Division, LC-USZ62-69544).

precedent for other West Coast communities, most notably Los Angeles. In Philadelphia, from 1885 onwards, surgeons were appointed in each police district and the city provided them with household telephones so their appointed station houses could contact them immediately. (This represented the ultimate in modernity at a time when less than one home in three hundred owned a phone.[15]) Philadelphia's police surgeons provided immediate attention to accident victims and serious medical emergencies in their districts and were to remain with the afflicted until an ambulance arrived. Their rates were previously agreed upon, subject to attestation by the district police lieutenant, and paid by City Hall monthly.[16] Similar programs existed in many other American cities, but, as in New York, the police surgeons gradually acceded their authority to rapidly expanding hospital and private ambulance services until, by the early 1900s, they had ceased to be a major force in public emergency care.

Today police surgeons are still very much in evidence, although their duties now revolve around providing physicals, documenting work-related injuries, and overseeing health initiatives. The role they once played in the development of ambulance and emergency services—training police ambulance crews, providing coordinated medical care at the scene, serving as administrators of police rescue squads—has been largely forgotten. From their challenging debut under the shadow of Tammany Hall to their ambulance heyday in the late 19th century, they represented the first attempt to create a professional force of dedicated emergency responders. While their contributions were important in laying the groundwork for the expansion of the ambulance, they were not the only contribution the police forces would make to the evolution of the ambulance. Indeed, from modest beginnings the patrol ambulance service was to assume the pre-eminent role in the ambulance story between the wars, leading the country in number of services, scope of care, and technical innovation.

Blue Cross: Police Ambulance Services

A hot day and an unfortunate vassal of the Newark Scavenger King introduce one of the most important stages in the history of the ambulance ... the neglected story of the Patrol Ambulance. In the summer of 1878 the Bellevue ambulance service had just celebrated its ninth anniversary, and *The New York Times* was still publishing daily temperatures according to the thermometer at Hudnut's Pharmacy on Broadway. The meteorological Big Ben registered 88 humid degrees at noon on July 3rd when *The Times* reported that a driver working for Henry "The Newark City Scavenger" Aherns had been "prostrated by the heat while at work on the Lister-avenue garbage dump. A Police ambulance was sent to remove him to the hospital, but before its arrival he was dead."[17] Across the river, in New York City, the city hospitals were fielding a fleet of hospital wagons, but in many towns like Newark fledgling police departments staffed ambulances, and they did so in numbers that soon put them behind a plurality of American rescue vehicles—until they were overtaken by mortuaries between the wars.

Driving this assumption of a medical role by the police were a variety of forces, some still obvious at this late date, others that time has rendered obscure. First, the patrolman on the beat was likely to be the first official on the scene of an accident, making it natural for them to provide elementary medical treatment. (In 1878 the St. John Ambulance Society initiated first-aid training for London's Metropolitan Police, graduating their first class of trainees from Scotland Yard on August 12th, and in 1883 Philadelphia patrolmen were given four lectures on first aid and provided with pocket sized manuals encapsulating the lessons, while nineteen police stations were provided with wheeled-stretchers called "hand ambulances."[18]) Secondly, as cities grew in the 19th century it became clear municipal authorities would need to abate nuisances that in a smaller town could be tolerated but when multiplied a thousandfold in a metropolis

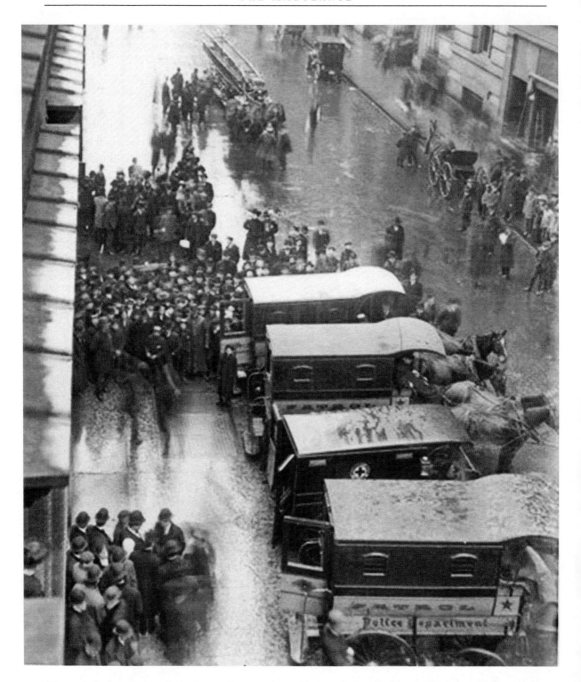

Turn of the century police wagons line up alongside hospital ambulances in Chicago. Patrol wagons, either with the addition of stretchers or without, supplemented existing ambulance services well into the 20th century.

made civil life unbearable. Not yet comprehending the size and complexity of what were entirely novel tasks, many cities simply turned to their new police departments and added public health to their portfolio. This "portmanteau" approach to police-work meant the original 1845 New York police manual put patrolmen in charge of privy inspections and investigating potholes and sewers, as well as fighting crime.[19]

Finally, there was the means: police departments had wagons. Starting in the middle 19th century police departments began acquiring patrol wagons to convoy officers to distant posts as cities grew past the bounds of a comfortable walk; they were also convenient to transport prisoners or deliver squads of patrolmen to scenes of riot. Still, it was not until the 1880s that patrol wagons became routine apparatus for the nation's police departments, and the decision by the Newark Police to provision a wagon for ambulance duty by 1878 may have been the first such innovation in the nation. While unquestionably practical as impromptu ambulances, police wagons were designed to transport several men at once and their stiff springs made hard traveling for the sick or injured, and the public awareness that such wagons were both frequently used as ambulances and also poorly suited to the job was reflected in the ideas submitted for humane combination patrol wagon/ambulances, some of which were patented.[20] Despite the problems, an imperfect patrol ambulance was preferable to no service at all, and by the early 1880s police ambulances were supplementing, replacing, or pioneering emergency services in communities of all sizes across the United States. Later, in a twist on patrolman as emergency responder, some emergency responders were made honorary policemen—for example, by 1900 New York ambulance surgeons were given the rank of acting police sergeant while on duty, allowing them to command whatever aid they required from the patrolmen on the beat.[21]

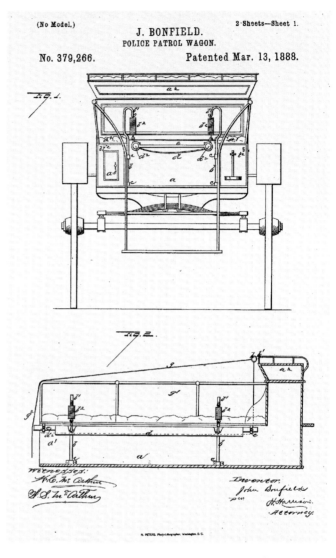

An 1888 patent shows how a stretcher suspended from the ceiling turns a patrol into an ambulance and spares the patient the up and down jolting of fast travel over uneven streets (United States Patent Office, No. 379,266).

Nor was the innovation confined to the United States. Across the horizon in England, the first large scale casualty ambulance service (as opposed to one set up solely to transfer the contagious sick) was organized in London under the auspices of the police department. The movement began in February 1882 with a large meeting at the Royal United Service Institution in Whitehall, presided over by the Duke of Cambridge in his capacity as president of the London Hospital. Attending were such luminaries as James H. Crossman, who had co-founded London's Hospital Carriage Society in 1867, and Dr. Benjamin Howard, the American physician and ambulance advocate who brought his latest hospital wagon with him to the proceedings.²² A half-dozen stem-winding speeches were delivered to the crowd, and in addition to the expected moral appeals there were the kinds of "pounds and pence" arguments that could actually persuade tough-minded Victorian capitalists to invest in the underclass. As Mr. Crossman of the London Hospital put it:

> There are probably 900,000 people engaged daily in manual labor [in London] and subject to serious accident at any moment. The value of health to those who have to maintain their families on weekly and daily earnings is as of great importance to the community as the quick restoration of wounded soldiers to an army in the field, and, therefore, the sooner a man is restored to health after severe injury the better for the State, and every means ought to be provided for the easy transference of the wounded man to the nearest hospital without any aggravation of the injury.²³

Such practical moralizing had the desired effect, and at the end of the evening a committee was formed with the goal of providing ambulance service across London by means of public subscriptions. Their first success came in July 1882 when Sir Edmund Henderson, Commissioner of Police of the Metropolis, approved fifteen police stations for the stabling of ambulance carriages—although it was left to the charitably minded to provide the vehicles.²⁴ The first of these "jitney ambulances" were delivered to the Bow Street and Carter police stations in October, thanks to the philanthropy of H.L. Bischoffsheim, and by 1884 there were Howard ambulance wagons at the Stoke-Newington, Fulham, and Lambeth police offices as well.²⁵ Unfortunately, the London constabulary charged between five and ten shillings for the ambulance,

In this 1895 patent illustration for a combination patrol and ambulance wagon the seats fold down to form a bed (United States Patent Office, No. 546,855).

no small beer in an era when menial laborers might expect four shillings a day and skilled tradesmen six.²⁶ As one observer noted, "the poor are completely unable to pay such a sum," and even many of "that struggling body who come from the lower middle class" lacked the means to make good the debt.²⁷ Billing practices aside, other London police stations had been making do with significantly less: as far back as 1860 a number of Metropolitan Police station houses had acquired simple wheeled litters, but others clung to their heavy wooden stretchers until an 1878 edict from the Metropolitan Police Commissioner ordered them retired in favor of an improved perambulating stretcher on outsized wheels.²⁸ Including a removable bedrest along with leather restraints firmly fixed to the iron frame of the cot, the stretchers were kept in service into the 20th century, before eventually being phased out in favor of automotive services.²⁹ (Meanwhile, the jurisdictionally distinct City of London, a square mile of real-estate with its own police force, lagged the rest of the metropolis, not retiring their ancient hand-litters until 1907, when they acquired an electric ambulance from Mayfair's Electromobile Company. Fashioned of mahogany panels on ash supports, this thoroughly modern machine was garaged in the Pathology Wing of the city's oldest hospital, St. Bartholomew's.³⁰)

Back in the United States, cities were embracing the police ambulance with considerable vigor. Rochester, New York underwent a modernization spell in 1886, putting in thirty police telegraph boxes around the city and acquiring its very first patrol wagon, which, absent any hospital ambulances, was sensibly equipped with stretchers for casualties.³¹ Both the telegraph and the patrol-wagon/ambulance were attributable to the reformatory zeal of Chief Joseph Cleary, another example of how the war turned laymen into post-bellum ambulance advocates. Before the war Cleary had been a nurseryman in Rochester's famed commercial gardens, but as a young lieutenant he found himself one of an estimated 3,000 wounded men left lying on the battlefield after the Second Battle of Bull Run, the majority of whom would die waiting for Dr. Bowditch and his colleagues to arrive with the ambulances days later.³² In the fullness of time it was *Major* Joseph Cleary who returned home to Rochester, but instead of once more

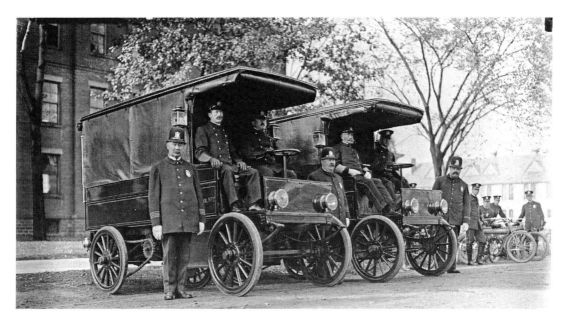

Patrol wagons in Rochester, New York, circa 1916. Equipped with stretchers, they could serve as simple ambulances when the need arose (from the Albert R. Stone Negative Collection, Rochester Museum & Science Center Rochester, N.Y.).

laboring in the famous nurseries of "The Flower City" he traded his officer's braids for a patrolman's stripe, rising through the ranks to become chief of police.[33] In 1886, twenty-four years after he laid on a bloody field wondering whether death or the ambulances would find him first, Chief Cleary gave Rochester its first ambulance service by placing stretchers in the city patrol wagons, and it would be difficult to believe his interest in creating a city ambulance service was not partly related to the horrible miseries he endured and witnessed from their want on that long-ago battleground.

Chief Cleary's telegraph boxes ensured immediate dispatch of the patrol wagon ambulances, but not everyone appreciated his efforts, as seen by the following anecdote. In the winter of 1890 the Reverend Copeland took ill, and his anxious friends sought aid. Although the city had recently acquired a separate, designated ambulance for such emergencies, the neighbors didn't know the number to call and rang for the police as of old. A patrol ambulance promptly appeared and ferried the Reverend to the hospital without incident, but neighbors peering through their curtains and seeing the prelate loaded into the paddy-wagon drew evil inferences about what business he had with the police. A letter to *The Democrat and Chronicle* implied that poor advertising of the city ambulance was to blame for the padre's ignoble departure, but tart correspondence in *The Union Advertiser* pointed out that the ambulance

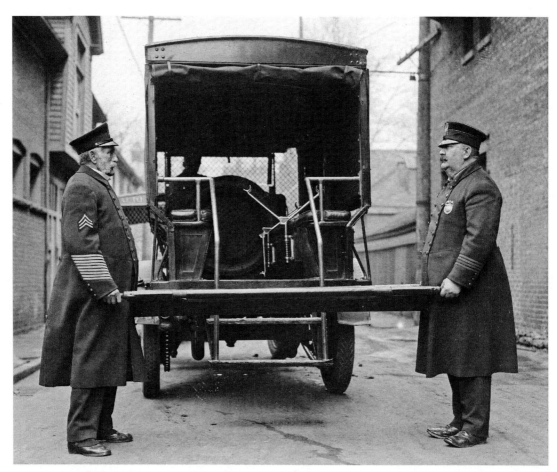

Rochester patrol wagon with stretcher, from 1916. The cot rested on an elevated frame, visible on the right side attached to the bench seat (from the Albert R. Stone Negative Collection, Rochester Museum & Science Center Rochester, N.Y.).

number was pasted on the covers of the city telephone directories, and the new vehicle was every bit as prompt as the patrol wagon which it had been intended to replace. Concluding on a tremulous note, the writer complained "the friends of humanity who gave toward the purchase of the new ambulance are hurt beyond expression at the persistence of those who send the patrol wagon instead of the proper conveyance in such cases ... (signed) HUMANITY."[34]

The Police Ambulance in Rochester: A Case Study

Rochester's patrol ambulance was typical of the nation's early police emergency services. As in New York City the ambulance was the brainchild of an ex-soldier exposed to military ambulance services; as in many other cities the police ambulance began with a monopoly on emergency transport and continued to play an important role even after more traditional services came on the scene; and, lastly, its operation foretold the national arc of initial enthusiasm slowly giving way to administrative exhaustion as police ambulance services appeared to draw funds and resources from crime fighting. Before looking at layers of evidence laid down by the nationwide flood and retreat of the police ambulance it will be useful to examine the process in miniature, and the records from Rochester's Proceedings of the Common Council give an unusually intimate accounting of how a police ambulance was handled, and ultimately disposed of, in a representative medium-sized city.

As mentioned, Rochester's first police ambulance was nothing more than a patrol wagon with a stretcher or two in the back. Two years later, in 1888, the city hired a police surgeon to attend any cases brought to the station, making the police bureau a free-standing emergency medical service, similar to what Mayor Wood had proposed for Manhattan in 1855. The police medical service achieved a new level of professionalism when, in 1890, the department bought a new patrol wagon for the princely sum of $525 and dedicated the old paddy-wagon exclusively to ambulance use. Since space was limited at the station, the new aid-wagon was billeted across the street at the *Standard Cab Coupe, Sale and Boarding Stable* for $25 a month.[35] In early 1892 the ambulance moved across the Genesee River to the newly opened Patrol House No. 2, and a few months later the service was completed by assigning patrolman Patrick Cummings full-time to ambulance duty at the standard roundsman's salary of $75.00 a month.[36]

CHAS. W. SHELLEY.   FRANK S. SHELLEY.

STANDARD CAB,

Coupe, Sale, and Boarding Stable,

19 to 29 South Fitzhugh Street,

Opposite City Hall.

Telephone, No. 139.   C. W. SHELLEY & SON.

1890 advertisement for the Standard Cab Boarding Stable, when it was the home of Rochester, New York's first modern ambulance.

(For his money Patrick Cummings, like the rest of the force, worked twelve-hour shifts with one day off per month and eight days annual leave.[37]) During fiscal year 1892 the Police Clerk began reporting income from the police ambulance service. A representative entry, showing the rate charged for the ambulance, appears in the Clerk's August report:

> Use of ambulance by H.P. Warner 2.00
> Sale of one load of manure 75
> Use of ambulance by R. Woodworth ...... 2.00 [38]

As the second item shows, Rochester's constabulary was resourceful when it came to financing their operations. As to the charges for ambulance service, the average wage of industrial and textile workers in 1892 ranged from $50 to $60 a month, so $2 was easily a day's wages.[39] Not surprisingly, Rochester's hardworking populace registered their opinion of the billing schedule in the usual way: after 278 ambulance calls between March 1892 and March 1893, the police department managed to successfully bill all of $58.00, a disappointing collection rate of less than 10 percent.[40] (On the other hand, they brought in $8.25 from the sale of manure.)

Police Emergency Services in the Northeast

> "Gentlemen: I have the honor to report to your committee the result of our visit and inspection of the police departments of the cities of Cleveland, Detroit and Buffalo...."

The dismal returns from ambulance billing could hardly have endeared the service to Rochester's Superintendent of Police, and when he embarked on a fact-finding tour of regional police departments in 1892 the police ambulance situation figured prominently in his report. Published in the *Proceedings of the Common Council*, August 23, 1892, it provides a rare glimpse of how a contemporary police administrator viewed the marriage of law enforcement and emergency medical services. Accompanying the Superintendent on the tour were representatives of the Committee on Public Safety and Charities, which operated a separate municipal ambulance principally for the benefit of the city's poor.

The no-nonsense Rochester burghers arranged to canvass three cities in four days, traveling by steamboat and train to Cleveland, Detroit, and Buffalo. In Cleveland they found that the police department had four wagons at its disposal, but no patrol ambulances as such: accident cases were handled swiftly by the paddy wagons, as best they could. Otherwise, "each undertaker in the city has an ambulance and answers all calls from the police departments, and it seems to give good satisfaction to the departments and the public." In Detroit it was much the same, with sick and accident cases brought in on the patrol wagons as required. This absence of a police ambulance carried little weight with the Rochester Hawkshaw, who found the Detroit police patrol system to be "as perfect as can be," with its force of 368 men and "6 patrol wagons on duty all the time ... lighter than ours, but they have a few heavier wagons on the reserve in case of riots or other serious trouble." Of Buffalo the report is brief, but favorable, with the Superintendent noting the city employed six wagons, but making no reference to ambulance services.

While, as we shall see, the absence of police ambulances was anything but universal, the selective view the Superintendent received of how things were being done in the "big towns" must have made his department appear provincial and their police ambulance service *infra-dig*. Still, it served an otherwise unmet need, and by 1895 the department was running a pair of ambulances in addition to two patrol wagons equipped with stretchers. Then, in 1896, a deputation from the city hospitals suddenly offered to take over all the city ambulance services in exchange for a yearly municipal subsidy of $1,000 per ambulance, with the expectation that ultimately the city's major infirmaries would provide a total of four ambulances.[41] Among the advantages to this arrangement was the hospitals' promise to staff the ambulances with physicians, as well as a potential savings to the municipality. As to these costs, the police department was spending upwards of $3,000 a year to maintain its ambulance service: $1,800 a year for the two patrolmen on ambulance duty plus $1,000 or so for the feed of the horses, wagon repairs, and medical supplies.[42] Meanwhile, the City Poor Department's simple ambulance service added some $700 a year, while the Board of Health was renting a vehicle as needed (mostly for contagious cases) at variable cost depending on the health of the city, but generally less than $200 a year.[43] All told, the hospital offer was calculated to exactly match the annual expense of the municipal services, while offering the embellishment of physician attendance. There being no objection raised in Council, the offer from the hospitals was cheerfully accepted, although the change was slow in coming (in fact, not until December 1896 did Patrolman Cummings descend to the ranks of the foot-patrol).[44] All were satisfied by the new arrangement, which persisted for the next fifty-four years until economic changes swept aside the old modes of ambulance service, in Rochester as well as elsewhere.

Police Ambulances Ascendant

Rochester's experience with the police ambulance would be recapitulated across the country in the decades to come, as police departments found the expense of providing this service increasingly burdensome and hospitals and private providers began asserting a more prominent role for themselves. Rochester was only unique in its precociousness, because even while it divested itself of police ambulance services in 1896 similar operations were *gaining* ground nationally. Out west, for example, Seattle's police department introduced the city's first ambulance in 1890, a fringed surrey with rubber tires that also functioned as paddy wagon and

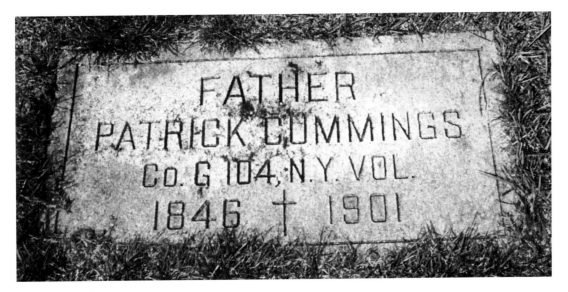

The gravestone in the Mount Hope Cemetery for Patrick Cummings, Rochester's first full-time ambulance attendant. He started out as a patrolman, an office he resumed after the police ambulance service was disbanded in 1896. A capable officer, he had worked his way to the rank of sergeant in the 4th Precinct at the time of his death.

mobile headquarters of the riot squad, depending on what crisis was uppermost at the moment: in 1906 it was replaced by a Knox Auto that also did triple-duty as ambulance, prisoner transport, or riot car, depending on the circumstances.[45] Boston, an early adopter, had six police ambulances by 1898, in addition to its twelve "patrol vans." Around 1900, The Massachusetts Emergency Society recommended that the Boston Police place rubber tires on patrol ambulances and wagons alike (to spare the bones of the injured) and outfit regular patrol wagons with "dust-proof first-aid packets."[46] At first, only ambulances carried stretchers, suspended from the ceiling to save the occupant from being bounced into the air with every bump. Any injured person unlucky enough to be transported in a patrol-wagon either sat on the bench seats or lay where they could, although simple mattress stretchers were, mercifully, quickly thrown in the rear of all patrol wagons: by 1901 Boston had nine ambulances and fifteen patrol wagon/aid-cars on call, staffed by a driver and attendant who each held a diploma for emergency first aid, and it was reported that no one in the city would wait longer than seven minutes for an ambulance after notifying a constable, a boast putting Boston's patrol ambulances in the nation's top rank in terms of speed of service.[47] By the early 1920s police departments were providing more ambulance services than any other group in the United States, outpacing hospitals and funeral homes, and dwarfing the still nascent volunteer ambulance crews and free-standing services who were only beginning to assume a measurable presence in the field.

In Cincinnati, where hospital ambulance service started back in 1865, the local police force acquired seven "Combination Cruiser/Invalid Cars" in 1935, each kitted out with two stretchers and a first aid kit. The sad impetus to this had been the untimely death of Motorcycle Patrolman Hicks, who had been thrown headlong into a metal pole after losing control of his bike during a high-speed pursuit. After being found by a local citizen some time later, he had lain on the cold ground for another thirty minutes before a patrol vehicle could reach him and remove him to the hospital.[48] His brother officers demanded, and received, the new "scout cars" in order to dramatically improve response times and ensure some minimal level of care for the stricken. Similar efforts were being made by police officers around the country during this time, and in retrospect the 1930s represented the high-water mark for patrol ambulances, when they represented a plurality of the total ambulance services in the United States and were integral parts of police-operated emergency hospitals around the country. After the Second World War the police ambulance services began to wane as enormous changes came to the emergency medicine field: for now, suffice to say that higher post-war crime rates diverted administrative attention from police medical squads, and the increased cost of new medical equipment and ever more elaborate service expectations made the police ambulance an expensive and distracting white elephant for many departments, one they were eager to be quit of. By the 1950s such services were much the exception rather than the rule, gradually yielding to mortuary ambulances and the beginnings of the large-scale private providers that would dominate ambulance operations by the end of the century.

The changing times did not eradicate the police ambulance, however, and in some communities they still fly on emergency runs, although changes have overtaken their service. For example, the Nassau County Police Department bought their ambulance in 1953, at a time when many other departments were selling theirs, and quickly developed a reputation for progressive operations. In 1970, with funding from the National Safety Bureau, they put defibrillator-electrocardiogram units in eight police ambulances (one in every precinct).[49] Each unit had a radiotelephone hook-up to the County Medical Center ER, and the transmitted telemetry allowed physicians to give directions to the responding officers (these were the first ambulances so equipped in New York and among only a handful in the country). In 1971 they fielded fifteen ambulances, staffed by 58 officers whose training was vastly superior to the majority of ambulance providers of the era—advanced first aid training and 104 hours of additional

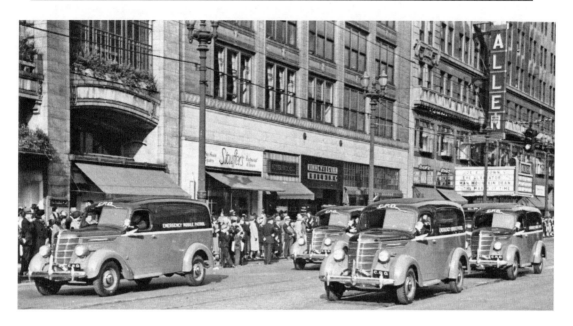

Cleveland Emergency Patrols on parade in the late 1930s (courtesy the Cleveland Police Museum).

training in cardiac care to complement their advanced telemetry equipment.[50] By 1995 the Nassau Police Ambulance Service was probably the busiest police medical response team in the country, responding to more than 42,000 calls, but the era of police emergency responders was ending, and the department now employs civilian EMTs in lieu of peace officers to staff its emergency vehicles.

One of the last all-police ambulance services is also one of the most celebrated, Maryland's State Police Aviation Command. Operational since May 1970, the Maryland program is America's oldest continually operating helicopter-based trauma evacuation service, preceding the military's widely known Military Assistance to Safety and Traffic (MAST) program by two months. Maryland's pioneering service has expanded considerably since those early days, but in the great tradition of the police rescue wagons each flying ambulance is staffed by elite Maryland State Troopers who, after completing tours of duty on the highways, undergo additional training to become certified flight paramedics.

Operations such as these, and the special Emergency Service squads discussed in later chapters, are the last reminders of those vanished fleets of police ambulances first appearing in the 19th century. While representing a tiny fraction of modern emergency services, operations such as Maryland's Police Aviation Command stand as vivid reminders of the magnificent medical services once provided by thousands of anonymous police surgeons and patrolmen in the backs of creaking patrol wagons in the age of gaslight, in harbor patrols chugging across oily rivers with attempted suicides shivering under a wool blanket in the stern, or inside sleek police ambulance cruisers between the wars. Police services were often a community's only emergency ambulances in the early days and, with their training programs, provided a forum for disseminating first aid practices at a time when such techniques were new. Finally, during the 19th century public skepticism of the new police forces ran high, and a quality police ambulance service was a powerful ally in winning public trust for the police department supporting it. From their inception the patrol ambulances were an irrefutable symbol of the police officer's commitment to public service, to protect and to serve, to safeguard the most helpless in their hour of greatest need.

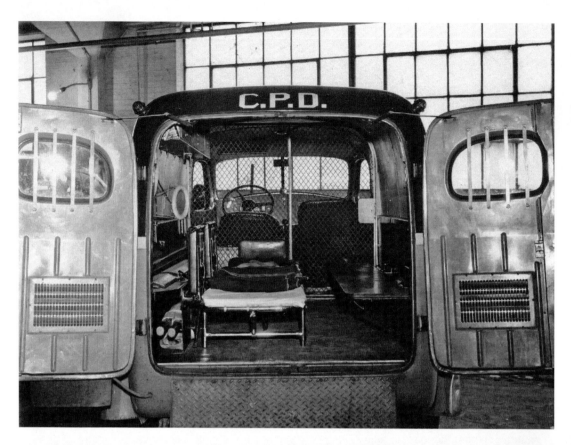

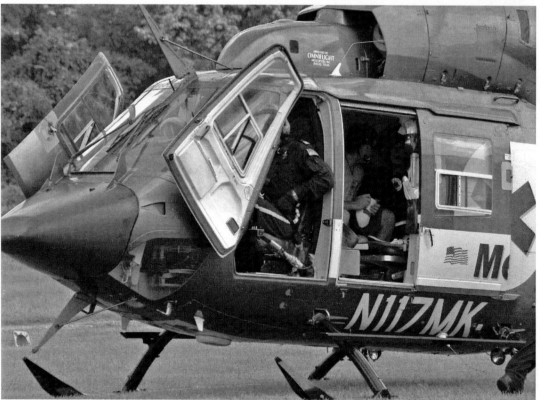

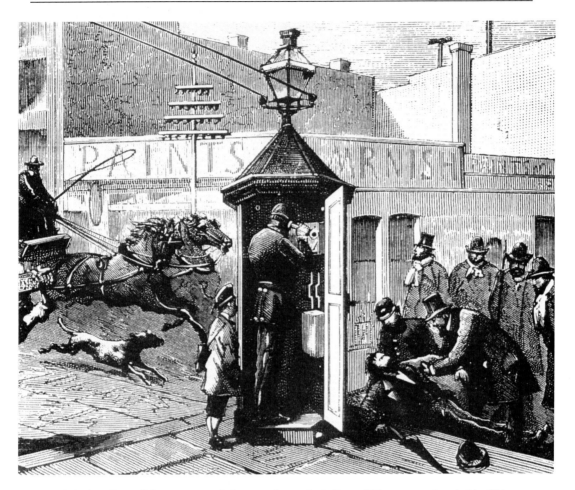

The original police call boxes were miniature telegraph stations. This one was located in Chicago, circa 1878, and its gabled roof and ornamental features were examples of high Victorian style.

Before 911

Of course, providing tangible medical services from the back of patrol wagons did not exhaust the contribution of the police forces to ambulance history. No matter how elaborately constructed or competently staffed, any ambulance in a stable or garage was of no use, and how to quickly and efficiently summon early ambulances to a single spot in a teeming metropolis was a vexing problem. Bells, tolling coded peals, had long alerted fire departments to emergencies in a particular district, trusting that the smell of smoke would direct the horses to the right block, but this would not suffice for an ambulance. The first solution to speed and particularity in dispatch came with the telegraph, but as soon as more than one ambulance service became available a central intelligence was required to ensure that the electric marvel didn't

Opposite, top: An interior of a Cleveland Emergency Patrol. At the time of their introduction in 1938 they were among the most advanced ambulances available, representing an early peak in police emergency medical services (courtesy the Cleveland Police Museum). *Opposite, bottom:* Civilian medevac helicopters like this modern rig in Columbus, Ohio, are the descendants of a pioneering program by the Maryland State Police Aviation Command which started in May 1970 — a few weeks before military units offered similar service in Texas (Kenn Kiser).

strike the various ambulance barns with the randomness of a lightning bolt. Making ambulance dispatch *effective* as well as rapid required centralized command and control, a task usually assigned to unflappable police telegraphers. Wherever such central dispatch was absent hospitals were sure to "poach" patients from one another's neighborhood and citizens were endangered when the multiple ambulances responding to a single call were unavailable for subsequent emergencies.

For one example among many, Rochester, N.Y., had four hospitals providing ambulance service by the late 1890s and, lacking a central call center, in the general tumult of a public mishap each infirmary would get a call from some passerby or another, resulting in all four rigs sparring over a patient. To tame the chaos the hospitals assigned themselves particular districts in 1899, agreeing that calls outside their neighborhood would be forwarded to the appropriate infirmary and happily predicting that this collegial scheme would "save much wear and tear on ambulance and horses, as now they have many needless calls."[51] What resulted from the collision of perfect plan with imperfect man? Let the reader see for themselves in these extracts taken from the City Hospital ambulance log of 1900:

> Aug 20—Hahnemann's beat us to Four Corners, & tried to get woman to go to their Hosp. (Call was sent [illegible] from Police Station). The woman left the ambulance & went home in street car.

> Nov 20—About 1 P.M. we received a call to Monroe & South Clinton Sts., which we transferred to Hahnemann Hospital [nearest to scene]. About 1:45 Miss Curtis [the Hahnemann dispatcher] telephoned that when their ambulance arrived there, they found the Homeopathic ambulance there. The Homeopathic ambulance took the patient to their hospital—Miss Curtis called Miss Allenton [at the Homeopathic] and said she would give them just 15 minutes to send the case to Hahnemann Hospital.[52]

(Given the confusion, it is small wonder that the woman in the first case gave up in disgust and went home in a streetcar.) With the voluntary zoning scheme an abject failure, the Department of Charities and Corrections ordered all ambulance calls forwarded to police headquarters for assignment, imitating the successful scheme followed in New York City. Similarly, by 1907 central police dispatch of ambulances could be found in Boston, Brooklyn, Baltimore, Albany, Cincinnati, Detroit, St. Louis, and Chicago, among other progressive cities, and the able work done by these pioneering police agencies prefigured today's 911 services.[53]

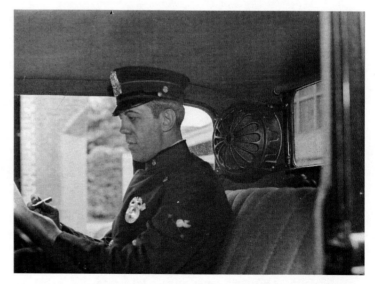

Police radio patrols like this one in Rochester, New York, pioneered central communication for emergency services, so ambulance crews quickly came to depend on police bureaus for efficient dispatch. By 1949 New York City's police-run ambulance call center took up two rooms painted a bilious green, with hospitals required to forward ambulance calls to the police for assignment (Richard Strouse, "Riding Bus with a Hospital Interne," *New York Times*, January 2, 1949, SM16). (From the Albert R. Stone Negative Collection, Rochester Museum & Science Center Rochester, N.Y.)

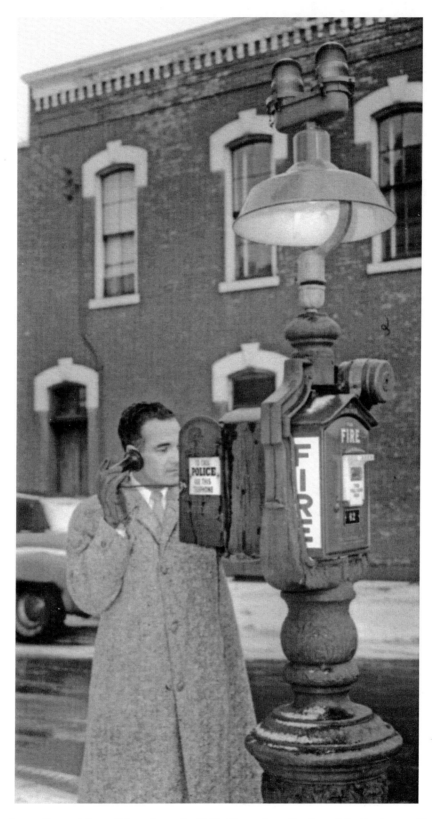

Combination police and fire call box, from the 1940s (from the collection of the Rochester City Hall Photo Lab).

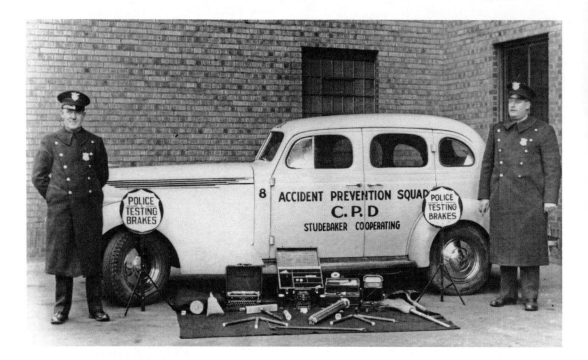

Eliot Ness created Cleveland's Accident Prevention Squad to assist prosecutions of driving offenses and cipher out factors contributing to roadway casualties. Shown alongside a yellow "canary car," these investigators predated similar national efforts in the 1950s and 1960s, when the highway safety movement began influencing ambulance development and design (courtesy the Cleveland Police Museum).

Even when the police were firmly in control of ambulance dispatch there was still the question of getting the message through to headquarters quickly. In the days before telephones the quickest method was telegraphy, leading directly to the innovation of the callbox — free-standing miniature telegraph stations placed at strategic points across a city that enabled patrolmen and citizens to summon aid without having to race to the nearest Western Union office or police precinct. Credit for realizing this scheme goes to Moses Farmer and Dr. W.F. Channing who, in 1852, gave the first call-boxes to the Boston fire department: setting the pattern for decades to come, each call-box sent a unique signal to the central station, which then telegraphed the firehouse nearest the alarm.[54] Keys were given to trustworthy individuals living near the box, with their addresses posted prominently on the device. Once opened, one had only to turn a crank, and "by this means any child or ignorant person who can turn a coffee-mill can signalize an alarm for his neighborhood with unerring certainty," which must have been a particular relief to the neighbors of ignorant underage coffee drinkers.[55]

These devices entered the history of emergency medicine with the appearance of police ambulances in the 1870s, prompting some precincts to deploy call-boxes with indicator dials allowing the officer to signal either an ambulance or a paddy wagon, as required. Chicago callboxes were among the most elaborate, offering patrolmen eleven different pre-set alarms, including *Accident*, *Riot*, and *Fire*, as well as *Forgers* and *Murder*.[56] Telegraph alarms were ultimately replaced by telephone call boxes, which, persisting well into the 1950s, allowed callers to provide details of the emergency to the dispatcher, particularly useful in ambulance calls in an age when interns were increasingly only being sent to the most serious cases. Today the call-box is all but extinct, although many colleges have posted them on their campuses for the security of co-eds out after hours, and some states still maintain a few scattered about major highways. Their once prominent role in summoning ambulances has been supplanted by two-way radio and the near ubiquity of the cell phone, but their place in the history of the ambulance, and that of the police services in general, is assured.

• 7 •

The Ambulance Surgeons

The queer places of metropolitan life become familiar. He knows the precinct station as well as his own room. Docks and garrets, cellars where sickness lurks neglected, streets unfrequented save by the outcast and the police, haunts of violence and crime, are included in his daily ride.
     —*The Hospital Review*, "With an Ambulance," 23(8):126, March 15, 1887

For the last two months the ambulance surgeons of this city have been going daily, and several times a day, to cases which they know might be, and many of which proved to be, typhus; and within a week one of them, called to such a case, saw every friend of the patient rush from the room when the dreaded word was spoken, and he was compelled to take him in his arms and carry him to the ambulance alone and unaided.
     —*The New York Times,* "City Ambulance Service: An Examination of the System, Which Admits Certain Imperfections in It and Asserts for It Manifold Merits"; March 28, 1892; p.9

After the initial rush of excitement had passed, the long hours and unpleasant working conditions made ambulance service unappealing to most established physicians. On the other hand, interns, eager for experience and conditioned to expect meager remuneration, made ideal candidates for ambulance duty. The life of these 19th century junior physicians was not enviable. Even as late as 1914 a third of medical graduates shunned internship in favor of starting directly in private practice, but the additional training an internship provided was often a passport to professional advancement.[1] While there was no mandated national curriculum, most programs averaged 16 months, with the intern rotating through posts as a junior medical, junior surgical, senior medical, and "house surgeon." A few programs were a year or less, some of the top programs could stretch out two years, but on virtually all of them the intern was expected to take their place on the ambulance.

"The Very Best of Their Age"

Ambulance surgeons were frequently junior surgicals, and, in addition to being subject to ambulance calls at any time, their duties generally included giving anesthetics at several operations a day, applying dressings (which might need to be changed at four-hour intervals around the clock), and handling those minor surgical cases which the house surgeon found too tiresome or trivial to bother with. An account of the life of an ambulance surgeon appeared in *The New York Times* on March 28, 1892, as a letter to the editor written by two surgeons supervising ambulance services in the city.[2] Mincing no words, they wrote:

> the life of the ambulance surgeon does not excite much envy: and when to it is added the constant exhaustion of exacting duties we can only feel surprise that men are willing to take the places. They

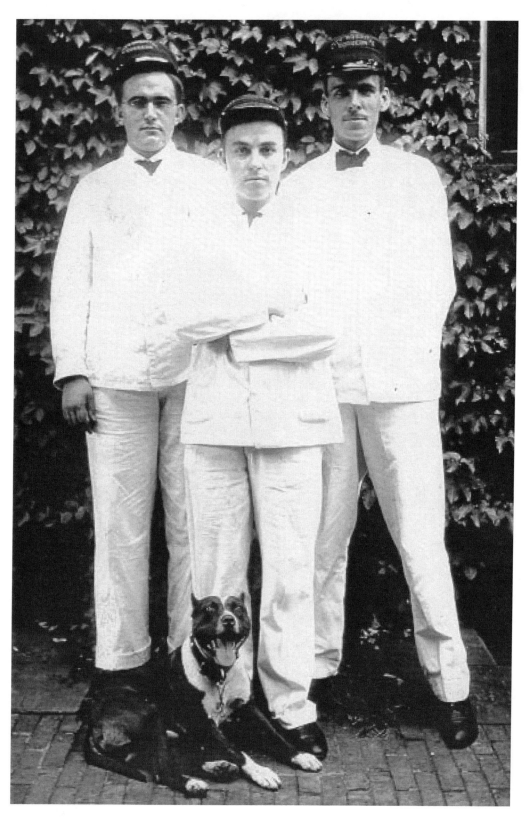

Intern Ambulance Surgeons, Genesee Hospital (Rochester, N.Y.) in 1907 (ViaHealth Archives Consortium, Rochester, N.Y.).

frequently fall ill from overwork or through contagion, and occasionally one dies. Look at the great tablet in Bellevue Hospital covered with the names of young men who have "died in the discharge of duty." These young men are the very best of their age in the profession: they have eagerly competed for the opportunity to assume their onerous duties, and they perform them with a fidelity and zeal that are rarely exhibited in other places, for their work is done under the stimulus of a desire for self-improvement, not for money.

At the time some argued that the expertise to handle the variety and severity of cases seen on ambulance duty required doctors with skills that only came from long experience: turning tyros loose on the ambulances struck the reform-minded as inviting error, malpractice, and disaster for those dependent on the city's ambulance service. Such concerns were swept aside on the grounds that the hospitals had no resources with which to buy wisdom, while animal strength was cheap. As our correspondents put it:

> older [physicians] of more experience and knowledge, and of equal ability, are not to be had. An older man who would accept such a position [as ambulance surgeon] for such a salary as a hospital could pay would be a self-confessed failure, and any expectation of better work from him would certainly be disappointed. Such extraordinary exertions as are made by the young ambulance surgeons in the performance of their duties can be made continuously only by the young, the vigorous, the enthusiastic. If they were not earnest and eager in their work they would not remain in the service a week. The elderly man of experience ... who should attempt to take the place of one of these young men, would at the end of a few days be in as pitiable a condition as if he had acted as a substitute on one of our college football teams.

Still, the situation in New York was poisoned by frequent newspaper stories alleging that some ambulance interns refused to take patients from outside their district, turned down patients as drunk who later turned out to be suffering from fatal skull fractures, and that ambulance

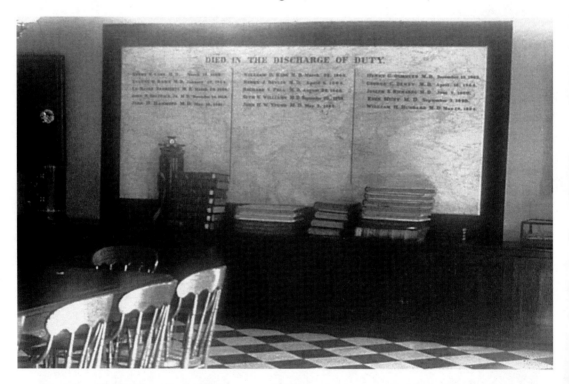

The "Great Tablet" inscribed with the names of Bellevue interns who died in the line of duty, including those who met death while serving on the ambulance (courtesy of the Edward G. Miner Library, University of Rochester Medical Center, New York).

surgeons in general were unprofessional and of dubious competence.[3] These claims were taken so seriously that a Grand Jury was impaneled in 1891 and directed to employ the full weight of its subpoena and investigative powers to expose the true scale of the abominations alleged.[4] As it turned out, the Grand Jury found otherwise on all major points of complaint, but, despite its report, relations between the ambulance crews and the New York public sank to a nadir, although the services were the target of fewer attacks as the years passed.

For their labors most 19th Century interns were given room, board, and free laundry, in addition to a token stipend ($5 a week if they were fortunate) to buy necessities. Despite the poverty, for most interns the ambulance service was unquestionably the most exciting portion of their internship, as outside the hospital gate they operated with complete autonomy: the evidence suggests that they were generally unsupervised after their first few runs, simply handed their bags and expected to function as fully credentialed members of the profession. (Not surprisingly, in their memoirs these ex-ambulance interns often admit relying heavily on the pointed "suggestions" of their vastly more experienced drivers.) This system proved a hardy one, almost as hardy as the interns it was built on. For eighty years the portion of the ambulance intern remained virtually the same—as did the economics, with interns subsidizing ambulance service with their abysmal wages. For example, in 1936 Bellevue interns were paid $30 a month along with room, board, and laundry services.[5] While many in the Depression might have jumped for such a berth, its terms were virtually unchanged since the 1880s. In fact, the Bellevue interns were lucky to be receiving even their dollar a day, as in 1935 one third of teaching hospitals paid no salary at all, only providing beds, meals, and clean clothes once a week. The remaining two thirds of hospitals paid monthly salaries ranging from a low of $4.60 to a high of $125, with the average salary coming in just under $6 a week.[6] The paltry pay reflected a longstanding belief that paid interns would be tempted to leave the hospital on occasion to

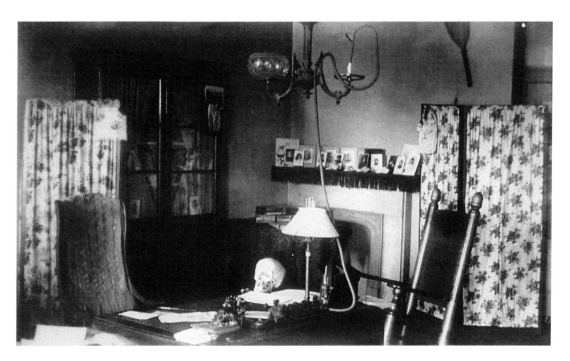

Bellevue resident's room in the 19th century: Post-Victorian ambulance interns faced more Spartan accommodations (courtesy the Edward G. Miner Library, University of Rochester Medical Center, New York).

spend their wages, whereas if they were kept destitute they'd be forced to stay indoors where they could always be found and put to constructive use. Others argued that since the purpose of an internship was to educate, the interns should be grateful that the hospitals didn't charge them tuition for the privilege of working twelve-hours a day.

Of course, the grueling hours, dismal pay, and an occasionally ungrateful public took its toll, and on some nights an exhausted intern might become selective in how they applied the Hippocratic Oath. In a 1939 WPA interview a New York City ambulance driver recounted one intern's strategy for dealing with a difficult patient:

> You've got to take plenty of abuse in the ambulance business, particularly on the night shift when you get the pie-eyes and psychos by the dozens, half of them boys they let out of Rockland and Islip to make room when it's overcrowded in them institutions, the guys with the shivers and shakes and snakes and goddamn hallucinations. But there's one kind I never can stand, the stiffs that started out with a hundred bucks at 8 P.M., and when you get them around 1 [A.M.] they got exactly 2½ ¢ and a big voice askin' for "de-looks soivice."
>
> One doc I was riding with, he hated them too, [and he] used to be a full-back from Alabama. One night we get a call for the front of the Rivoli [Theater]. We drive up and there's a big stiff in all his glory abusing about 3,000 innocent people while he [urinates] on a taxicab. We pick him up and get going up the street, and the first thing he does is look the doc straight in the eye—and toss his cookies. A sad sight that brave guy was. All the guts out of him and on the doc's white suit. Boy o' boy! the doc just took ... and heaved him right through the back window. Like a bird he flew—but he didn't land like a bird. I hate to think of it. "Now he'll need an ambulance," the doc said. "Just keep going."[7]

Last Call

While an intern on ambulance duty was buying a ticket to the greatest show in medicine no matter where they were stationed, from the 19th century through the late 1930s Bellevue's

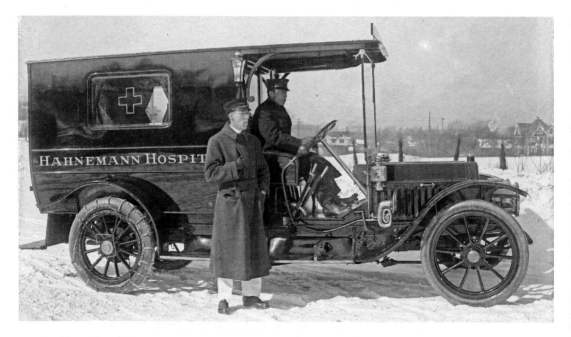

In this undated photograph, an ambulance surgeon and driver with the Hahnemann Hospital in Rochester, New York, pose beside their gleaming rig in bitter winter weather. In lieu of a siren, the ambulance features an elaborate, bulb-operated brass horn (from the Albert R. Stone Negative Collection, Rochester Museum & Science Center Rochester, N.Y.).

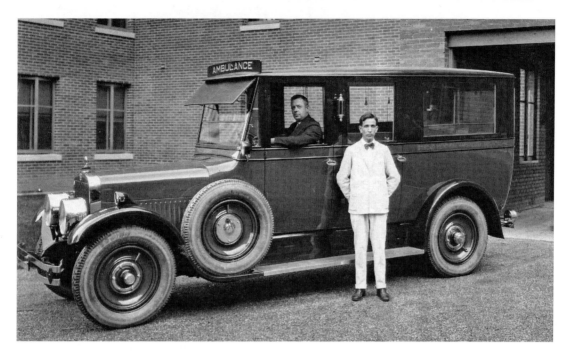

Driver Dave Muckle and Dr. Ernest Arena pose beside an ambulance shared by Strong Memorial and the Rochester Municipal Hospital, in 1926 (courtesy the Edward G. Miner Library, University of Rochester Medical Center, New York).

ambulance service continued to be among the nation's busiest and remained an eagerly sought appointment among northeastern medical graduates. Decked out in a stiff blue hat like that worn by train conductors and dress whites, the Bellevue interns could expect a variety of cases worthy of the city during their month on service. One wrote that on his first day "riding the bus" in the 1930s he covered nineteen calls, including heroin withdrawal, a human bite of the hand, chest pain, psychosis, gall bladder disease, and a woman whose leg was caught in an elevator.[8] Among the macabre customs of the Bellevue ambulance (and many other hospitals around the country as well) was one dictating that anyone returning to Bellevue with a DOA patient had to buy a round of beer for the other interns.[9]

Still, whatever its advantages in teaching and as a means of guaranteeing a trained physician at the emergency scene, not all hospitals could operate intern programs and those that did could not always spare them for ambulance duty. By the middle 1930s ambulance calls were generally billed, if at all, at around $5 to $10, making it more economical for most hospitals to staff an ambulance with an orderly and keep the intern on the wards performing more lucrative procedures. Indeed, by the outbreak of World War II interns had become the exception rather than the rule, a trend hastened by the dramatic physician shortage occasioned by military service. When the war-time doctor shortage compelled New York City to withdraw physicians from ambulance duty Mayor La Guardia delivered the news to the populace in a 1942 radio address, explaining

> This change in practice has been brought about by the shortage of internes due to military requirements and the necessity of eliminating unnecessary calls so that ambulances may be available in the event of a real emergency. Now, in making such change, New York City has returned to the standard practice of almost every large city in the United States. We went above the standard for several years in order to provide people with the best possible ambulance service and placed an interne on each ambulance, and the use of this has been abused quite a bit.

> The purpose of an ambulance is not to send out a doctor to administer care but only to bring in a patient who is in need of hospitalization. The custom has developed to send for an ambulance just to get some medical care. In the past approximately half of the calls made by city ambulances, or 250,000 calls a year, were on cases where hospitalization was not required.[10]

Warming to his theme, the Mayor warned that those who had come to rely on this "de luxe service" to bring a doctor into their living room for "a case of, oh, just a little stomach ache," had better get used to visiting hospital outpatient departments or phoning the family doctor and paying for the service. (This was hardly a novel complaint: from the beginning of the Bellevue service citizens had, faced with the temptation of a free house-call, never hesitated to ring for an ambulance, so for "trifling injuries, for bruises received in a drunken altercation ... horse, driver, and surgeon are brought out to put on a piece of court plaster."[11] In one of countless examples from around the country, during a 1900 March blizzard in upstate New York a factory-worker phoned in a "hurry call" for morphine poisoning, but when the ambulance at last breasted through the drifts at the factory gate the young woman confessed that she only wanted a ride home through the storm, and didn't want to spend the money for a cab.[12] Not surprisingly, this escapade prompted a local flurry of activity to make unfounded ambulance calls a misdemeanor, akin to phoning a false fire alarm.)

Despite some alarmist concerns, the use of non-physicians on the ambulances did not result in wholesale death and disaster, and after the war ended there was a national reluctance to put interns back on the ambulances. Not only had non-physician attendants proved their worth during the war, but all the economic incentives ran against putting the interns back on "the bus." It was no surprise, then, that New York City's Hospital Commissioner, Dr. Edward M. Bernecker, announced in 1948 that attendants would continue to staff municipal ambulances in lieu of interns. Declaring ambulance service to be more "efficient and perhaps more satis-

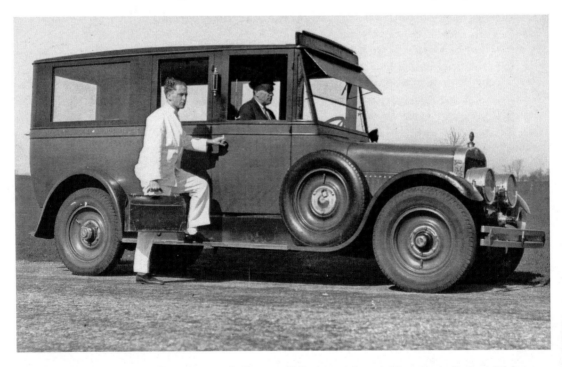

Intern poised to dash off on an errand of mercy: Like as not, he would arrive to find a trivial case attempting to finagle a free house call. Such abuses hastened the end of the ambulance surgeon (ViaHealth Archives Consortium, Rochester, N.Y.).

factory" than ever, and noting the decrease in ambulance calls from those merely seeking "convenient and free medical service at home," the Commissioner anticipated concerns by noting that physicians would be routinely dispatched on maternity cases, to disaster scenes, and in any instance where the police requested their presence (recall that ambulance dispatch, as always, was being handled through the police communications bureau, which took the particulars of the call before relaying it to the nearest hospital).[13]

This reform didn't last long, however, and by December 1948 the interns were back on most of New York's city-owned ambulances. The precipitating event was an ambulance attendant pronouncing a woman dead, who later turned out to be quite alive.[14] The episode was a nine-day wonder, and thirteen city-run hospitals felt enough pressure from the public relations fallout to put doctors back in their ambulances. Happily insulated from the political pressure of appeasing voters who read the papers, the city's private hospitals quietly continued their use of non-physician attendants, and by 1949 just 15 percent of the city's private hospitals staffed ambulances with physicians, a statistic consistent with the national trend.[15] Professionally, the medical community was of two minds about this shift in staffing, with many, including overworked interns tired of riding out at three in the morning for a sore throat or a drunk call, feeling the practice was a waste of everyone's time, to say nothing of money. Other onlookers

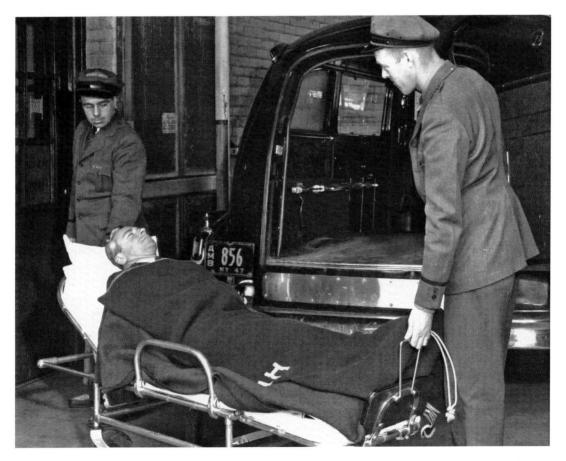

Two ambulance crewmen pose with a mock patient in this publicity photograph for Strong Memorial Hospital in 1947. By the end of the 1940s most private hospitals had given up trying to recruit interns to staff ambulances and were relying on lay attendants to operate their aid cars (courtesy the Edward G. Miner Library, University of Rochester Medical Center, New York).

firmly believed ambulance duty created independence in young doctors and gave them a chance to see the real conditions under which patients lived—and as the house call receded into history, it was unlikely that these physicians would ever again visit a patient's home and see the environment that might contribute to the ailment or interfere with its resolution.

These debates aside, hospitals had another reason to take doctors out of the ambulances—it dramatically reduced the number of frivolous summons from those looking for a free house call (hospitals only charged for transportation, and if the patient wasn't sick enough to be removed they could usually cajole the intern into giving a diagnosis and leaving a prescription behind, or perhaps even some free medicine). For example, as physicians left New York City's ambulances during the war years the number of ambulance calls had decreased from nearly 500,000 a year in 1942 to something over 300,000 in 1948—a better than 30 percent drop *despite* a small increase in the city's population.[16] It surprised no one when the return of the interns precipitated a corresponding increase in ambulance calls: as the *New York Times* put it "the New York public has been alert to distinguish between doctors and attendants, and has indicated a preference for the doctors."[17] According to the article, the busiest ambulance service in the five boroughs, Harlem Hospital's, saw its daily dispatches jump *49 percent* during the first month interns were back on the ambulances, and absent evidence that north Manhattan was in the grip of the bubonic plague the only explanation was that word had gotten out that once again a free-house call could be had by calling the ambulance desk.

In addition to these economic arguments the practical issue of attracting staff was soon added. By 1950 interns were voting with their feet, and those hospitals still requiring ambulance duty were seeing applications fall off: in that year there were 9,124 internships available nationally, but only some 7,000 interns to fill them: the sharp competition meant, for the first time ever, the interns were in a position to get what they wanted—short of better pay, that is.[18] (In 1950 fully 85 percent of the most selective hospitals paid under $50 a month, and among the less attractive non-teaching hospitals only half paid more.[19] Amenities, such as freedom from ambulance duty, were one currency hospitals could still trade on.) Still, even when interns were excused from routine duty it was not uncommon for hospitals into the late 1950s to provide physicians on particularly serious calls, either replacing an attendant on the run or taking a taxi or a police cruiser and meeting the wagon at the scene.[20] (This practice was most common where the hospital itself still provided the ambulance, and rarely did they participate when a third party operated the aid car.) Some places held out for a longer time, with the Newark municipal hospital not replacing its ambulance interns with first aid–certified attendants until 1960, when it too succumbed to an intern shortage.[21] As it became clear that interns weren't essential on ambulances, increasing numbers of hospitals decided the ambulance service itself was superfluous: if an ambulance wasn't going to chauffeur an intern, let it be garaged someplace else, with some other entity paying the insurance and dealing with the staffing issue. This divestiture of hospital ambulance services gained momentum in the 1960s, as we will see in a later chapter, and by the end of the decade the ambulance intern become a memory. Having debuted in 1869 the American ambulance surgeon didn't survive their centennial, but the work of these young physicians ensured that the civilian ambulance service was built upon a foundation of excellence that would support and inspire future reformers as the ambulance was continually re-invented in the decades to come.

"She'll Do": Emily Dunning, Ambulance Surgeon

Before leaving the intern behind, however, there is another aspect to consider: the struggle of women to be given their chance riding "the bus."

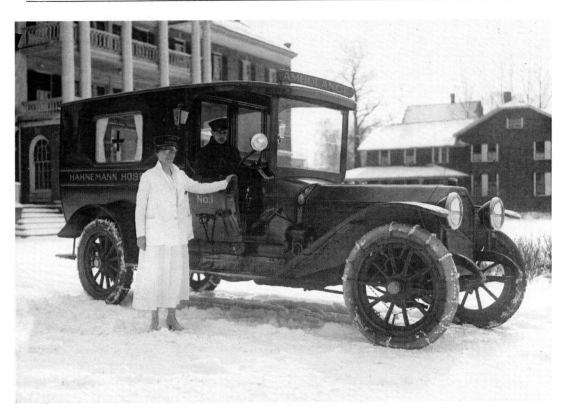

World War I, which pulled men into uniform, created openings in civilian hospitals for women physicians. Dr. Mary Foley became Rochester, New York's first female ambulance surgeon in 1918 (from the Albert R. Stone Negative Collection, Rochester Museum & Science Center Rochester, N.Y.).

History does not record when the first woman climbed aboard an ambulance to tend the wounded, but among the nameless medieval camp-followers trailing their men into battle there were unquestionably many tending casualties in the back of early, jarring ambulance wagons. By the 19th century French nuns were commonly serving on military ambulances, with one, Sister Marie Theresa, knighted for her forty years of heroic service under fire, and the Civil War saw American women taking their place on the ambulances as well.[22] Notable among the Civil War veterans was Anna Etheridge, twenty-one years old when she volunteered with a Michigan Infantry Regiment at the outbreak of the Civil War. In its August 20, 1864, number *The Christian Recorder* described her as "quiet, modest, and unreproachable in deportment ... 5 foot 2 inches in height, complexion fair though now much bronzed, hair light and cut short, and altogether decidedly good looking." Etheridge rode hard, braving cannon and musket to attend the wounded wherever the battle was fiercest, frequently riding alone where no male surgeon dared.[23] Her work with the ambulances was credited with saving countless lives, and her grateful commander awarded her a special Cross of Valor. Shamefully, when she was granted a veteran's pension in 1887 it was set at one-half the rate of a man's, but in death she was given the due denied in life, being interred at Arlington National Cemetery in 1913.

Despite these examples of valor, antiquated ideas about suitable jobs for women kept *civilian* ambulance surgeon work an all-male preserve until July 1903, when Dr. Emily Dunning (later Barringer) climbed aboard New York City's Gouverneur Hospital ambulance wagon and ended the male monopoly, and no history of the ambulance can overlook the difficulties facing Dr. Dunning and her successors. When Dr. Dunning finished medical school in New York City in 1901 it had been fifty years since Elizabeth Blackwell became America's first licensed female physician in 1849, but women doctors were still rare—although not rare enough to suit many of their male colleagues. The few women earning medical degrees were restricted to postgraduate training in specialty hospitals catering to women and children: the country's "general" hospitals all adamantly refused them internships, citing the unwillingness of male patients to tolerate female physicians (the preference of female patients was apparently of less concern) and the lack of separate living quarters for female interns (all interns were expected to live at the hospital—from whence the term "resident" for doctors in training). At that time New York's municipal hospitals offered the nation's premier internships, two-year terms including up to eighteen months on the ambulance service. Appointments to these coveted positions, with their promise of professional advancement, were by competitive examination only. With the active support of forward looking male colleagues, Dr. Dunning (then in her final year of medical school) was able to persuade the Board of Governors of the Bellevue and Allied Hospitals to open the intern qualifying exam at a single hospital—Gouverneur—to female candidates in 1901. Despite facing forty others from the finest medical schools in the nation, Dr. Dunning confounded her critics by placing first on the exam.

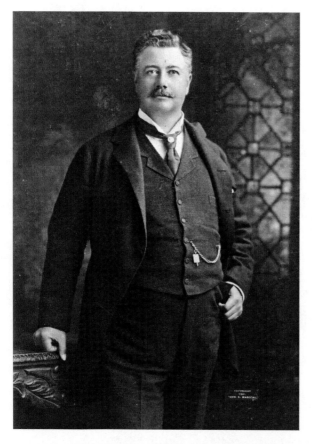

Mayor Seth Low, whose support for women's rights paved the way for equality on the ambulance services (portrait by Theo Marceau, 1901: Library of Congress, Prints and Photographs Division, USZ62-13124).

Success brought no victory: she was summarily refused a place. As she recounted in her memoir, she and another female doctor who had scored well on the examination arranged a meeting with the chief commissioner of the Hospital Board to plead their case. Despite their demonstrable qualifications and personal advocacy they were rebuffed by Commissioner J.W. Keller, who told them "I will not ratify your appointments. I will not be responsible for having a young woman doctor out on that ambulance service and have her break her neck."[24] Despondent at not being allowed to risk her neck as she pleased, Dr. Dunning spent several months working with an established female physician until the political climate changed with the election of the reformist mayor Seth Low. Sympathetic to woman's rights, Mayor Low appointed a new hospital board which announced that internships at Gouverneur Hospital, with its hectic ambulance service, would finally be opened to female physicians.

Dr. Dunning submitted herself to the exhausting test once more—a full day of written work canvassing everything from basic anatomy to the latest germ theory, with high scoring candidates summoned by telegram the next day for an examination of their practical technique. She placed fourth overall and was instructed to report for duty on January 1, 1903, at Gouverneur Hospital, hard by the waterfront. (Originally built as a general infirmary it had evolved into an "Emergency Hospital," its ambulance service kept busy with a high percentage of trauma cases from the docks and rough neighborhoods of lower Manhattan.) Her next obstacle was obtaining a uniform. Even in these waning hours of the Victorian era women of her social status were expected to greet the public well-covered from throat to toe. Since the male surgeon's coat and trousers would have been as unthinkable as reporting to work in a bathing suit, the hospital simply gave her a sum of money equal to what it spent to purchase a man's uniform and bade her to come up with something suitable. As it happened, the Boston tailors V. Ballard and Sons volunteered to create an outfit gratis, accepting payment in honor and publicity. In consultation with their tailors, Dr. Dunning devised a pocket-rich plain-cut jacket worn over a divided skirt (this last provided the convenience of trousers with the respectable appearance of a dress), the outfit rendered in heavy blue serge, satin lined, with the only ornament a simple red cross sewn onto one sleeve. To keep her surgeon's cap in place her mother cut the standard foot-long hat pins in half, so that they would not protrude like antennae above her crown.[25]

After six months of ward duty Dr. Dunning was assigned to her first ambulance call, a routine transfer case accompanied by as much public interest as the promenade of a sitting president. According to an account in the *New York Times*, on the evening of June 29th the hospital superintendent asked Dunning to accompany a woman and infant on their transfer to Bellevue Hospital, with a stop to pick up a third patient at Beth Israel along the way.[26] Conscious of the historic nature of the occasion, a swarm of doctors and attendants surged out to the ambulance shed to watch her departure: as she approached the wagon some of her male companions stepped forward to assist her into the back, but the cheerful young surgeon waved them away with a "Never mind, that is easy!" and, mounting the step, cleared the backboard with a spring.[27] For a moment, all antipathy towards the "intrusion" of the female surgeon into the ambit of the male physicians was swamped by the novelty of the occasion, and she rolled out to a resounding cheer. When in due course she arrived at Bellevue with her charges she encountered a crowd of well-wishers at the hospital gate, her beaming mother foremost in their ranks, and they greeted her lustily even as boys in the street ran alongside shouting, "Get a man!"[28] Having proved she could ride, she was given a day off before assuming her role as a full-time ambulance surgeon on July 1, 1903, a day whose arduous schedule would prove far more representative than the leisurely promenade she enjoyed on the warm summer evening when she had made her historic first trip.

Tipped off in advance, the local papers were ready to pounce on her travails, and she was accompanied by a bevy of reporters to record each momentous utterance and jot down every telling action. Her adventure started, of course, with a misadventure for the patient doomed to be the unwilling supporting player in this medical drama. It began early in the day when a peanut vendor was pushing his cart along Park Row. As he stepped around the corner into Chambers Street, he was struck by a brewery truck. In an instant the massive wagon threw him to the pavement and a heavy wheel ground his right leg into the very bricks, and as the miserable wretch lay there writhing in gore a flock of newsboys dashed over and began snatching up the feast of peanuts strewn about the wreckage of man and cart.

A passing patrolman soon scattered the urchins and assisted in laying the casualty in the shade of a boot-black's stand as word was sent for the Gouverneur ambulance—which arrived along with a reporter for the *New York World* to record the "gasp of amazement" that escaped the policeman and the milling crowd when they looked up at the somber ambulance and watched as a "natty feminine figure in blue skirt, jacket, and a cap set jauntily on a wealth of light hair swung off the vehicle."[29] Unfazed, Dr. Dunning set to work immediately, kneeling beside the terrified man and giving what was likely her first order as an ambulance surgeon: directing her attention at the still gaping policeman she pointed to the patient's right foot, below the mangled leg, and said, "Officer, please take off that shoe." In quick order she had cut the bloody pants leg away, ascertained that the peddler had suffered a compound fracture, palpated the wound above and below where the jagged femur jutted like a glistening white harpoon above the tortured flesh, splinted the leg expertly, supervised the patient's transfer to stretcher and into the ambulance, and, as the gong sounded and the rig pulled away, the mob shook off its surprise and sent up a rousing cheer.[30] Watching her ride off, the constable told a reporter from the *Sun:* "Well, I'll be darned.... Never saw anything more businesslike. She'll do."[31] A quote from the doctor herself was impossible, since the Hospital Board had placed her under a gag order, but her driver suffered no such limitation and cheerfully gave his opinion of Dr. Dunning's first day: "She's all right and she's got nerve enough for anybody. Smart woman, too. I'd rather have her treating me than any of the young doctors in the house—and say, if anyone insults her or says anything she resents while I'm driving her, I'll knock his head off."[32]

Dr. Dunning's day didn't end with the maimed peanut vendor, of course. In her inaugural twelve hour shift she also used the ambulance to bring in two inebriates, a demented woman detained at a police station and remanded to the hospital's care, a case of sunstroke, and a workman who put a hole in his foot: in addition, when not on ambulance runs she was responsible for whomever walked into the hospital's casualty department—on this day, some sixty ambulatory patients.[33]

In all she spent eighteen months as an ambulance surgeon, and though the drivers and nurses took a shine to her, her fellow interns did not: they fretted that her presence would interfere with their jolly collegiality; would prompt chivalrous colleagues to relieve her of the most disagreeable calls, resulting in a disproportionate distribution of work; and, perhaps most to the point, would inevitably lead to the day when she, a woman, would be giving orders to junior males.[34] So dire was the prospect that resident physicians at the Bellevue, Gouverneur, Fordham, and Harlem Metropolitan Hospitals all signed a petition to the commissioner of charities demanding that Dunning's job offer be rescinded immediately.[35]

The commissioner ignored the petition, but after her arrival at Gouverneur the four senior residents scrupled at nothing in their efforts to discredit and discourage her. In mockery of their pious claim that having a woman on service would mean extra work for chivalrous men obligated to take her place for the worst of the ambulance work, she was routinely assigned *extra* shifts on the wagon, sometimes riding "the bus" for more than sixty hours without relief, while on numerous occasions her supervisors violated policy by leaving her alone in the hospital—in the hopes that she would make an error justifying her dismissal (that a patient might die was apparently of less consequence to them than that this experiment in gender equality should fail). With endless variety they made it clear that they were "bent and determined to get me off the staff ... in their selfishness and youthful arrogance they gave no thought to the argument that, given the same education and preparation, [I] had as much right to be there as they."[36] No matter how egregious their conduct became, she refused to make a report, feeling to do so would be an admission of weakness. Ultimately, she proved herself not only a competent surgeon, but a courageous one, as when she answered a call at the collapse of a tenement house and straightaway plunged into the debris looking for survivors, heedless of the literally tons of rubble held above her by a few sagging timbers—a feat that a veteran reporter considered symptomatic of her "characteristic recklessness in seeking to save lives."[37]

While her male physician colleagues may have tried to avoid her, she had the opposite problem when it came to the gentlemen of the press. Her position made her an instant celebrity, and when she stepped into the role as America's first female ambulance surgeon there were no fewer than fifteen major dailies competing for New York City's nickels, explaining the lengths

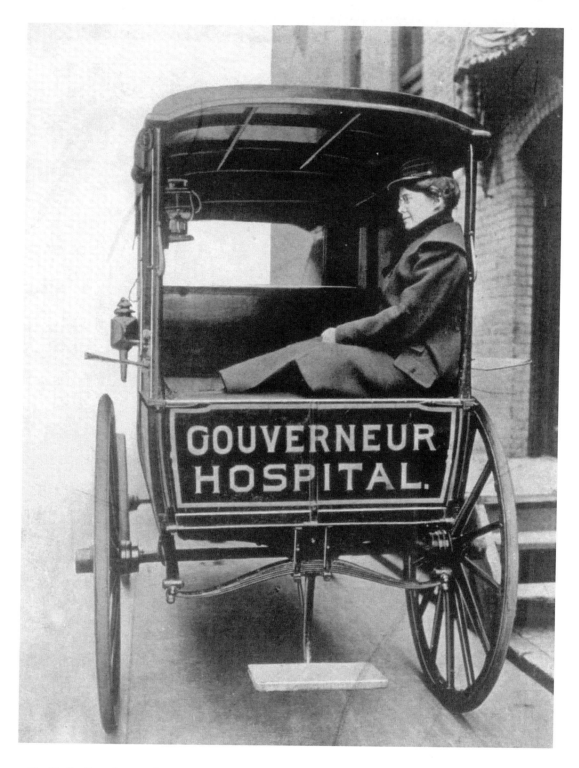

Dr. Emily Dunning on the Gouverneur ambulance in 1903. Ambulance surgeons commonly sat crosswise on the rear seat, using their feet to brace themselves against the opposite side during a swift gallop over uneven streets (courtesy the Connecticut Women's Hall of Fame).

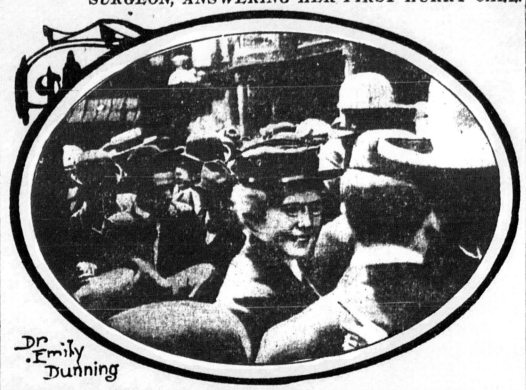

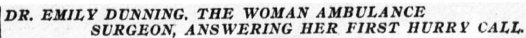

SCOLDED, LITTLE GIRL RUNS AWAY

She Was Strained by Hard Study, and in Her Supersensitive State Brooded Over Her Mother's Chiding.

Chided by her mother for not attending to her household duties, Helen Isabel Kaffler, a thirteen-year-old school girl, of No. 362 West Thirty-sixth street, disappeared from her home and a general

WOMAN SURGEON HAS FIRST CALL

In Natty Uniform Dr. Emily Dunning Hurries on Ambulance to Attend Broken-Legged Peddler in Chambers Street.

Dr. Emily Dunning had her first ambulance case to-day, and the manner in which the bright-faced young woman who rides on a Gouverneur Hospital ambulance ordered policemen from the

FOUND WEDDING VERY CATCHING

So Mr. Waltjen and Miss Marie Keem, After Being Best Man and Maid of Honor, Got Married Themselves.

School Trustee John N. Waltjen, of Hoboken, is being congratulated by telegraph to-day by his friends, who have just learned of his marriage to Miss Marie Keem, of No. 331 Spring street,

The *New York Evening World* gave Dr. Dunning's debut the full treatment—on its society page, placed among the articles pitched to its distaff readers.

one newsman went to secure her picture for the rotogravure section of his paper. After Dr. Dunning refused to pose for him, the enterprising gentleman came up with a scheme to catch her unawares. He grabbed a photographer and rushed down to the East River, determined to throw himself in and be "rescued" before Dunning went off duty—thus guaranteeing eye-grabbing pictures of New York's most celebrated ambulance surgeon in action when she arrived for his resuscitation. The plan started well, as he had no trouble making the sudden transition from pier to river, where he proceeded to flail about and, in the words of a bemused report by a rival paper, "made as much noise as a ferryboat."[38] This commotion attracted the attention of a policeman named Quinn who threw caution aside along with his helmet and jumped in to make the rescue—unfortunately, it quickly became apparent that the reporter was the better swimmer, and he wound up dragging the constable back to the pier, where the officer was unceremoniously hauled onto dry land by a gang of workman and a stout rope.[39] Undaunted, the reporter resolved to tread water until Dunning arrived to supervise his rescue and revival, but while he was busily churning up the East River and waiting for his chance, the enterprising workman succeeded in lassoing him and quickly hoisted him onto the dock with more force than care.

It was a sore and soaking scribe who looked up gratefully when the Gouverneur ambulance clattered down the planks, but to his dismay it wasn't Dr. Dunning who leapt out, but a burly male surgeon who had just relieved her.[40] When his unwitting co-stars failed to see the humor in the scenario the ersatz patient was hauled into Police Court on a charge of attempted suicide. Ultimately the magistrate turned him loose with a reprimand, but his city editor was not so forgiving, and the soggy newshawk found himself without a picture, without a story, and without a job.[41] The only one who appeared to profit from the transaction was Officer Quinn, who collected a medal and a commendation for his daring rescue attempt.

For the remainder of her term on the ambulance Dunning periodically made the papers with her adventures, but as the months went by she became an accepted part of the East Side scene, increasingly noteworthy for her abilities as physician rather than the novelty of her gender. In due time she was promoted to chief of staff, an honor her rivals and opponents could not deny she had wholly earned by merit, but after her two year internship ended she decided to forego a career in the public hospitals and instead chose to celebrate her marriage to a fellow physician, Dr. Benjamin Barringer, by entering private practice. On a chilly December evening two days after she had formally resigned, she was enjoying a solitary evening at home, free for the first time in months from the jangling summons of the ambulance bell and at last guaranteed an unbroken night of sleep, when a summons at the front door brought her into the hall. Opening the door she found herself faced with a delegation that filled the stoop and spilled down to the sidewalk: at the head stood her two ambulance drivers, Tim Murray and Tom White, while behind them were police captains from the Seventh, Twelfth, and Thirteenth precincts, and a constellation of local politicians, patrolmen, hospital attendants, and shop owners and businessmen from her ambulance district.[42]

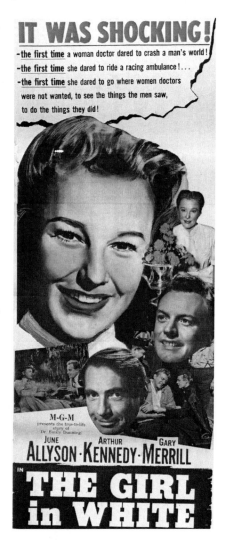

June Allyson played Dr. Emily Dunning in this 1952 MGM biopic. Despite eye-catching taglines the film only made a modest impression on the box office, with a script that played up a fictitious love-triangle over the historical realities of her work (Metro-Goldwyn-Mayer, Inc., all rights reserved).

With due solemnity the assemblage swept into the entryway, the drivers carrying between them an enormous parcel that, when unwrapped, turned out to be a heavily framed set of illustrated "resolutions" extolling her virtues as a physician. In the center was a sketch of Dunning wearing a mortar board at her medical school graduation, and at the foot was a beautiful portrait of Stockings, her ambulance horse, standing between the shafts of the rig and forming a proud blaze of white next to the dark paneling of the wagon in whose cabin she had spent so many hours, and in which she would never ride again. Scarcely had she time to begin reading the inscriptions when the school inspector, Mr. Williams, stepped forward to deliver the oration the occasion demanded. It was reprinted in full a few days later in the *Sun,* and beneath the high-flowing rhetoric a human warmth pulses, conveying through the muffling prose the plain affection in which Emily Dunning was held. He told her:

> It is our humble opinion that you, by your courage, hard work and independence, have broken down a prejudice which has existed for centuries and have attained a place in the front rank of the vast army of prominent physicians of this country....
>
> These resolutions, to our minds, embody your career as we know it for the past two years. The paper is the foundation, yourself; the wording your work and achievement; the glass, [the] plenty opposition which served to display your qualifications to a better advantage; the beading, a narrow strip of sunshine and a sense of gratification at duty well performed; the frame of oak represents the

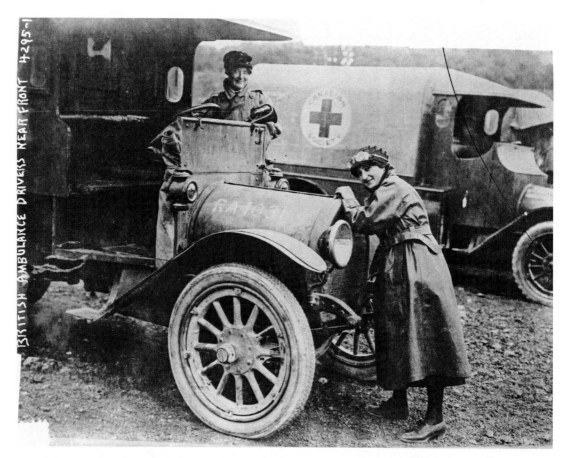

While Dr. Dunning was the first female ambulance surgeon, women had a long tradition of service on military ambulances. In this undated photograph, drivers with a Canadian ambulance squad pose with their machines during World War I (George Bain Collection, Library of Congress, LCB2-4295).

sturdy men and women who watched you with pleasure as you advanced step by step until you reached the high position in the medical profession which you have recently resigned and so ably filled.⁴³

Visibly overcome with emotion, Dunning required a few moments to compose herself, and then thanked all present for their gift and their kindness. Their duty done, the deputation wheeled and tramped back into the night, and as the last of her admirers stepped into the cold, the career of Emily Dunning, ambulance surgeon, ended with the click of a latch and the closing of a door. The momentum of her life's work was not to be arrested by stepping off the ambulance: she went on to become one of America's foremost OB/GYN surgeons and for the rest of her life remained a strong voice on issues affecting women in medicine, including lobbying for the legislation allowing women to be commissioned as medical officers in the armed forces. She will always, however, be known as America's original female ambulance surgeon, a woman of spirit and courage who, despite the most vicious efforts by her supervising residents, completed her job, leaving behind no doubts that a woman could hold her own on the ambulance service—or anywhere else in the medical profession. As her friends told her in their farewell speech the night they paid tribute to her career as both America's first female ambulance surgeon and its first female chief of staff in a general hospital, "you came among us unknown and, as we thought, doomed to failure; but to your credit and our delight you have surmounted all petty and adverse criticism and gained the goal for which you strove..." and in so doing she put the same prize, and many even more wonderful, within reach of all her sisters.⁴⁴

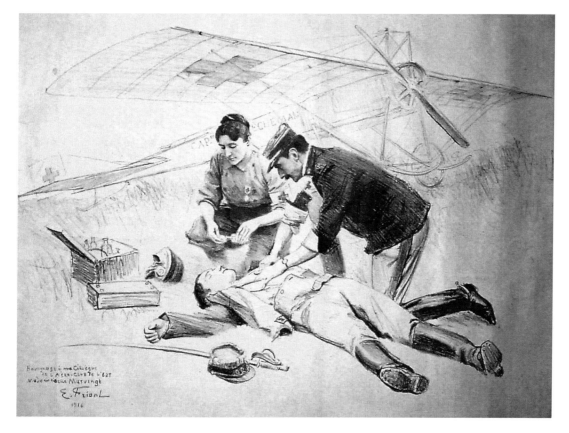

Sketch of Marie Marvingt with a rendering of her proposed aero-ambulance: Unfortunately, her factory manager embezzled the operating funds and her plane was never built (Emile Friant, 1914).

The Dove

While Dr. Dunning was making history in the United States, another woman in Europe was preparing her own outstanding contribution to ambulance history, but her name would be written on the air. The Frenchwoman Marie Marvingt, born in 1875, earned the sobriquet "the fiancée of danger" with her lifelong passion for high-risk sports, including alpine climbing and trench-warfare (she disguised herself as a man and served briefly on the front lines of the First World War). Naturally the risks of early flight were irresistible to her, and she became one of the first women in Europe to earn her wings—but it was her dedication to the air ambulance that secures her place in medical history. Just seven years after Kitty Hawk, in 1912, Marvingt designed France's first aero-ambulance, but production was aborted after her factory manager absconded with the capital.[45] Short on funds but long on zeal, she continued to proselytize, happily seeing her dreams realized when the French military debuted mercy-flights in the 1920s. In 1932 she helped develop the original aviation nursing program, the Corps des Infirmieres de l'Air, and was its premier diplomat in 1935.[46] Somehow she simultaneously found time to write, direct, and act in the 1934 documentary *The Wings Which Save*, which toured European cinemas thrilling popcorn munchers from the Pyrenees to the Rhine with stories of air ambulances and making the case for their widespread adoption. Charming, fearless, and indefatigable she worked for the improvement of medical evacuation until her death in 1963, and her contribution to the sky-ambulance is recognized by the inscription on her tomb at Nancy: "Marie Marvingt ... the founder of medical aviation."[47]

War Opens a Window

The coming of the First World War created an opportunity for Marie Marvingt to champion her aero-ambulance, but it created incalculably greater opportunities for women on the ground, when large numbers of male physicians enlisted for military service. For the first time there is anecdotal evidence of women assuming civilian ambulance duties in significant numbers, women like Dr. Mary Foley, of the Hahnemann Hospital in Rochester, N.Y., who was the city's first female ambulance surgeon. Women were also represented in the ambulance service at the front lines. One of the first American women to go overseas in this capacity was the singer Mary Carter, who told a *New York Times* reporter in 1915 that she had volunteered with the Allies in January. In an article appearing September 13 of that year, the 26 year old told how she had been originally assigned to driving a three-ton truck for the British Transport Service but had later been given charge of an ambulance—a change in commission that began inauspiciously, as she confessed "the first time I started it I knocked down a soldier because the machine jumped so quickly, and I had become accustomed to the slow movement of the three-ton truck." Serving alongside many women from the Commonwealth and the Allied nations she wound her course through the battle lines, at one point looking up to see zeppelins passing overhead, showering the landscape with bombs. The intrepid *Times* reporter caught up with her as she steamed into New York to prove to her family in Long Island that, despite the efforts of the Hun zeppelins, she still lived, but she assured the reading public that she would be retuning to the front, and her ambulance, after a few weeks of rest.

Similarly, after Pearl Harbor a sudden depletion of available men opened up new opportunities on the nation's ambulances for women. Stepping squarely into the gap was the American Women's Voluntary Services, founded in 1940 by Manhattan socialite Alice Throckmorton McLean, who during her annual hunting trips in Britain had seen firsthand the outstanding war work done by Great Britain's Women's Voluntary Service.[48] After initially limiting itself to placing a smattering of female ambulance drivers at willing hospitals, in October 1942, the AWVS announced that it would train all-woman crews to replace the interns on ambulance duty at the Flushing Hospital and Dispensary in Queens.[49] Female volunteers demonstrating what a magazine article described as "good health, intelligence—and nerve" were given the Red Cross Basic and Advanced First Aid Courses along with three weeks of lectures covering the most common ambulance calls, such as ear infections and obstetric cases.[50] After two weeks probation working alongside a male ambulance intern the successful candidates were assigned their own rigs, ready to "immobilize a fracture, revive victims of collapse, handle 'psychos,' or even help the stork," in the words of a *Colliers* article.[51] The experiment proved a runaway success, allowing the dwindling number of draft-age interns to devote their working hours to hospital work instead of riding "the bus," and by 1943 twelve hospitals in Manhattan were relying on the AWVS to keep their aid-cars running, while by war's end literally thousands of AWVS volunteers staffed ambulances nationwide.[52]

After the war the overwhelming majority of women relinquished the ambulance services to their returning masculine counterparts, and by 1947 the sight of a female ambulance surgeon was once again rare enough to rate a feature article like one appearing in the Rochester, N.Y., *Democrat and Chronicle*:

> If you've been at the scene of an accident lately or watched the Genesee Hospital ambulance speeding down one of Rochester's streets, you may have seen a young, attractive girl sitting next to the ambulance driver.
>
> No, she isn't a friend of the driver just going along for the ride, or a nurse or hospital aide. She's DOCTOR Barbara A. Wood, the only woman interne at Genesee Hospital and one of the few woman internes in the city who has ridden the ambulance in emergency calls.

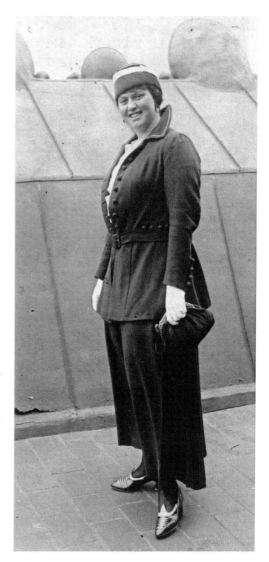

Twelve years after Emily Dunning started her career as an ambulance surgeon, Mary Carter (Mrs. Bartlett Boder) became one of the first American women to drive an ambulance during World War I, chauffeuring a British ambulance truck at the front lines in 1915 (Library of Congress, Prints and Photographs Division, LC-USZ62-103935).

The article went on to astonish readers by reporting that this intrepid "brunet doctor" had delivered babies on the side of the road, trudged through snow drifts when the ambulance bogged down in a blizzard, and that she had even put herself in harm's way after a locomotive plunged into the Genesee River. The article assured readers her gender brought with it no privileges and she was just as ill-used as her male colleagues, particularly on the interminable weekend shifts when she reported to the Emergency Room on Saturday morning and worked straight through until late Monday night, snatching what sleep she could between ambulance calls and

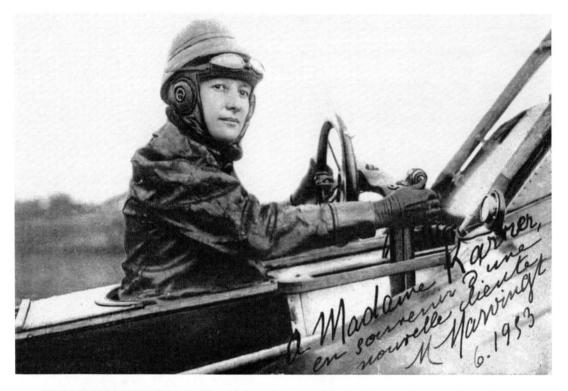

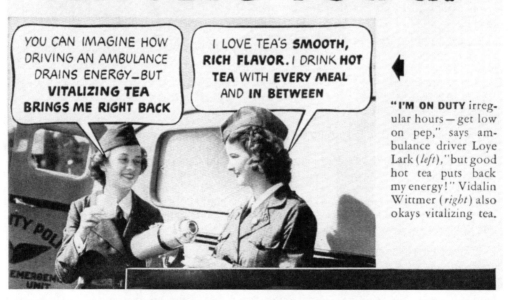

Top: Marie Marvingt in the cockpit of her plane, around 1916. She later became the first person to be certified as an aviation nurse, in 1935. *Bottom:* In this 1941 advertisement from the tea industry, a municipal police ambulance is staffed by a female crew fueled by a "delicious, vitalizing, economical" brew promising pep in every cup.

patient work-ups. Little wonder that when asked what she did for recreation she replied that she read, went on dates, but "mostly, and she emphasized this: just SLEEPS."[53]

Women like Dr. Wood continued to enlist in the various medical disciplines in ever increasing numbers, particularly after the early 1970s, and by 2001 it was estimated that women accounted for 31 percent of all emergency medical technicians employed in the ambulance services.[54] When Dr. Emily Dunning climbed aboard the horse-drawn ambulance at Gouverneur Hospital there was only one woman in charge of an ambulance in the entire world—ninety-nine years later, in 2002, there were over *fifty-five thousand* female ambulance workers in the United States alone.[55] That exponential progression vindicates the efforts of one woman and her determined allies in turn of the century New York, efforts guaranteeing that future ambulance services would profit from the complete spectrum of human talent and compassion, not only one arbitrary half.

• 8 •

First Aides: Early Ambulance Attendants and Emergency Hospitals

While ambulance surgeons dominated hospital-based services until the Second World War, and receive the bulk of attention in ambulance histories, non-physician attendants were crucial to the development of early ambulance services, and their gradual ascent towards professionalism mirrored their assumption of primacy in care delivery. We have already seen the role that police officers and female wartime volunteers played in the emergency services, but there were other lay providers breaking trail on the way to the modern ambulance, and their story, improbably, arcs from the blood drenched sands of 11th century Palestine to British railway terminals and funeral parlors across America. In a slightly later but parallel development, the emergency hospital movement helped lay the foundation for improved ambulance services by providing well-equipped safe-harbors for trauma cases: the need to deliver patients capable of profiting from the interventions available at these specialty hospitals demanded improved interventions at the scene, hastening innovations in training and equipment.

The St. John Ambulance Society: Pioneering First Aid

While formal first aid-training for civilian ambulance attendants goes back at least to 1866, when ambulance cars were added to Swedish passenger trains and guards were given what one observer described as "the elements of surgery," the most important of these efforts was started under the auspices of the St. John Ambulance Society, a league of Victorian gentlemen whose antecedents were warrior monks plying sword and scalpel with equal fervor in the days of the Crusades.[1] To appreciate the debt owed by ambulance professionals to 11th century Crusader clerics we must consider the history of the group that became the Sovereign Knights of Malta.[2] The story begins in 600 A.D., when Abbot Probus established a hostel, or charitable house of refuge, for pilgrims visiting Jerusalem. The hostelry stood a few doors down from the Church of the Sepulcher (a popular destination reputed to stand over the empty tomb of Jesus), offering rest, meals, and simple nursing care for any pilgrim who found their threshold. This benign purpose didn't save it from being destroyed in 614 by invading Persians, however. In 638 the hostel was revived, passing to the Benedictines in the 9th century, only to be leveled again in 1005 by El Hakim, caliph of Egypt and sworn enemy of all religions save his own. Sometime after 1033 wealthy merchants from the Republic of Amalfi on the Italian peninsula bought the site and helped rebuild the hostel, and by 1070 the reconstructed sanctuary was dedicated to St. John the Baptist and came under the direction of The Blessed Gerard.[3]

By 1118 The Hospitallers of Saint John had received Papal recognition and, under the leadership of Raymond du Puy, operated a string of hospitals along the pilgrim route from Europe.

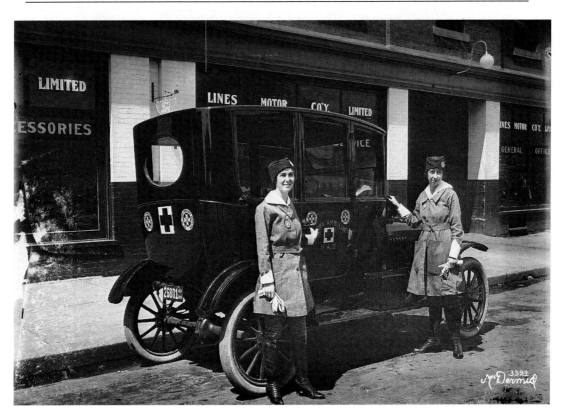

Nurse members of a St. John Ambulance "Voluntary Aid Detachment" pose beside their ambulance in Edmonton, Alberta, in 1918. Nurses with the VAD were assigned to the Royal Army Medical Corps during the war, where many served in ambulance services both at home and abroad (McDermid Studios, 1918, courtesy the Glenbow Archives, NC6-3393).

It was du Puy who considered the number of times the order had been sacked and toppled by Islamic counter-crusaders and decided that while there was grace in *aiding* the weak and helpless, it was tiresome *being* weak and helpless. Emulating the warrior Knights Templar he reorganized the Hospitallers as a military religious order, divided into three classes: monks, serving brothers, and knights. All three took vows of poverty, chastity, and obedience, and glorified their deity with medical and charitable acts—the knights further exalting their god by taking up the sword when the hospital or the city was threatened. In the words of poet Samuel Rogers, "that Hospital sent forth its holy men in complete steel ... the cowl relinquished for the helm."[4] In 1160 a visitor described a fortified hospital accommodating two-thousand patients—without prejudice to faith or disease.[5] One hundred twenty four stone pillars buttressed its lofty walls, and groin arches opened into spacious apertures on all sides. When all beds were occupied the mortality rate could reach fifty souls a day; they were interred in a charnel house on the grounds. Two churches and a convent for nuns were also found in the complex. By 1170 the sick were being given eight ounces of white bread a day, and, in a gesture towards preventive medicine, inmates were given boots and a cloak to wear when walking to the latrines. The hospital's expenses were partially paid by the taxes assessed on two small towns, and that this medical order had the power, both temporal and moral, to command the taxes of entire communities allowed it to preserve itself during the reversals of fortune which were swiftly to come.[6]

Resources, local opinion, and force of numbers were all in favor of the Islamic armies, and a series of defeats pushed the Hospitallers of St. John north and westward—first to Acre,

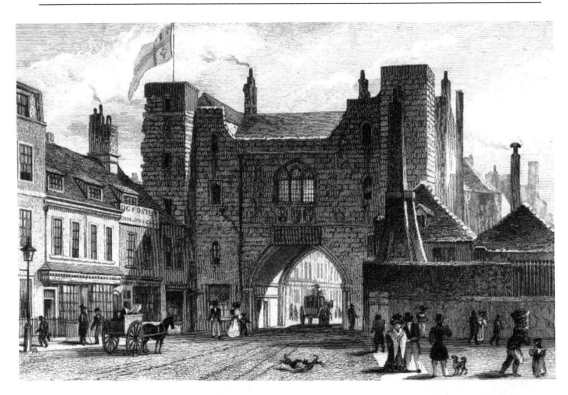

19th century sketch of St. John's Gate in London, the historical headquarters for the Order of St. John of Jerusalem in England.

then out into the Mediterranean from Cyprus to Rhodes and, finally, to Malta in 1530. In 1792, Napoleon, who did so much to inaugurate the modern ambulance, evicted the Hospitallers from Malta, and they decamped to Rome, where to this day they remain as the Knights of Malta, a sovereign government without a country. After the Bourbon restoration revitalized the Hospitallers in France, the Knights celebrated their resurrection by scheming to reclaim Rhodes and Malta by force of arms. To strengthen their little army they sought to enlist the descendants of the long dormant English Hospitallers, whose order had been dispossessed by Henry VIII and Elizabeth I. After years of negotiation between the prodigal British order and the Vatican the Holy See decided the prospect of *Protestant* Hospitallers was too appalling to contemplate: nonetheless, the idea of a resurgent order had taken hold in Albion, and in 1858 the Order of Saint John of Jerusalem of England declared itself formally independent of Rome and henceforth a self-governing, independent body.

By now, there was no more talk of invading Rhodes and Malta, and, absent a new Crusade, the British order found itself with a name and a flag but no purpose. For a few years it limped along as little more than an exclusive gentleman's club until, in 1872, some members considered their order's inception as an aid to the afflicted and persuaded their fellows to donate £100 to establish a simple ambulance service in the Midlands mining and pottery districts.[7] Apparently inspired by initial results, in 1874 the order invited the Army's Surgeon General to address the General Assembly on the best methods of handling industrial injuries in mines and factories.[8] His remarks found an eager audience, and a year later members unveiled a new ambulance litter resembling a stretcher mounted between spoked wheels, a simple device that was cheaper than any ambulance wagon and comfortable and convenient for both patient and rescuer: over the next three years they sent one hundred of these hand-ambulances to various mine pits, police stations, depots, hospitals, factories, and docks across Britain.[9] In retrospect, the Surgeon General's remarks were a fulcrum on which the order's fortunes were to pivot: prior to them, the order had limited itself to the distribution of apparatus, with little attention to the circumstances in which they would be used, while after the lecture many members began to see that without distribution of practical medical knowledge their ambulance depots were little more than a closet with a stretcher. With the addition of skilled lay attendants, however, the ambulance depot would become a source of actual assistance, not merely a healthier substitute for a wheelbarrow or a rough-riding cab. At the same time, other members were keenly interested in creating a sort of "medical national guard'" that could supplement the deficient military medical forces in time of war. Many members had hoped that the recently activated British National Aid Society, the forerunner to the British Red Cross, would have committed its energies towards creating civilian medical reservists, but they had been bitterly disappointed when the aid society declined to cooperate with military authorities in this aim.[10] For these members, then, the Knights of St. John, with their proud tradition of warrior-healers, would be a natural training ground for the hoped for civilian reservists.

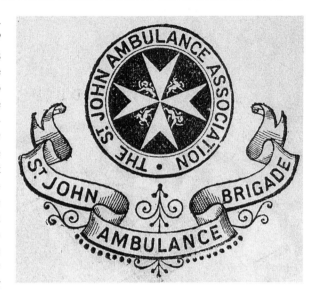

19th century version of the Maltese Cross (common to many fire and ambulance insignia). Originally the design likely honored the nearly identical Badge of Amalfi worn by the ancient Italian benefactors of the Jerusalem hostel. (Of note, the Amalfi emblem was not a religious symbol, taking its shape from four arrow heads arranged point to point.) (Courtesy the Order of St. John, St. John Ambulance Society.)

While the question of whether the order would be an extension of the armed forces or an independent charity devoted to civilian aims would ultimately have to be decided, there was general agreement that public first aid training was a worthwhile object of the order's efforts, and in the spring of 1877 a meeting was convened at the ancient St. John's Gate to put the issue before the members. After an evening of high-flung oratory the members voted to establish the St. John Ambulance Association, whose mission would be to create and deliver a public curriculum in first aid to all who wished to learn. In addition, they pledged £1,000 to finance a series of ambulance centers across England, centers equipped with the organization's own design of wheeled stretchers and staffed by successful graduates of their lecture series.[11] The premier training course was given in January 1878, at the London suburb of Woolwich—a location that was hardly coincidental, since the town industry was wrapped up in the enormous arsenal kept there, and accidents were distressingly common. (Those who hoped to see the St. John Ambulance Association work closely with the military also found the site a natural one for recruiting medical reservists for Her Majesty's armed forces.) Overseeing development of the course were two army officers, Colonel Francis Duncan and Surgeon-Major Peter Shephard, aided by Capt. John Furley. In the event, they didn't have to wait for the commencement of hostilities to go to work, as just six months after the first course had been completed a catastrophic collapse of a massive storage shed trapped a hundred arsenal workers in the debris. Instantly the Woolwich St. John Ambulance Corps rushed to the scene, conveying the injured to the local military hospital with their wheeled litters and providing essential first-aid. The

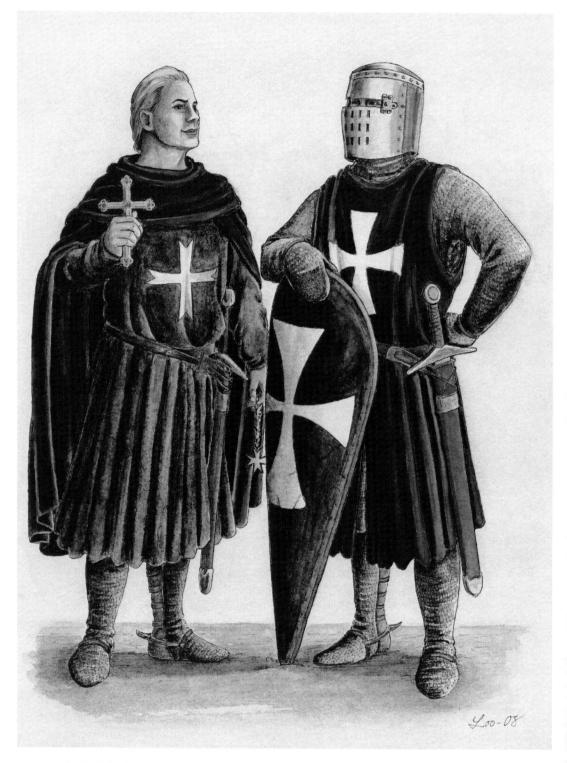

Hospitaller Knights of St. John in the 13th century. In addition to knights obligated to defend pilgrims and the hostel, the order included serving brothers whose principal labors were medical (Ann-Cathrine Loo).

Daily Telegraph crowned their efforts with grateful praise, noting "had it not been for the promptitude of the assistance thus rendered many of the wounded must have remained some time in a position which would have reduced their hope of recovery to a minimum."[12]

The experience was a revelation to many who had supported confining the organization's efforts to a military auxiliary, bringing most of them across the aisle to join those who had always aspired to create a popular movement for universal education in emergency medicine: accordingly, class organization was quickly ramped up at sites considered particularly prone to accidents, as with the popular series offered at Paddington Railway Station. By September, 1878, just nine months after starting, Major Duncan boasted "[w]e have ... taught soldiers, policemen, railway porters, miners, professional men, idlers, women of all ages and degrees, and many of the young of both sexes, to the number now in all of about 2,000, how to handle the injured until medical aid can be obtained."[13] By 1880 there were no fewer than four hundred courses being offered in various communities across the United Kingdom, and nearly twenty thousand certificates had been awarded to working men of all classes, to say nothing of idlers and women.[14] From this point forward there would be no more talk of limiting the association's efforts to the military, and the St. John Ambulance would always belong to the nation as a whole.

Initially, the men's course consisted of five weekly lectures, ninety minutes long, with an extra lecture on general nursing and preparing the sick room offered for women only. The lectures began with basic anatomy before focusing, broadly, on the immediate

Aid to the Injured.

ORDER OF
ST. JOHN OF JERUSALEM
IN ENGLAND.

PROCEEDINGS
OF A
PUBLIC MEETING
HELD ON
WEDNESDAY EVENING, FEBRUARY 6TH, 1878,
AT THE PALL MALL RESTAURANT,
REGENT STREET, LONDON,

SIR EDMUND A. H. LECHMERE,
BART., M.P.,
(Secretary and Receiver of the Order)
IN THE CHAIR,

TO DESCRIBE THE SYSTEM OF INSTRUCTION NOW BEING CARRIED OUT AT VARIOUS PLACES BY THE ST. JOHN AMBULANCE ASSOCIATION, IN THE PRELIMINARY TREATMENT OF THE SICK AND INJURED, EITHER IN PEACE OR WAR.

PRICE SIXPENCE.

WOOLWICH:
PRINTED BY A. W. AND J. P. JACKSON, LIBRARY, THOMAS STREET.
1878.

At the time of this meeting, the society's ambulance classes were only a month old, but were already extremely popular. The unexpected response prompted a spirited debate that night over the direction of the society—to pursue public first aid training as an end in itself, or focus more narrowly on creating a military medical auxiliary?

treatment of broken bones; control of bleeding; relief of the apparently drowned or asphyxiated; coping with the most common minor traumas and nuisances of Victorian life, including burns, scalds, frostbite, and "lime in the eye or vegetable matter in the ear;" and, naturally, various strategies to remove the injured.[15] Finally, after absorbing the equivalent of a two-year nursing degree in four hundred fifty minutes, participants could sit for an exam. Passing required demonstrating how to treat fractures and hemorrhage, along with either artificial respiration or patient removal, and scoring at least fifty percent on a brief oral examination (a few years later a written component was added). In order to keep the material firmly etched in the disciple's mind, candidates could return at one year intervals and, by retaking the examination, qualify for progressively higher levels of certification, from voucher to medallion to label.[16]

Recognizing that even the best trained personnel required equipment to put their talents to fullest use, the order organized a companion to the ambulance association—the St. John Ambulance Society, charged with acquiring and distributing equipment for ambulance stations, the first of which was an outpost underneath the steps at the southwest corner of St. Paul's Cathedral.[17] While these locales were at first only equipped with wheeled stretchers, by 1882 John Furley had invented two new ambulance carriages, a larger one for deployment at collieries and industrial areas and a smaller, two-patient ambulance for city use.[18] In July of that year Furley wrote the *Times* urging caution in the debate over whether to establish a formal horse-ambulance service in London, as was being urged by Mr. Crossman, Dr. Howard, and other members of the London Ambulance Society.[19] Furley mentioned that in the preceding forty-eight hours he had received five applications for ambulance service at his Seven Oaks Ambulance Centre, and in each instance "the light two-wheeled [hand] litter was found better adapted for the purpose than a carriage drawn by a horse." Ultimately, however, the privacy, the protection, and the suitable platform for providing care en route that could only be delivered with an ambulance carriage won the day, and the initially reluctant St. John Ambulance Society finally organized its own Invalid Transport Corps in 1884, staffed by four attendants, two rolling litters, and one horse-drawn ambulance: lacking suitable publicity and an efficient means of summons, it was only called seventy-eight times in its first year.[20]

An important milestone came in 1887 when the service provided carriages and hand-ambulances during Queen Victoria's extensive Jubilee celebrations, an effort advertising its utility to the huge section of the public attending the various events. Still, the society had its public relations problems, and despite smart-looking black and white uniforms the early ambulance men were often jeered as "Body Snatchers.'" In 1893 Edward, Prince of Wales, patron of the Order of St. John, famously requested an honor guard from the organization to attend him at the dedication of a memorial to the Duke of Clarence, who had died of pneumonia after some ill-advised hunting in terrible weather. Making sure that he had the full attention of the press, the prince put his hand on the shoulder of the commanding officer and said, "Gentleman, this is a good uniform. I believe much good will come of it," a bit of royal P.R. that did much to elevate the stock of the ambulance men in the field.[21]

As good work upon good work elevated the program in the general esteem, graduates of the St. John Ambulance spread out across the commonwealth, bringing civilian ambulance services to Australia in 1883; Bermuda, the Bahamas, Bombay, Gibraltar, and Hong Kong a year later; New Zealand in 1885; and even the island of Borneo had its ambulance center in 1887.[22] Bringing the movement full circle, Jerusalem, the original home of the Order of St. John, opened an ambulance center in 1886, with the Jerusalem Ophthalmic Hospital of St. John overseeing medical operations and the Turkish Governor of Jerusalem (political descendant of the Saracens who had evicted the Order from the holy city) standing as the first president.[23] Closer to home, Scotland welcomed the St. Andrew's Ambulance Association in 1882, founded in Glas-

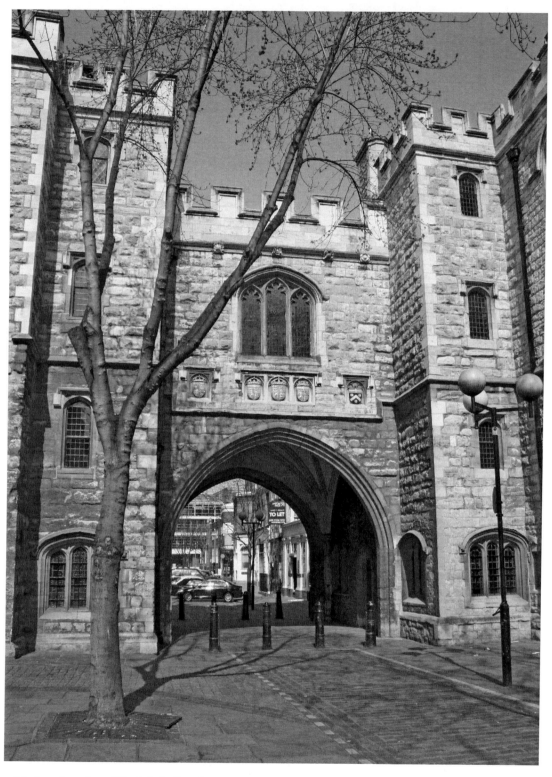

Modern day view of St. John's Gate in London, the historical headquarters of the Order in Britain and still the center for their ambulance activities.

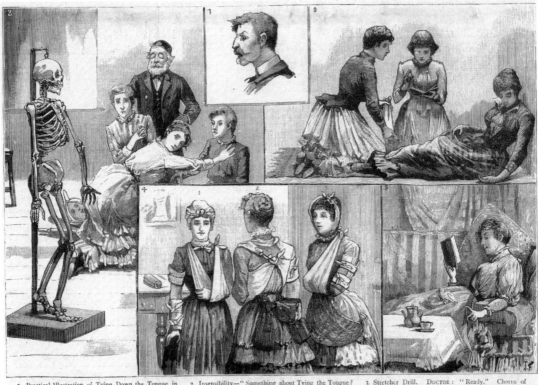

Vignettes from a St. John's Ambulance Society training class for women. In addition to the material covered by male recruits, the women's course included training in setting up a sick-room and preparing meals for invalids (*The Graphic*, October 1, 1887).

gow and following the same lines of its southern cousin.[24] Of course, there were some in the medical profession who saw the ambulance as a threat. In 1882 *The Lancet* noted

> [t]here are not wanting members of the profession who discountenance the whole [ambulance] scheme, as it tends to interfere with practice. This is especially the case in the vicinity of some of the larger works, factories, and ship-building yards, in connexion with which numerous accidents occur every year, entailing the disbursement of considerable sums to medical men for "first-aid." [25]

The fear was not entirely unjustified: the development of ambulance services did deliver more accident cases to the hospitals, in the process facilitating the dramatic transition from home-based care, dominant for centuries, to the current model of inpatient care. As one disgruntled British physician noted, after volunteer ambulance training became commonplace each large training first-aid class in his neighborhood meant another £50 out of his pocket in lost calls.[26]

Overall, such enmity was too diffuse and too unmistakably self-serving to have any chance of swaying either public or political opinion. Accordingly, the order continued to expand its influence in the United Kingdom and the overseas possessions and soon sparked European reforms as well. The first continental offshoot appeared in Germany, after Dr. Johannes Frederich Von Esmarch, an old friend of St. John pioneer John Furley, was so impressed by a Lon-

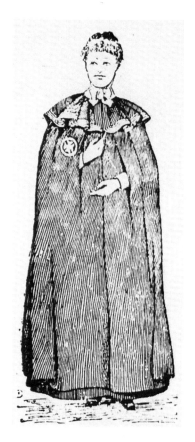
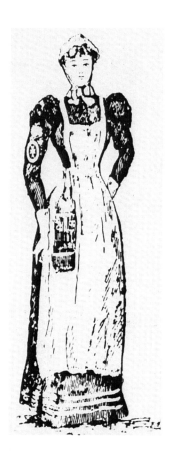
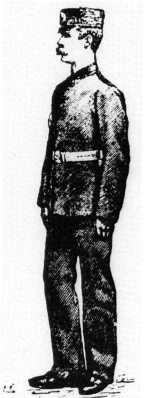

Top and left: Early sketches of the St. John Ambulance field uniform, for men and women (courtesy the Order of St. John, St. John Ambulance).

don demonstration of the chapter's work in 1879 that he returned to Kiel and organized the "German Samaritan Association'" to teach first aid and advocate for municipally funded "accident stations'" across Germany.[27] These *Unfallstationnen*, staffed by full-time physicians and often equipped with horse-drawn ambulances, inspired similar efforts in France and other European nations.

Overall, America was slower swinging aboard the first aid express, although some volunteer societies had been teaching first aid and publishing manuals since at least the Civil War (for example, the First Aid to the Injured Association of New York's eponymous *First Aid to the Injured* in 1882). Clara Barton, who formed the Red Cross in 1881, appears to have been the first to deliver first aid training on a national scale in America. While her interest

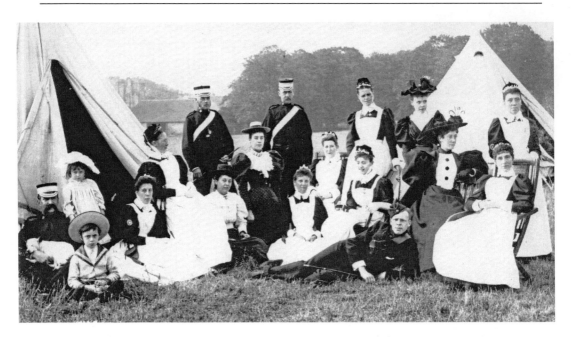

St. John Ambulance crew members relax on an outing, circa 1890 (courtesy the Order of St. John, St. John Ambulance).

in the field started during her tenure as president of the American Red Cross, her forced resignation in 1904 gave her the opportunity to pursue the matter full time, and she immediately organized the National First Aid Association of America, which published manuals, taught classes, and distributed improved first aid kits.[28] The organization was absorbed into the Red Cross around 1909, after which time the Red Cross made medical training one of its core missions: it was in that year the Red Cross started its celebrated public first aid courses, quickly allying itself with the Y.M.C.A. (The Y.M.C.A. had been offering a lecture course called "First Aid to the Wounded" in larger cities since at least 1895, with the series sometimes used to train police ambulance crews: the addition of swimming pools to many Y's in the 1880s also created opportunities for lifeguards to develop practical experience in resuscitation, a skill they brought with them to the joint Red Cross first aid program.[29])

While a smattering of innovative police surgeons had been providing abbreviated first aid courses since the late 1880s, both police and fire departments were quick to pursue first aid training in large numbers when it became available through the Red Cross. By expanding the reserve of people with the training to effectively staff non-hospital ambulances, the first aid movement represented a dramatic stride forward in the evolution of American mobile emergency services. At the same time, American industrial plants and mines were fielding increasingly sophisticated ambulance crews and rescue squads, aided by this relative profusion of new training resources. On both sides of the Atlantic the First World War created a demand for civil defense and emergency preparedness that stimulated a small boom in first aid training, a process repeated on a much larger scale during the Second World War a generation later. By the early 1940s the civilian first aid movement, which had begun as an offshoot of an ancient caste of warrior monks in dusty Palestine, had become an established part of civil life in America as well as the Commonwealth. Nonetheless, even as the Red Cross taught basic first aid to American ambulance attendants and the St. John Ambulance Association evolved into the largest and most respected medical charity under the British flag (ultimately providing provincial and statewide ambulance services in Canada and Australia), it would fall to a later generation to

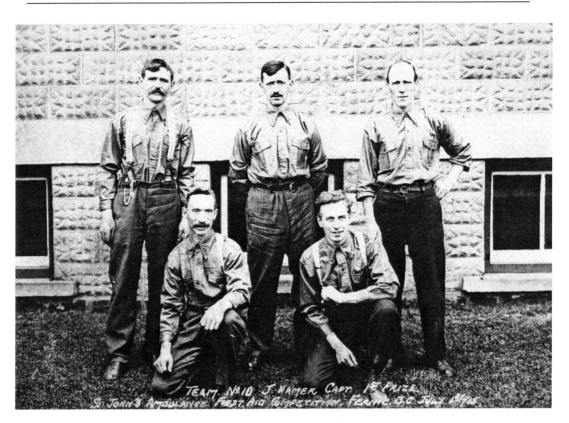

An enduringly popular method to keep St. John Ambulance graduates in trim were the annual competitions between ambulance companies, with the victor usually being given a commemorative cup or plate to hold for the year. In a 1915 competition in Fernie, British Columbia, Team 10 from the Coal Creek Colliery took top honors (J.P. Spaulding, Courtesy Glenbow Archives, NA-3663-21).

imagine transforming the ambulance from a vehicle for improved first aid into an instrument of advanced medical intervention.

Emergency Hospitals

Another aspect of the democratization of the first aid movement was the development and proliferation of the emergency hospital. From the opening of Bellevue's satellite hospital on Centre Street the ambulance was intimately associated with the reception hospital movement when, seeking to reduce the travel time for the seriously injured, municipalities like New York City and Boston erected small but well equipped receiving hospitals adjacent to their industrial districts and naturally included ambulance services in their designs. Especially important in the development of these emergency hospitals were the police departments: as the police were the first responders to most crises it became routine for police surgeons to treat urgent cases brought to the station house by patrol wagon, and while Mayor Wood's scheme to install surgeries at police precincts foundered in the 1850s, the continuing importance of the police ambulance led many departments to open their own small emergency hospitals for the better receipt of such casualties, especially if the community as a whole lacked efficient hospital or private ambulance services, or if the city's own charity hospital was far removed from the population center (such municipal hospitals usually took in the bulk of trauma cases, as

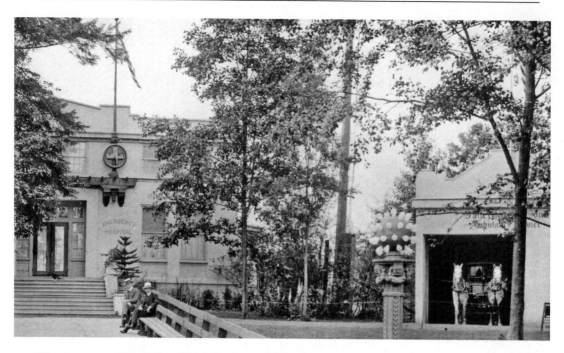

The emergency hospital at Seattle's Yukon-Pacific Exposition in 1908, with the ambulance barn alongside (Frank Nowell, University of Washington Libraries, Special Collections, x2365).

grievous injury was more likely to befall the impoverished wage-slave than his plutocratic employer).

The impetus for such police emergency hospitals was the rapidity with which police surgeons hit the limits of what they could accomplish at the station-house, as well as the growing number of police ambulance services which needed some place to deliver their patients. For example, Portland, Oregon, in 1907 was like many other communities in relying on the police to transfer minor cases to the station house for evaluation by the police surgeon. In April of that year the evening paper carried a story about a young woman who fainted downtown and was brought in by patrol wagon, where, to the disgust of the editors, she became only the latest citizen to be "compelled to lie on a dirty stretcher in the foul-smelling station, exposed to the gaze of the morbidly curious."[30] This sordid event was considered by the paper to be yet another "forcible illustration of the absolute need for an emergency hospital." Nationally, many other municipalities agreed, and the prevalence of police ambulances and their role in emergency services created such pressure for police receiving hospitals that by 1913 a West Coast editorial proclaimed "such institutions [are] one of the most important divisions of the police departments in many ... cities."[31] As things evolved, local influences resulted in the police hospital becoming pre-eminent on the West Coast, while further east satellite receiving stations were more likely to be opened under the auspices of city hospitals, and in England they usually represented the outpouring of private philanthropy, as with the great Poplar Accident Hospital serving the East India Docks from the mid–1800s.

San Francisco's Influential Idea

When Bellevue's Centre Street/Park Hospital opened in 1870 it was the earliest example of an integrated specialty receiving hospital and ambulance operation, but it was a modest con-

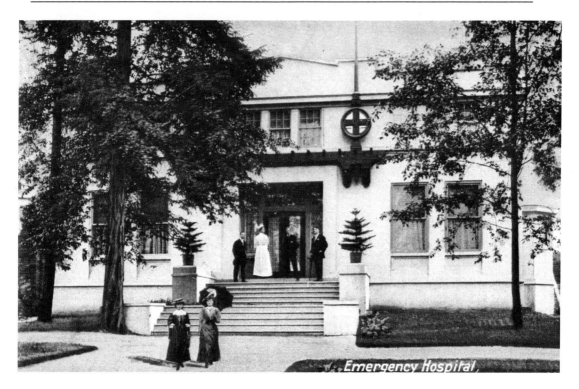

Emergency hospitals like this one at Seattle's Yukon-Pacific Exposition in 1908 inspired new innovations in ambulance dispatch and promoted the expansion of emergency medical services.

tribution and must yield pride of place in scale and influence to the service assembled in San Francisco just a few years later, an entity influencing similar operations from Los Angeles to Portland, Oregon. In the earliest days those seeking emergency medical aid in San Francisco were likely to turn to a pharmacy (some of which were open all night), following a practice common to large cities in the early 19th century. City pharmacists, like the medieval barbers, frequently found themselves doubling as emergency physicians in the absence of anything more formal, and in the Bay City the most famous of these institutions was a drug store known as "The Port of Broken Heads," on the Barbary Coast. It had opened for business sometime before 1875 and was open around the clock, not only to sell to liniment, compound medications, and dispense nerve tonics, but to deliver basic medical care to a steady stream of unfortunates—with the emergency trade being most active from midnight to the hour just before dawn. In 1910 an owner explained how things went, and how they had been going for over thirty-five years at the little shop:

> You find all nationalities around here—Hindus, Filipinos, Syrians—all peoples. Would you expect them to live in harmony—always? Of course they fight; but impromptu fights in general—you can tell by the weapons—a penknife sometimes, or a beer bottle. It is quite remarkable the many different kinds of wounds a beer bottle can make![32]

Night after night they stumbled in or were dragged over the threshold, four or five emergency cases a night: not only assault and accident victims, according to the proprietor, but "they lug the suicide cases in here, too ... somebody gets a bit tired or disgusted and swallows a dose of wood alcohol or an antiseptic tablet—and then rushes in here." The apothecary staff handled what they could, sent the most serious off to the hospital by whatever means was most expedient, then mopped the floor and waited for the next customer. So things went until 1876, when the police opened a single emergency hospital under the direction of a departmental surgeon to handle the "rush"' cases that couldn't wait for the haul up to the municipal infirmary. At first the patrol wagons delivered the casualties, a good number of them collected from the floors of all-night pharmacies like the "Port of Broken Heads," and in time the paddy wagon gave way to a fleet of specially built police ambulances as more hospitals were added to accommodate the growing city. The service stayed with the police department until 1894, when the city decided the enterprise had grown sufficiently large to demand specialty management and transferred the police emergency hospitals and ambulances to the Health Department.[33] The department inherited five hospitals and made sure that each was staffed around the clock by an experienced physician (no interns), a nurse, and an ambulance driver and medical steward who had each been trained in emergency medical care (of the five infirmaries, Mission Emergency Hospital, serving the Barbary Coast and the city's skid row, was the busiest, requiring two full-time ambulances to collect the mangled dregs washed into the gutter from one bucket of blood or another).[34] The ambulances continued to be operated free of charge, including transfer from a receiving hospital to San Francisco General if necessary for treatment: individuals insisting on being transferred to a private hospital were invited to hire their own commercial ambulance for the ride uptown.

After picking up its first auto ambulance in 1913 the service never looked back, and by 1932 its drivers were averaging five calls a day (three out of five as emergency runs, the balance transfers to home or other hospitals); that year its Central, Harbor, Mission, Potrero, Park, Ocean Beach, and Insane Detention Hospitals took in 56,497 admissions, or 1.7 patients per bed, per day.[35] Central Emergency was always a hotbed of activity, and press photographers routinely tailed the ambulances on their calls, hoping to grab a picture that would land above the fold on the evening edition.[36] The excitement kept most ambulance stewards loyal to the work: in 1952 a veteran driver loosened the collar of his navy-blue Eisenhower jacket and confessed to a reporter that the job was "like circus work; it gets in your blood. Here you see life, and sometimes, brother, it's sliced right down the middle."[37] The ambulances served the city through wars, earthquake, fire, and the Great Depression, until their duties were finally assumed by the fire department in 1997.

From the beginning the success of the system did not go unremarked, and in Los Angeles the municipality was operating its own Police Receiving Hospital by the early 1890s.[38] As in San Francisco, police patrol wagons were the earliest ambulances, but by 1906 the department had at least one horse-drawn ambulance, which was soon joined by a 1908 model Studebaker "Electric Patrol Ambulance."[39] These L.A.P.D. ambulances, receiving hospitals, and station houses were intimately associated, often sharing quarters in the same building, and the most famous of the lot was the Georgia Street Receiving Hospital. Built in 1915 as a juvenile detention facility, a police receiving hospital was installed on the third floor in 1927, replacing an earlier infirmary on 1st and Hill.[40] At its peak in the 1930s fifty doctors and fifty nurses handled seven admissions per bed per day, from anonymous drunks pulled from a brawl to celebrities like wrestler Terrible George Zaharias, brought in by a police ambulance after a 1934 drubbing at the ham-sized hands of Man Mountain Dean.[41] While Georgia Street Hospital was introduced to a nationwide audience through radio crime dramas set in Los Angeles (on "Dragnet" Joe Friday was a frequent visitor, calmly collecting victim statements at the bedside), fame couldn't guarantee immortality, and the last ambulance left Georgia Street on July 13, 1957, when services were transferred to the county-run Central Receiving Hospital on West 6th Street.[42] Of course, Georgia Street had just been the largest of the Los Angeles police infirmaries, and in its heyday the L.A.P.D. ran fourteen ambulances to serve its receiving hospitals. By the 1920s each rig was staffed by a police driver along with a doctor or nurse, but in time the work devolved to a non-police driver and an ambulance

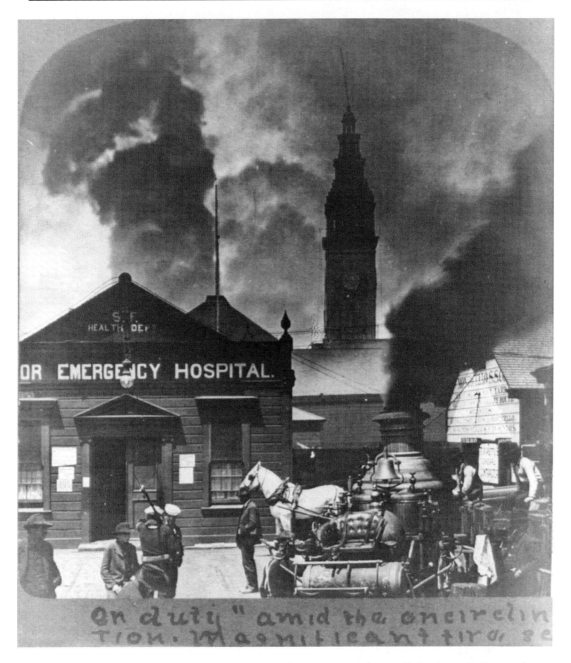

In the wake of the San Francisco 1906 earthquake, flames threaten to engulf the city and a fire truck is seen outside the Harbor Emergency Hospital, operated by the Department of Health and served by its own ambulance service. (C.L. Wasson, "On Duty," July 21, 1906. Library of Congress, Prints & Photographs Division, LC-USZ62-33523.)

attendant, and in the late 1960s the police had been reduced to providing garage space in their precinct stations for ambulances staffed directly by the county.[43] Finally, the fire department took over operation of the ambulance service in 1970, and after eighty years of service the last remnant of the Los Angeles police ambulances and their emergency hospitals went dark forever.

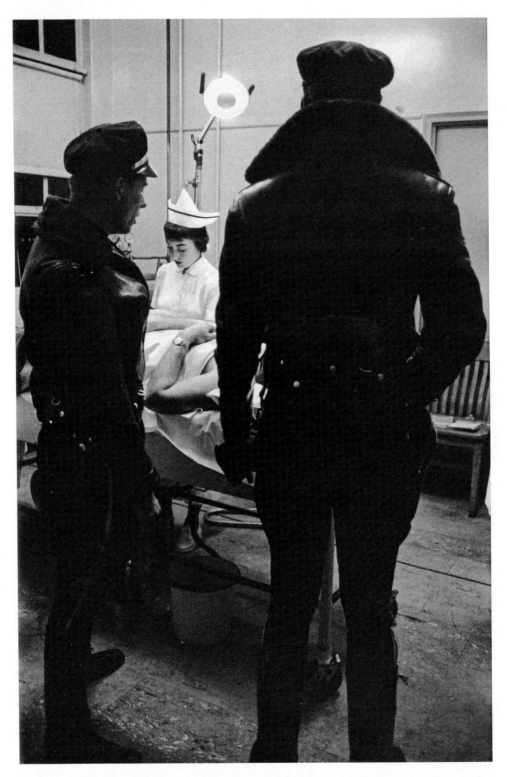

Police officers stand guard at Georgia Street Receiving Hospital in 1956 as a patient is examined by a nurse. Operated by the Los Angeles Police Department, Georgia Street was one of the largest emergency hospitals on the West Coast and was served by a fleet of police ambulances. (Robert Vose, photographer. Library of Congress, Prints & Photographs Division, Look Magazine Photograph Collection, LOOK-Job-56-4133.)

Beyond the Golden Gate: Emergency Hospitals Outside California

While California's Queen Cities represented the apex of ambulance and emergency hospital integration, their influence was felt elsewhere in the West and was reproduced, if faintly, in other regions of the country as well. To the north, Portland long lagged its southern neighbor in civic amenities, a fact not lost on a cantankerous local press that frequently criticized the absence of a receiving hospital system of the kind found in their rival, San Francisco.[44] Instead, the Rose City maintained contracts with two local hospitals to receive accident cases and relied on the patrol wagon to deliver them, on an alternating, "share and share alike"' basis. When, in late 1913, the decision was finally made to open a municipal emergency hospital, the proposal called for its installation on the fourth floor of Police Headquarters, with staffing by three interns working consecutive eight-hour shifts—at forty dollars a month.[45] When told of the proposed salary the City Health Officer told a local paper that he doubted any sane doctor would work for such a pittance, but was pleasantly astounded to find "many young physicians willing to serve" for the meager wage offered.[46] These willing public servants were detailed not to the police department, but to the municipal health bureau, and on February 14, 1914, they took possession of twenty cots, a small pharmacy and laboratory, and a one bed operating theater.[47] The little emergency hospital was listed in the city directory for almost sixty years, only closing in 1973 when it yielded its share of the suddenly stricken to newly consolidated city hospitals with modern emergency rooms and full complements of staff and equipment—emer-

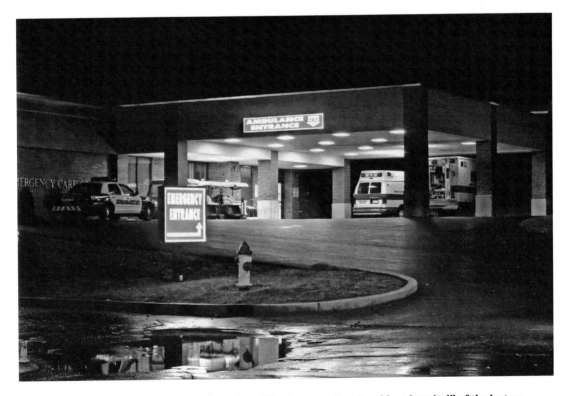

Modern emergency rooms ultimately replaced the free-standing "accident hospital" of the last century, as improved trauma medicine required ever greater investments of capital and staffing (photograph by William Mahar).

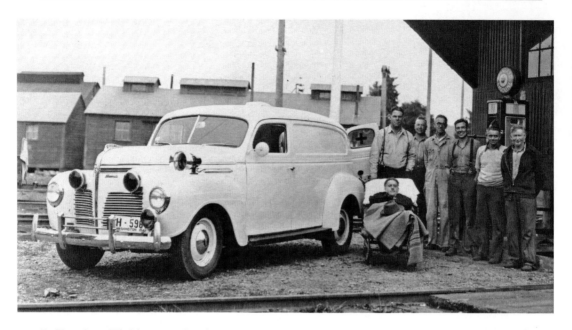

In Hoquiam, Washington, a logging company's volunteer ambulance crew stands next to their Plymouth ambulance in 1943. Many industries supported such on-site emergency squads, equipping them with aid-cars and even providing emergency hospitals (University of Washington, Special Collections, C. Kinsey 2855).

gency rooms that were themselves the spiritual and clinical descendants of those few rooms on the fourth floor of the police headquarters.

If painful comparison with southern rivals goaded Portland into better medicine, proud Boston hadn't bent its stiff neck to look around for some time, a complacency leaving it with woefully inadequate emergency service long after the modern ambulance had its Bellevue premiere. Interestingly, when Boston had built its new city hospital in the deserted South End back in 1864 the city fathers discussed including an ambulance service linking it to the city proper, an innovation that would have put Boston at the forefront of American ambulance development. Nothing came of the brave scheme, however, and it wasn't until 1892 that the scandal of the injured and ill being driven miles in the backs of wagons or hacks en route to the public hospital forced civic leaders to fund a public ambulance service. The eleven horses and twelve men of this ambulance squad were stabled together in a former smallpox hospital on Albany Street downtown, in order to at least halve a long commute that could only be prejudicial to the injured, and surgeons only rode along for serious "crush'" cases (in order to perform immediate amputation if required), while lesser injuries were simply loaded up and carted south to the city hospital.[48] Finally, in 1900 Boston opened a centrally located "City Hospital Relief Station'" in Haymarket Square. Essentially a freestanding emergency hospital, Haymarket Station had its own ambulance squad to handle the steady torrent of casualties from the rapidly growing industrial district surrounding it.[49]

While Boston's experience belatedly recapitulated Manhattan's 1870 construction of Park Hospital to intercept Bellevue-bound cases from south of Houston Street, nationwide a variety of factors were contributing to the expansion of emergency hospital and ambulance operations. The largest industrial plants began building receiving hospitals for injured employees, often with an in-house ambulance service attached: in 1935 the Pullman Emergency Hospital in Illinois had twenty-five beds for its employees, for example, and similar facilities could be found in Pennsylvania steel mills and large northern timber companies.[50] Photos taken of these outfits invariably show the emergency ambulance crews to be made up of regular employees, and here we see the influence of the first aid movement in creating the human capital that encouraged development of these infirmaries. Taken together, by the late 1930s police reception hospitals, municipal emergency infirmaries, and industrial accident stations were supporting a sizable fleet of ambulance services nationwide. During a time when most hospital emergency rooms were staffed by community and hospital physicians on a rotating schedule without regard to their specialty (so a pediatrician might abruptly find themselves confronted in the middle of the night by an elderly patient with a heart attack), emergency hospitals were important community triage centers.[51] Ultimately, the increased professionalism of hospital emergency rooms, along with the newly recognized specialties of trauma surgery and emergency medicine, made the old emergency hospitals redundant. Further undermining their viability were changes in the economics of health care making it harder for minor providers to stay solvent as medical equipment was becoming more advanced and more expensive every year. Still, these hospitals, usually small operators in their own day and forgotten in ours, contributed greatly to the success of the young ambulance movement by ensuring that the patient in the back of a clattering police wagon or a speeding aid car was guaranteed a fighting chance at the end of their ride.

• 9 •

From Horses to Horsepower

The second decade of the 20th century oversaw the ambulance's traverse from the horse-drawn era to the motor age. Though the transition was remarkably brief, the high cost of automobiles as an initial outlay, as well as questions about their maintenance costs, brought the business side of ambulances into sharp relief. For some time the ambulance was caught between two epochs as medicine shifted from a low cost art practiced in charity hospitals and private homes to a high cost economic leviathan built out of profit and loss centers. Additionally, each advance in medical technology required new investments in training and material, and relatively underfunded police departments, city hospitals, and fire departments found themselves struggling to keep pace with developing interventions in mobile medicine.

The era of automobile ambulances started in 1899 with an electric ambulance acquired by the Michael Reese Hospital in Chicago. A year later St. Vincent's Hospital in New York City acquired a nearly identical vehicle resembling a boxy milk-wagon with only a stubby ledge over the driver's bench to protect him from the elements: steering wheels were a bit avant garde in those early days, and like its predecessor in Chicago the steering was done with an "L" shaped lever. (Manhattan's Roosevelt and Presbyterian Hospitals acquired their own electric ambulances in 1902, recreating the first wave of ambulance purchases some thirty years before, when the acquisition of a rig by one institution led competing private hospitals to quickly follow suit.)[1] While the typical horse ambulance might weigh six hundred pounds, this vehicle was a staggering two tons, in good part owing to its reliance on massive lead batteries swimming in acid: the advantage of the extra mass was that it guaranteed a fairly smooth ride despite the absence of pneumatic tires—to hold up its weight it depended on stout wooden wheels upholstered with solid rubber rims measuring three inches thick.[2] Its proud makers, Frederick R. Wood & Son of Bridgeport, Connecticut, were enthusiastic about their contribution to medical science, telling a local paper "An ambulance of this kind possesses many advantages over its horse drawn prototype. A greater speed is attainable; there is more ease and safety for the patient; [and] it may be stopped within its own length when running at full speed."[3] With its four horsepower motor it was capable of up to thirteen miles an hour going forward (and six miles an hour in reverse), but although it was rated for approximately twenty-five miles traveling on a single charge, the time it took to replenish the batteries once that radius had been exhausted was considerable, a defect contributing in large part to St. Vincent's decision to abandon their electric ambulance around 1905.[4]

The United States Army, always a conservative institution, bided its time before gingerly experimenting with automotive ambulances. Their first effort came in 1905 when the medical department deployed a gasoline ambulance with the Camp Roosevelt infirmary in Mount Gretna, Pennsylvania. Built on a truck chassis with wood slat walls covered by folding canvas tarps, it could cart four litter patients on the floor with two more swinging from the ceiling, or a total of fourteen ambulatory patients sitting on its benches.[5] The cost was considerable—$3,600, or

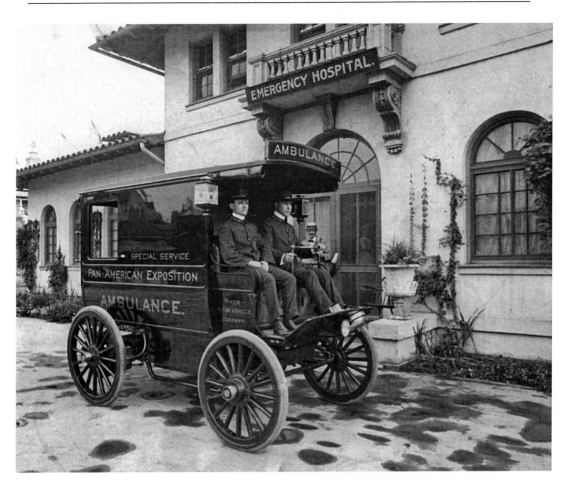

Shot by a would-be assassin, President McKinley rode this electric ambulance to the Pan-American Exposition Emergency Hospital where clumsy probing of his wound led to his fatal sepsis. As emergency medical techniques improved, better ambulance services were required to deliver patients who would be able to benefit from such innovations (courtesy the National Library of Medicine).

over $65,000 in 2006 dollars — but for their money the army got a vehicle that could travel six times as fast (on reasonably level ground, at least) as the standard issue ambulance drawn by four mules.[6] (During one of its "shake down runs" the flying ambulance made such good time blasting through a dusty hamlet outside Harrisburg that its panic stricken town marshal was chased off the street: he immediately laid hands on the nearest telephone and told the next town over to put up a road block for the rogue machine, which was accomplished by having that town's constable stand in the middle of the dirt road flapping a red bandana. The ambulance driver obligingly pulled up short but, being the only one who knew how to drive, he convinced his "patient" to give himself up to the law while he drove back to camp to arrange bail.)[7]

The electric automobile took an early lead in the sales race, but within five years of its debut it was already facing stiff competition from steamers and gasoline ambulances: for example, when Brooklyn Kings County Hospital emptied their stable in 1908 it hedged its automotive bet by taking on two horseless ambulances, one steam powered, the other gasoline fueled, while at the same time an ebullient Commissioner Hebberd, chief of public charities for New York City, prophesied:

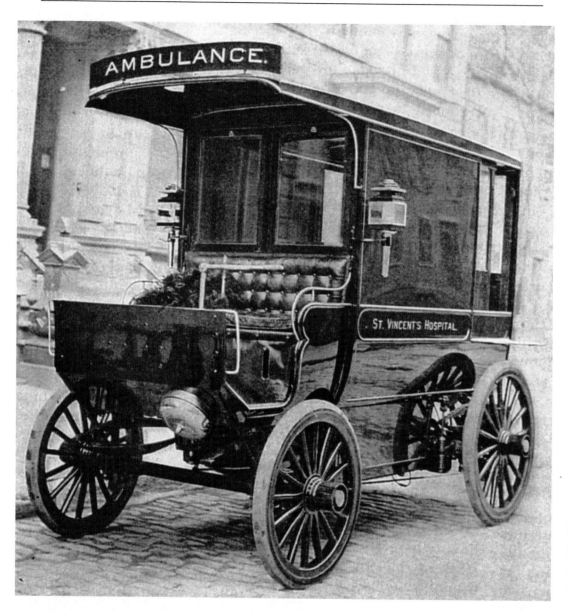

The first automotive ambulance in the United States was an electric vehicle acquired by the Michael Reese hospital in Chicago in 1899. The St. Vincent hospital in New York acquired its model, seen here, a year later (courtesy the National Library of Medicine).

It may confidently be asserted that the power ambulance, because of its marked efficiency and comfort, has come to stay. A very important consideration is the fact that the use of the automobile ambulance in place of the horse ambulance improves the sanitary condition of the hospital by doing away to a great extent with the nuisance of the stable, including the pest of flies ordinarily to be found there.[8]

(While smog and automotive pollution are now justly condemned, during Commissioner Hebberd's era over one hundred thousand horses deposited some 2.4 million pounds of manure *every day* on New York's streets—and flushed the gutters with at least three hundred thousand quarts of urine.[9] Flies proliferated in numbers that, today, would bring comparison to a bibli-

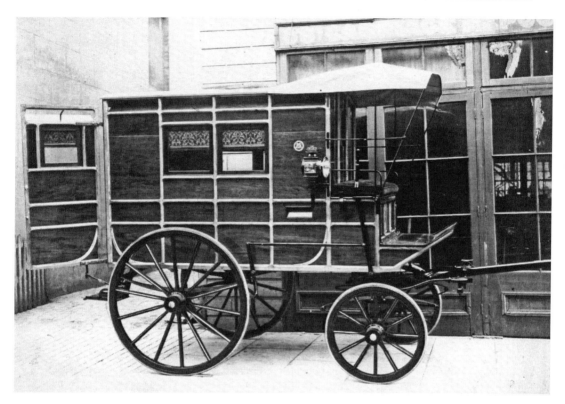

British ambulance wagon, circa 1893 (courtesy Order of St. John, St. John Ambulance Society).

cal plague, and behind that twenty-four pounds of manure per animal per day were multitudes of city granaries, doubling as pasture for rats. All of this meant that hospitals entailed a great deal of extra work in maintaining a sanitary environment while stabling horses on their grounds.)

While the automobile looks inevitable in retrospect, when the first motorcars hit the streets not all commentators agreed with Commissioner Hebberd that they were certain to replace the horse-drawn ambulance. In January 1915 the following confident appraisal regarding the future of the equine ambulance appeared in a national hospital journal:

> [T]he time should never come when the horse will be entirely discarded. This statement may seem strange when the economy and speed of motor equipment are compared with the slower and more expensive horse ambulance, but during last winter's blizzard in New York the horse saved the service. High-powered cars were helpless in the drifts, but horses working in teams pulled through ... and for two days the horse ruled the situation.[10]

The writer was a poor Nostradamus as eleven months later, in December 1915, the last horse ambulances in New York City were retired, the hospitals citing efficiency and economy.[11] The rest of the country was swift to follow, and by 1919 the horse-drawn ambulance was finished.

And That Ain't Hay: Choices and Costs

While the citations above support the view that the auto was cheaper than the horse, early experience frequently pointed otherwise. In fact, although automotive ambulances provided a faster and smoother ride than horse drawn vehicles, their adoption was often delayed by the

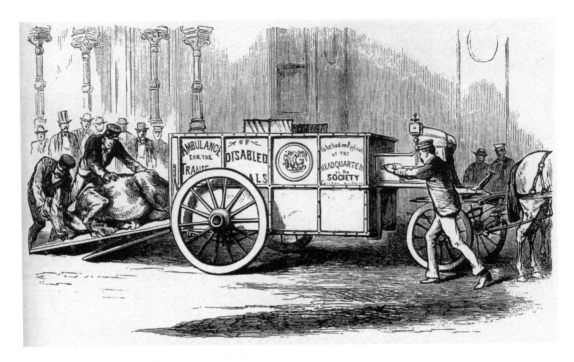

Considering the horse's role in early ambulance services, it only seems fair that the first horse-drawn ambulance in New York City was a service for ... other horses. In 1867 the American Society for the Prevention of Cruelty to Animals introduced the world's first regular horse ambulance service, two years before Bellevue offered a similar benefit to humans.

initial capital expense and fears of high operating costs—although as Margaret Moore, Superintendent of the Jackson City Hospital in Michigan, pointedly noted when discussing the topic, "[t]he primary consideration in hospital service is the saving of life and not of money."[12] Admitting that laudable principal, a hospital that couldn't pay its bills wasn't going to stay in the business of saving life for very long, so hospital boards across America took an active interest in the relative costs of the various automotive ambulance options versus the humble steed.

At the dawn of the automotive age a motor ambulance, be it gas, steam, or electric, was nothing cheap, with a ticket price anywhere from $2,500 to $4,000 versus $1,200 for a quality ambulance carriage and a horse, and the autos were costly to maintain when subjected to hard usage. For example, Manhattan's Polyclinic, serving an upscale clientele north of 42nd Street, treated socialites to an all gasoline-ambulance service starting in 1912. In addition to the $7,950 spent on the three vehicles themselves, there was another $1,000 for liability insurance, an annual repair budget of $2,900, and $900 more for gasoline, oil, and incidentals.[13] By comparison, maintenance for Mt. Sinai Hospital's electric ambulance was $700 a year when nothing broke down and $1,700 when it was overhauled and had the batteries replaced. Meanwhile, a contemporary horse ambulance required a mere $400 a year of upkeep, plus another $100 for the forage and some lesser sum for tack and blacksmithing.[14] Even allowing for the assumption that a motor ambulance could replace two horse ambulances (since cars didn't need to rest after making a long run or a swift "hurry call"), the horse ambulance was still relatively cheaper when simply comparing the price of hay to spark-plugs. The equation soon shifted, however, when the cost of motor ambulances began to tumble: prices for gasoline motors fell first, thanks to Ford's assembly line innovations, and the Model T went from $800 in 1908 to just $440 in 1914. Although the sedan and truck models needed for ambulance work

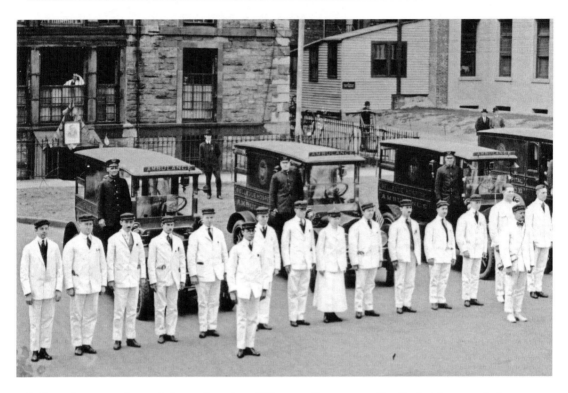

Bellevue's automotive ambulance fleet circa 1918, some three years after the last horse ambulances were retired in New York City (courtesy Ehrman Medical Library, NYU Medical Center).

were more expensive than the Tin Lizzies, mass production would quickly reduce prices for all but the hand-crafted luxury models.

Some idea of what a hospital actually got for its money in these early days of the automotive ambulance comes from the pages of *Carriage Monthly*, a trade magazine whose May 1909 issue introduced readers to the latest offering from James Cunningham, Son & Co., in Rochester, New York. The Cunningham gasoline motor ambulance's three speed gear shift put the driver in charge of a thirty-horsepower engine (for comparison, today you can buy riding lawn mowers with twenty-horsepower). Patients floated above the roadway on an array of springs; a gong beneath the toe-board served as a siren; and the exhaust was piped through the cabin inside heating elements. Four electric dome lights illuminated the linoleum floored patient compartment, with its suspended cot and seating for two attendants, while the rear step and running board were finished off with pyramid-textured rubber to avoid slips. This exemplary ambulance weighed an appreciable 3,434 pounds and sold for $4,000 ($3,200 to dealers).[15]

Hospitals willing to enter the machine age had the option of purchasing a complete ambulance like the Cunningham, or they could buy a chassis and have the body built to spec by a local carriage maker. The latter approach was often significantly cheaper (the army, by 1917, was buying chassis for $360 and contracting the ambulance body at $225, while navy spendthrifts were laying out $2,200 for a stock ambulance, delivered).[16] In a time when carriage makers were still clinging to relevance in their carpentry shops, many hospitals opted to commission custom bodies for their ambulances, often drawing on their practical experience to produce uniquely efficient designs. For example, at the suggestion of their ambulance chauffeur, Thomas McGann, the Massachusetts Homeopathic Hospital commissioned a side-opening ambulance limousine that allowed a pivoting stretcher to be loaded or unloaded at any

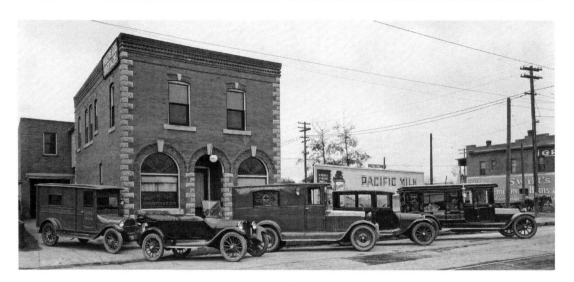

A funeral home in Edmonton, Alberta, shows off its fleet in 1921, including an elaborate hearse and a modern ambulance rig (courtesy Glenbow Archives, ND-3-1104).

convenient angle, avoiding the necessity of having to back straight into the curb or carrying the patient into the street in order to shovel them in over the tailgate.[17] (Incidentally, the same scheme had been used on Larrey's original ambulance carriages.)

Once the decision was made to acquire a motor ambulance, and by the late 'teens they had become de rigueur, the question got back to whether to purchase a steam, an electric, or a gasoline model. Electrics could only maintain a top speed of twenty miles an hour since their massive arrays of batteries almost anchored them in place, while a gasoline auto promised forty or even fifty miles an hour: of course, in a major city, with allowance for traffic, actual travel speeds were usually identical. In rural areas, however, the gasoline auto was at a decided advantage, and even in a city electrics were hampered by their limited range. While accounts of the day allege they could be trusted up to fifty miles over bad roads on a single charge, on a busy day they might need to be decommissioned after several runs for recharging, a threat dissuading some from their purchase.[18] On the other hand, there were unique advantages to an electric ambulance, such as *stealth*, since they were virtually noiseless. While this meant little to patients, it had its benefits for the staff, as described by Dr. Janet Travell who rode the New York Hospital's electric ambulance during her internship;

> Happy [the driver] liked to sneak along the sidewalk silently and then suddenly sound our gong close behind unsuspecting pedestrians. Scarcely believing their eyes, they jumped aside into doorways or into the street—startled marchers, secure, they thought, in the status quo.[19]

Ultimately, electric ambulances were done in by their limited range and comparative expense: because they were never produced in the numbers of the other models they could not capitalize on economies of scale, and the batteries, requiring periodic replacement, were costly. Likewise, steam ambulances, while initially popular, acquired a reputation for unreliability, required time and labor to bring the boiler to full steam prior to starting, and, ultimately, no manufacturer of steamers was ever able to match the volume savings achieved by the makers of the combustion engine models. Nonetheless, throughout the early teens many hospitals relied on a combination of vehicles, as in New York City where several hospitals, up through 1915, used horse and electric rigs for their short trips and sent out a steamer or gasoline ambulance to race around the vastness of the Bronx and the wild and undeveloped expanses of farthest Queens.[20]

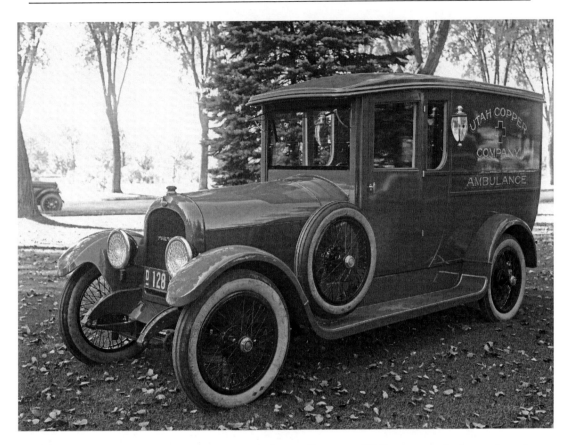

A 1916 Marmon ambulance owned by the Utah Copper Company. While an expensive luxury brand, a Marmon won the first Indianapolis 500 in 1911 and broke the transcontinental speed record in 1916, a desirable reputation for an emergency response vehicle (William Shipler, Photographer; used by permission, Utah State Historical Society, all rights reserved).

By 1917 gas powered ambulances were, even by the standards of the day, inexpensive to run. With standard models averaging 20 miles to the gallon, federal accountants estimated the gas and oil cost of a typical army ambulance ran a mere 2 cents a mile, a figure presumably comparable to civilian costs.[21] It was no surprise, then, that electric and steam ambulances had become anachronisms by 1920. Still, even when gasoline autos had cinched the market, there was the question of style and make. In accordance with human nature, experts on automobile ambulances made themselves easy to find as soon as the market took shape. One of the earliest guidelines was "Hints About Buying Motor Ambulances," published in *The Modern Hospital* in 1916. With keen insight into the spirit of charity, the author warned:

> There is a tendency just now for hospitals to change from horse-drawn to motor-driven ambulances.... It usually happens that some member of the board has a very good touring car or limousine that he would like to exchange for a new one ... and he immediately considers how he can save the hospital some money and at the same time make a sale of the automobile.[22]

The author notes that most such "pleasure vehicles" are poorly suited to the demands of ambulance service since the axle of a typical saloon car was only three or four feet to the rear of the driver, putting it squarely under the vertebrae of a recumbent patient and ensuring every jolt and shock would be immediately and painfully felt by the invalid. Instead, hospitals were encouraged to invest in a three-quarter-ton truck chassis riding on plump, pneuma-

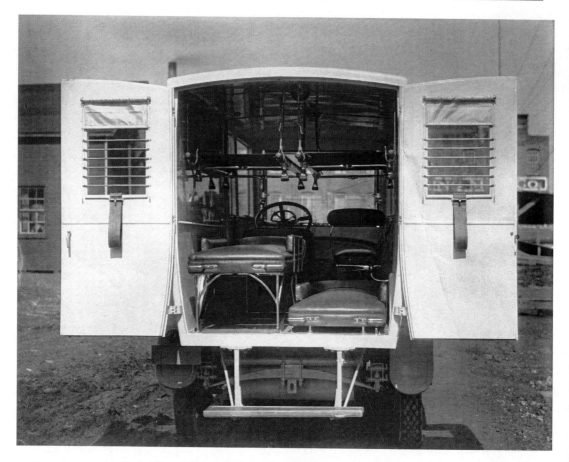

Interior view of the Steptoe (Nevada) Valley Hospital ambulance, in 1918. Its ceiling stretchers gave it a four patient capacity, a patient load that would have been nearly impossible for the common single horse ambulance of only a few years earlier (William Shipler, Photographer; used by permission, Utah State Historical Society, all rights reserved).

tic tires, with at least six and a half feet between the rear axle and the driving compartment. (Not all hospitals were quick to follow this excellent advice. As late as 1951 the average Manhattan ambulance was built on a traditional sedan chassis and needed its front end replaced every six months. In May of that year some New York City hospitals finally got around to unveiling new truck chassis ambulances — riding on airplane shock absorbers, since struts that could cushion a Pan-Am Stratocaster at least had a chance against New York City potholes).[23]

Private Ambulances Come of Age

While mortuaries had provided ambulance service from the backs of their funeral coaches since the Grant administration, freestanding commercial ambulance services awaited the introduction of the automobile ambulance. In large part this depended on simple economics, as after the sticker price of automobiles dropped below the four-digit mark it was considerably easier to make a profit with a motor ambulance than it had ever been with a horse-drawn one. After all, animals required feeding whether there was work or not, in addition to taking consider-

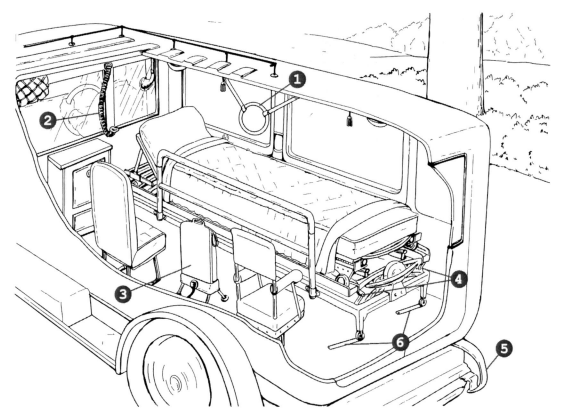

This 1929 Daimler ambulance was considered the acme of luxury, down to its horse-hair and wool stuffed mattress. Other features included: 1) handhold; 2) speaking tube; 3) heater; 4) cot adjustment; 5) grip; 6) caster tracks (Ann-Cathrine Loo).

able attention during the day, while automotive ambulances could be parked and forgotten between jobs, freeing the entrepreneur to pursue other work. In fact, if *any* freestanding horse and wagon ambulance firms existed it would be difficult to prove from the record, versus the steadily expanding roster of such concerns in the automotive age, such that by the 1930s private automotive ambulance services were common in virtually every moderate and large city in the country. In communities where hospitals had previously dominated the market the new private services often bridged the transition by requesting interns to ride along on complicated cases. For example, when the city of Seattle contracted with Shephard Ambulance Service in 1925 to provide local emergency services the municipality agreed to loan out interns from the City Hospital downtown, just as it had been doing for the preceding police ambulance since 1909.[24] While many saw the loss of hospital ambulances as guaranteeing a decrease in the quality of medical attention, particularly in the majority of communities where no regulations governed attendant training or equipage, in some instances the hidden hand of the market stirred up competition enough to inspire a breakthrough in services as a means of increasing market share. For example, Scully-Walton Ambulance, a private firm in the crowded New York City market, joined forces with Colonial Air in 1929 to create America's first civilian air-ambulance service.[25] Another notable innovator was the Buck Ambulance Company, of Portland, Oregon, which in 1942 became the first large scale ambulance operation to provide oxygen in all vehicles (an innovation driven by the high number of men succumbing to fumes while working at the city's shipyards).[26] That decision, while common sense today, was a decade ahead of leg-

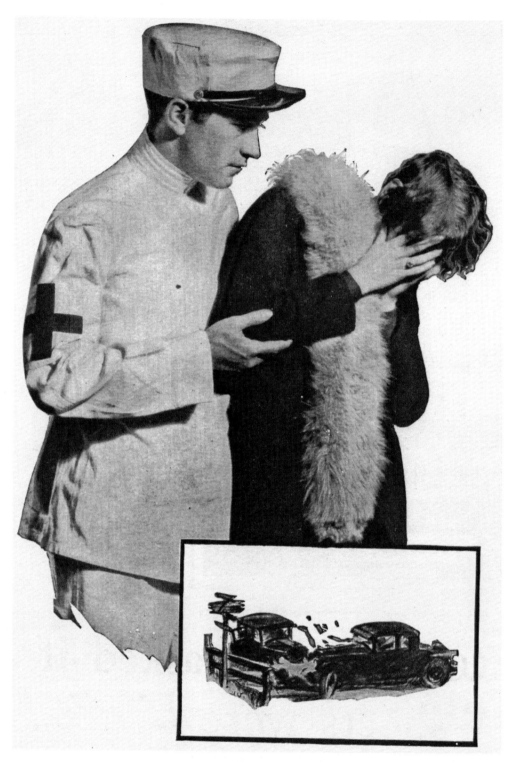

In 1936 one of America's most prominent neurosurgeons advocated that all filling stations be equipped with first-aid materials, in recognition of their natural proximity to the 1,285,000 individuals injured in roadway accidents that year. A similar logic, along with the potential for profits, soon inspired many service stations to add ambulance services to their repertoire ("First Aid," *Time*, November 9, 1936, www.time.com [accessed February 2006]; H. Kauffman and J. Goodrich, "Byron Stookey," *Neurosurgery* 40, no. 2 [February 1997], 383–87).

islation anywhere in the country requiring this fundamental equipment and put competitive pressure on rivals to meet the new standard.

Just as mortuaries had sought to recoup their investment in a hearse by using it for ambulance calls (perhaps later buying a separate vehicle with less ominous overtones for their ambulance work), other businesses began to examine if *their* inventory didn't lend itself to such dual use. Thus, in addition to new, proprietary ambulance services, by the 1920s medical gas providers frequently provided ambulance service as well, realizing that, with the moderate investment of a new car, they could provide a fee paying service using up their surplus oxygen tanks. A more ominous trend, from the hospital's standpoint, began when limousine companies started offering their cars for the use of lucrative "transfer" cases, taking convalescent patients home from the hospital or transferring the frail but not urgently ill in for a scheduled admission. Formerly such jobs, which required payment in advance, helped subsidize the poorly reimbursed emergency calls made by hospital ambulances, and the loss of business was keenly felt by administrators. On the other side, all a private service needed to commence operations was a comfortable car and an advertisement, since private nurses could be hired as needed and billed to the patient, sharply reducing overhead. Such glorified limousines satisfied a demand in the time when car ownership was rarer than it is today, but they also deprived hospital ambulances of easy revenue. Whether it was a saloon car ferrying invalids, a medical gas company offering oxygen-supported transport, or a new private ambulance company advertising everything from emergency service to a ride home after a stay in the maternity ward, the automobile, by lowering the threshold cost of the trade, was opening the ambulance business to new generations of entrepreneurs destined to inherit the office of emergency services in the decades to come.

One of the most significant of these automotive ambulance pioneers was Mary Storer Crane, ambulance entrepreneur, astute businesswoman, and a practical mechanic of no mean ability. In 1897 she and her husband co-founded the Crane Oxygen and Ambulance Company (one of the earliest ventures in that once common combination of medical enterprises), and in 1901 she filed for a patent on an improved ambulance horse carriage. After her husband's untimely death she remarried, and in 1909 it was as Mrs. Mary Heydecker that she applied for the first American patent on an automotive ambulance (while self-propelled ambulances had first appeared in 1899, they had been non-patented superstructures placed on proprietary machines). Mr. Heydecker came and went, but the Crane Oxygen and Ambulance Company and her patented ambulance carried on. It was in 1951 that a supposedly retired Mary Crane went into the office to do some work and succumbed to a massive heart-attack at the age of 73.[27] Her contributions to the ambulance field would be remarkable regardless of her gender, but the difficulties she overcame in an era when women of her brio and ability were seldom welcomed made her work especially noteworthy.

Dobbin's Last Run

Marvelous as all these automotive developments were, something was lost when the last harness was hung on an ambulance barn wall and a sputtering auto backed in as a horse was led out. Therefore it is fitting that we close this survey of the auto ambulance by giving the final word to the one who made the first ambulances possible — the noble steed.

Old Dobbin was an ambulance horse in Rochester, New York, and was said to have pulled the city's first hospital ambulance, back in 1895. By 1904, he had been put to pasture — a pasture standing alongside the City Hospital, and a reporter observed that "[e]ver since Dobbin was retired from daily service he has been eager to answer 'calls.' He knows the sound of the bell for the ambulance as well as do any of the doctors. If he hears it ring when he is in the lot he almost leaps the fence."[28] One hot summer's day Dobbin got his wish, when the entire stable of the City Hospital was out on calls and the alarm bell echoed in an empty barn. The word came down that an ambulance was needed, urgently needed, several miles away at Rigney's Bluff, overlooking Lake Ontario, and as a local paper put it:

> The horse that ran for the first time not less than twenty years ago was hitched to the oldest ambulance on the premises, the only one to be had. In thirty-two minutes he made the run to Charlotte. Several other ambulances were called at the same time, but Dobbin beat them all. The driver said he did not urge him once, for, said he: "Dobbin knows a hurry call as well as any man."[29]

Let Old Dobbin's heroic race, then, close that chapter in the history of the automotive ambulance.

Mercy Flights

While the internal combustion engine wrote ambulance horses out of history, it created entirely novel avenues for patient transport by opening the skies, and the ambulance was swift to take wing. Or at least swift to *try*. In 1910, seven years after Kitty Hawk, Capt. George Grosman of the Medical Corps and Lt. A.L. Rhoades of the Coastal Artillery attempted to convince the War Department to fund an experimental aeroambulance, but the top brass declined the opportunity.[30] It wasn't until 1913 that *The Modern Hospital* could announce success, when a small piece under the headline "An Aerial Ambulance" noted that a biplane "emergency ambulance" had recently taken flight in Aldershot, England. At this early date flying still struck many as a dubious, not to say foolhardy, activity, probably explaining why the editors concluded their brief sketch by noting, primly, "[e]ven so thoroughly a conservative a journal as the Hospital makes the

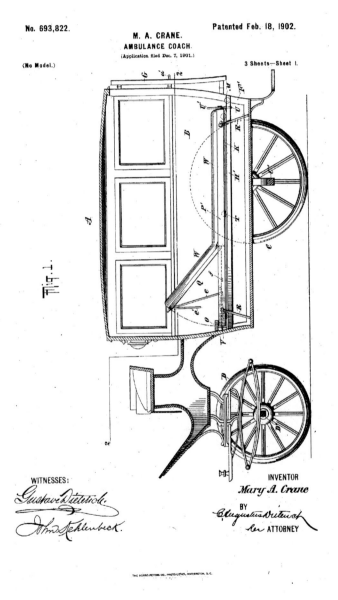

Mary Crane was the first woman to receive a patent for an ambulance design (a modified carriage), and the first American to patent an automotive ambulance (United States Patent Office, 693,822).

announcement as merely a chronicle of the day."[31] While the notice described how the float plane had been carefully kitted out with a folding operating table, anesthetics, instruments and dressings, it made no mention of the passenger compartment—because there wasn't one. Instead, the designer, an expatriate American named Samuel Francis Cody, simply tied a volunteer to a stretcher before lashing him onto the lower wing of the enormous craft. Unfortunately, the stretcher worked itself loose in mid-flight and began slipping inexorably towards the gigantic, rear-mounted propeller. Luckily, Cody was able to maneuver a landing before the advance of the aero-ambulance was interrupted by having its first patient "serialized."[32]

The jinxed plane seemed determined to claim a victim, however, and three weeks later it fell to pieces in mid-flight, sending Cody to his death—but others carried on his experiments and learned from his mistakes. During the Great War the Serbians were likely the first to use airplanes to evacuate the wounded, piling a number of casualties into unmodified aircraft during a retreat in 1915 and flying them eighty kilometers to safety.[33] In 1917 the French assembled an aerial ambu-

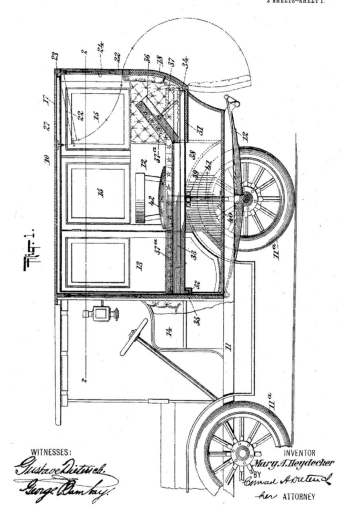

Mary Crane's patent for an automotive ambulance (United States Patent Office, 980,780).

lance capable of transporting two recumbent patients, and by 1918 they could claim a model fully equipped with a compact stove, x-ray equipment, surgical kit, and a small tent: nonetheless, no firm evidence has surfaced of this, or any other, specialty aeronautic ambulance being deployed in combat during the war.[34]

While the aero-ambulance may have been missing in action over the Western Front, it made its debut in the United States in February 1918, when the pilots and mechanics at Gernster Field in Louisiana sent aloft a JN4 modified to carry an invalid in a special seating compartment behind the cockpit. The unusual topography surrounding the airfield was the motivating force behind the innovation, since frequent crashes left wounded flyers stranded in nearly inaccessible swamps around the aerodrome, hours or even days from conventional rescue. After a few months of active service, the Jenny was further modified to permit a patient to lie flat during

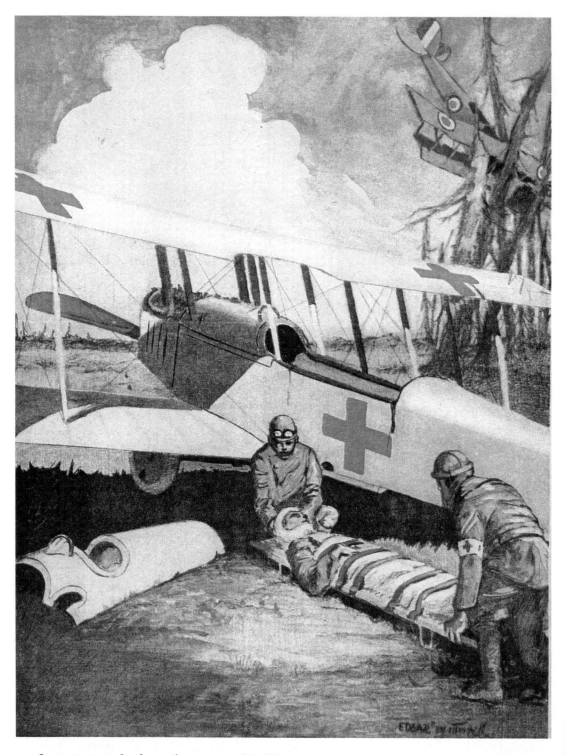

In contrast to the dramatic scene on this 1918 magazine cover, purpose built aero-ambulances were not deployed in combat during World War I, although when this magazine was going to press they had already made their appearance on army airbases in the United States (*Scientific American*, 1918).

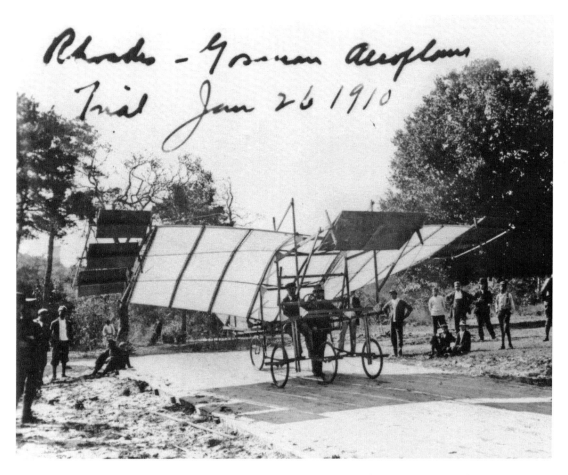

After Captain Grosman and A.L. Rhoades built this airplane in 1910 they unsuccessfully lobbied the Army to fund an experimental aero-ambulance. It would be eight years before the United States military adopted their idea and launched its first ambulance aircraft (Col. Albert Truby, "History of the Airplane Ambulance," courtesy the National Library of Medicine).

transport, a signal improvement in design that became the standard model for such craft through the early part of World War II. The successful experiment at Gernster Field eventually caught the attention of the director of the Army Air Service and by 1919 all military airfields were under orders to provide their own aero-ambulances, with enterprising mechanics around the country knocking together a variety of models in the absence of any mandated pattern.[35]

Ultimately, the military specialty flying ambulance didn't make its combat debut until 1920, during the United Kingdom's struggle to hold Somaliland against the patriotic forces of Sayyid Muhammed Abdile Hasan. In that fierce campaign modified DH-9 DeHavilland biplanes carried British wounded in a coffin-like fuselage compartment behind the cockpit.[36] Civilian air ambulances were swift to follow, and one of the earliest was a custom JN4 modified for ambulance use by two young ex-servicemen living in the Oklahoma oil-patch town of Ardmore, a country where industrial accidents were plentiful, distances vast, and hospitals sparse among the derricks and the dusty plains.[37] Operational sometime prior to 1922, the plane carried patients in a canopied compartment built into the fuselage behind the observer's seat, just aft of the open cockpit, and could make eighty miles an hour with its huge Liberty motor. Following this successful demonstration others were quick to deploy their own flying ambulances, and in 1923

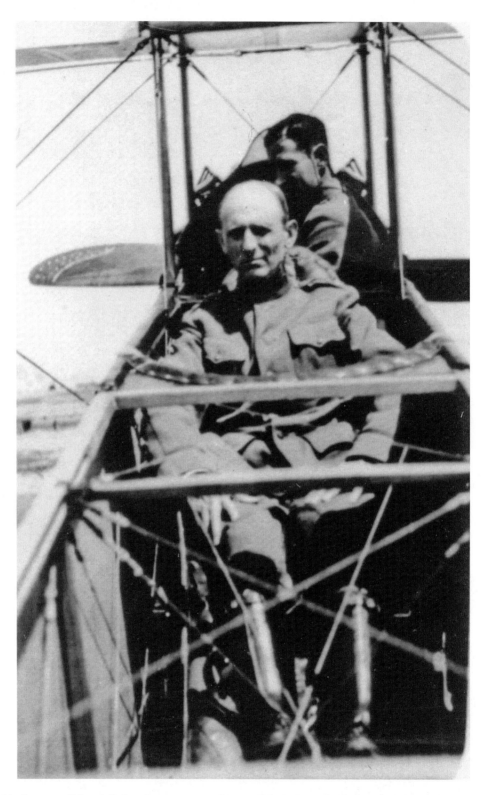

Air Surgeon Colonel Ocker demonstrates the somewhat uncomfortable ride offered by America's first ambulance aircraft, a converted JN4 deployed at Gernster Field, Lake Charles, Louisiana in February 1918 (Col. Albert Truby, "History of the Airplane Ambulance," courtesy the National Library of Medicine).

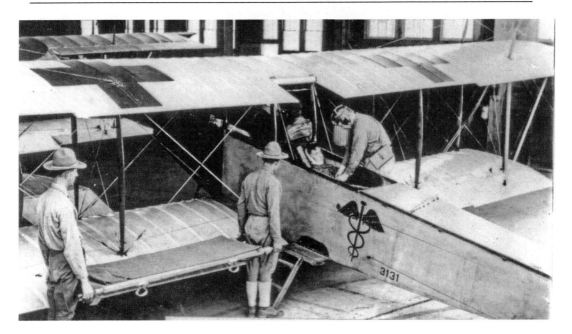

Within a month of its debut the Gernster Field aero-ambulance had been modified to permit recumbent travel for the patient (Col. Albert Truby, "History of the Airplane Ambulance," courtesy the National Library of Medicine).

The Modern Hospital revisited the topic of aero-evacuation with considerably more enthusiasm than they had a decade before. Quoting a breezy article in *The Survey*, it proclaimed: "Galloping hoofs no longer herald the ambulance bound on its errand of mercy. The modern Mercury may arrive even without the clanging of bells, amid the b-r-rrr of an airplane engine."[38]

Of all the early air ambulance services, the most successful is also the longest lived: Australia's Royal Flying Doctor Service, delivering medical services across the Outback since 1928. The service began with the work of the Reverend John Flynn, the director of the Presbyterian Church's Australian Inland Mission, which was involved with establishing clinics and hospitals in Australia's countryside shortly after the turn of the century. Since many settlers were scattered in remote hamlets too small to support even a modest aid station, simply building hospitals wasn't going to suffice to meet the medical needs of those in the most remote locations. In 1917 Flynn received a letter written by a young flier who was sailing on a troop ship to the Western Front. Lt. Clifford Peel suggested that the missionaries put their energies into organizing an air service that could deliver medical aid to wherever required, and set out his ideas on how planes could be converted for air ambulance use and the sort of support network required based on the range and speed of the available aircraft—in all, a well designed scheme that instantly recommended itself to the enterprising Flynn.[39] (Unfortunately Lt. Peel would not live to see his idea made real—he died when his plane was knocked out of the air over the German lines in 1918.)

What followed were ten years of fund raisers, public speeches, and recruitment drives as Flynn attempted to raise support for his "Aerial Medical Service." Finally, in 1928 he had put together sufficient resources to rent a DeHavilland DH-50 at two shillings per mile flown (approximately six U.S. dollars in today's currency), and after the first flight on May 17th the service flew a total of fifty sorties—and covered twenty-thousand miles.[40] When summoned by radio, the service would fly a physician out to render on-site care, and if necessary would fly patients to the nearest hospital in a cot located in the fuselage behind the

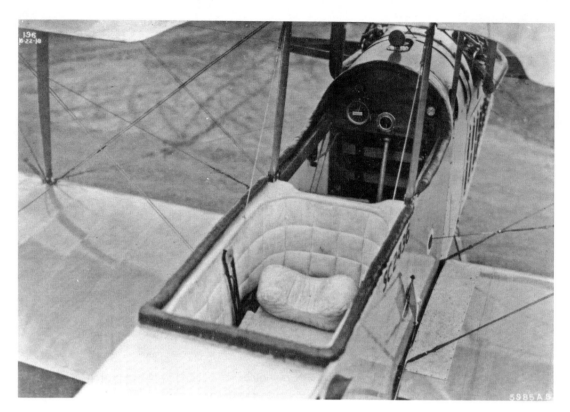
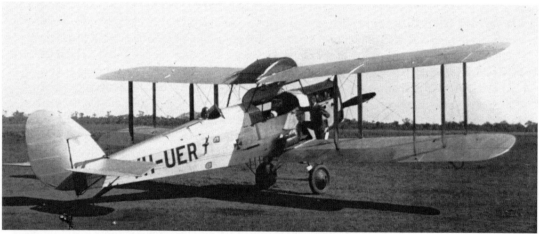

Top: After the success of the aero-ambulance at Gernster Field, the Army ordered all of its aerodromes to provide similar craft. With no mandatory pattern to follow and no commercially available airplane ambulances to purchase, individual mechanics were free to improvise their own versions (Col. Albert Truby, "History of the Airplane Ambulance," courtesy the National Library of Medicine). *Bottom:* The Flying Doctor Service used this De Havilland DH50, named "Victory," from 1928 through 1934. During its years as an air ambulance it flew 110,000 miles, carrying patients in a small cabin in front of the cockpit (courtesy the National Library of Australia, PIC 850-233b).

cockpit. In addition the AMS flew a regular circuit to visit remote areas without resident physicians and provided radio consultations in less urgent cases, or when requested by a local doctor.

While originally staged from a single center at Cloncurry, Queensland, by the early 1930s there was considerable interest in spreading the service across the continent, and despite the

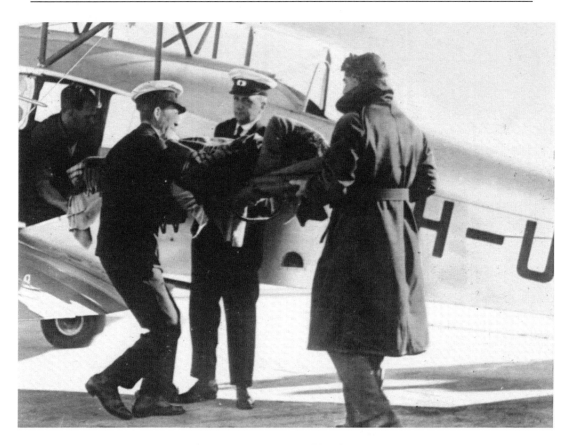

A patient is loaded aboard the "Victory" in the early 1930s for transportation to a hospital. During the 1930s the Australian Flying Doctor Service steadily expanded its aerial fleet as demand for its services increased (courtesy the National Library of Australia, PIC 244-51277).

crippling economic depression the service was duly expanded through a combination of government support and public contributions. In 1942 its name was changed to the Flying Doctor Service, and in 1955 it was granted the honorific of "Royal." A popular innovation of the service was the distribution of standardized medical chests to remote stations, boxes containing numbered bottles of medication and equipment. In this way a physician could diagnose a complaint over the radio and instruct the patient to be given so much from bottle number six, for example. A popular legend tells of a station manager instructed to give his wife a "number nine tablet." When the doctor radioed in later to see how the patient was progressing, her husband told him "We'd run out of number nines, but I gave her one five and one four and she came good right away!"[41] While this anecdote may be historically suspect, the success of the Royal Flying Doctor Service of Australia is not. It is not only the oldest continually operating air ambulance service in the world, it continues to be one of the most successful, averaging ninety-six patient transports a day in 2007, and serving almost a quarter million patients annually.[42]

From beginnings that ranged from the merely humble (pestilent Louisiana bayous where wayward aviators were wont to crash land) to the inarguably inauspicious (the untimely death of air ambulance pioneers in mid-air crack-ups), the marriage of wings to mercy was ultimately consummated in the years immediately following World War I, when a jerry-rigged surplus war-bird flew over the Oklahoma scrub and a network of radio relays across the Australian

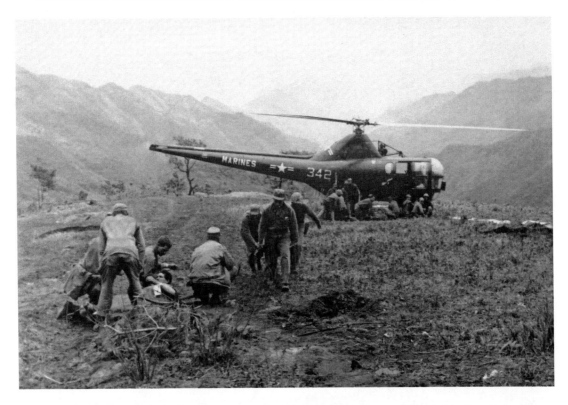

Navy corpsmen prepare wounded Marines for helicopter evacuation on Kari San Mountain, May 1951. The Korean War was the first conflict to rely on helicopter medical evacuation, setting the stage for a revolution in aerial ambulance services (N.H. McMasters, United States Army Archive).

outback summoned a patient-ready DeHavilland DH-50 to the remotest cattle station, each one signaling a new epoch for the air ambulance.

Rotor Rescues

Important as the fixed wing aircraft were to the development of the air-ambulance service, the most successful and versatile aircraft ambulance was ultimately the helicopter. While Leonardo da Vinci famously sketched a design for an "air screw" in the 15th century, practical helicopters didn't appear until Soviet pilots unveiled the first rotary-winged aircraft capable of controlled flight in the 1930s. A decade later an inspired decision by Bell Aircraft Corporation in Buffalo, New York literally launched the helicopter ambulance at a time when their bulbous appearance and hovering locomotion were a novelty.[43] The first use of a helicopter to effect a medical evacuation had occurred in 1945 when a Sikorsky R-4 was sent to airlift a wounded American pilot from his crash site in the Burmese jungle, and it was just a few months later that Bell Aircraft put its machines on 24-hour standby for emergency calls in the Niagara region of upstate New York, a largely rural area whose few municipalities were strangled by inadequate roadways frequently buried under snowdrifts that could top ten feet during a severe storm. Even under the best conditions ambulances often had to travel long miles to reach injured hunters or campers. Bell's helicopters, nicknamed "egg beaters," traveled faster than any ambulance and delivered medical care places no vehicle could even approach. Most often the mercy-flights involved airlifting in a physician to stabilize the patient on the scene while the tardy ambulance chugged along behind, but occasionally a patient made what one commentator called a "Buck Rogerish" ride to the hospital when speed was essential or the locale was inaccessible by road, as with water rescues of stranded boaters or evacuations from remote camping sites.[44] A year later, in 1946, the United-Rexall Drug Company installed a helipad on the rooftop of their Los Angeles headquarters, for the use of a new Bell 47 helicopter "mercy ship" outfitted with first-aid and rescue equipment, including a plastic version of the iron lung for transporting polio patients.[45] Rexall's acquisition marked the first civilian sale of a heli-ambulance, inaugurating what would become a critical addition to the ambulance armamentarium.

While the Rexall airship appears to have ultimately been more useful as a publicity device than a working ambulance and the Bell helicopter service was largely ad hoc, a critical turning point came in October 1954, when Kenmore Hospital in Buffalo opened a twenty-foot square heliport for emergency business.[46] Located just outside the ambulance entrance to the hospital, the landing spot was painted green and sported a bull's-eye for the benefit of the flight crew when swooping in for a landing. A burly war ace and ex-test pilot named Bill Gallagher

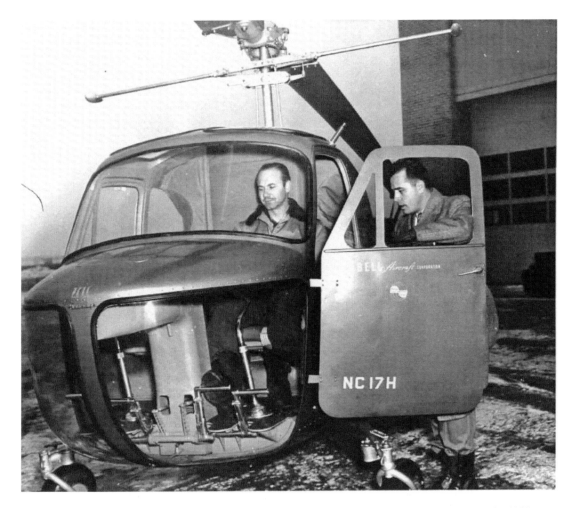

Albert Luke sits at the controls of a Bell 47-B helicopter, the model sold to Rexall Drug in 1945, when it was the first civilian operated "mercy ship."

took the controls of the first machine, specially equipped with two heated litter compartments arranged "pontoon" style above the landing struts. Swearing that "If I can see, I can fly these things," Gallagher proved that sometimes seeing was superfluous, flying in zero visibility conditions by hovering a few feet off the ground and drifting slowly forward while the prop pushed aside another few feet of swirling murk.[47] Notably, while Buffalo had pioneered the general use of helicopters for rescue in the 1940s, the first civilian hospital heli-ambulance actually belonged to the Santa Monica Hospital, whose rooftop helipad saw its first action in September 1954, a mere month ahead of Kenmore.[48] In both cases the civilian operations owed much to the use of helicopters to evacuate the wounded during the Korean War, when upwards of twenty-five thousand casualties were airlifted to safety using the unmatched speed and versatility of the rotary-winged aircraft.

Scaling Up

By the mid–1960s the track record of the original scattered helicopter services combined with public exposure to the aircraft's use in the Vietnam War to inspire a dramatic increase in their emergency medical use. In 1965 the Chicago Fire Department inaugurated what might be the nation's first municipal helicopter ambulance service, at the instigation of Fire Commissioner Quinn, both a dedicated reformer and a licensed pilot.[49] At first the Fire Department leased a Bell 47-G from Chicago Helicopter Airways, with special modifications for its intended role as air ambulance and rescue vehicle. It was fitted with pontoons for use on Lake Michigan, where boating accidents were relatively common, and carried steel and canvas litters that could be covered over and lashed to the pontoons for patient transport (while efficient this mode of travel must also have been deafeningly loud, with the canvas shroud snapping in the wind and the roar of the rotors overhead). The 47-G didn't provide much space in the cabin, so sacks hanging off the side were stuffed with a first aid kit, various resuscitation devices, and a six-man life raft that could be cut loose and dropped into the water.[50] In addition to water rescues the helicopter was also dispatched to pick up critically injured victims of highway accidents who, after receiving first aid at the scene, were airlifted to area hospitals.

After a year of trials, Fire Commissioner Quinn was sufficiently impressed to seek authorization for the purchase of a Bell 47-G4 in 1966, formally committing the department to the new service. The addition was kept tolerably busy in its first year, responding to two hundred thirty nine boating accidents, eighty expressway accidents and an equal number of operations that have only come down as "miscellaneous."[51] In 1968 the small Bell helicopter was replaced by a larger Jet Ranger capable of transporting several litter patients inside the cabin, which must have not only made for a more pleasant trip but permitted crews to deliver medial care en route: as one Chicago flight paramedic said at the time "Helicopters are the emergency unit of the future."[52]

Other states began to catch on as well, with Pennsylvania's State Police launching a one year feasibility study in November 1967, using a Bell J-2A modified for in-cabin stretcher transportation: it responded to one hundred twenty-eight traffic accidents in its twelve months of operation, transporting thirty eight patients, plus two non-traffic accident cases.[53] While finding that helicopter use decreased travel time by at least 50 percent and sometimes by as much as 84 percent, the program encountered resistance from some of the ninety-four "ambulance clubs" operating in its area, who felt the aircraft would compete with their own efforts and was, due to the limitations of cabin space, ill-equipped to render aid en route.[54] The initial reviewers of the program admitted that it was not clear from the data collected whether the most seriously ill patients wouldn't be better served by stabilization at the scene and a slower trip to the hospital with more intensive supportive therapy en route—while being airlifted, the necessity of seat belts and the cramped confines made CPR, starting an IV, or even clearing an airway difficult to accomplish successfully. Still, the potential for effective use—perhaps with specially designed aircraft equipment and more commodious cabins—was evident to the researchers, and the use of the helicopter for other police work such as search and rescue, traffic, and major crime scenes was rapidly discovered (for example, in addition to the one hundred forty-odd medical cases handled, the helicopter was also dispatched to fifty-five criminal cases, frequently bank robberies, where it was useful in tracking get-away cars and fugitives).[55]

The Department of Transportation continued to fund local uses of helicopter ambulances throughout the sixties, with increasing success as the earlier results were combed for clues to guide improvement. By the time Arizona's Highway Patrol began a DOT funded program in May 1969, there was a considerably deeper bench of knowledge to draw from since the day just four years earlier when the Chicago Fire Department began tying stretchers to the pontoons of a stubby Bell 48. The Arizona program started with eighteen months of planning and mock runs to work out the kinks and went into action with a leased Fairchild-Hiller FH 1100, chosen for its comparatively roomy interior, which permitted a litter patient to be worked on by crewmembers equipped with supplemental oxygen, resuscitators, vacuum suction, and all the recommended minimum equipment for a land ambulance, including standard first aid supplies, air splints, airways, and so forth.[56] Crewed by veteran troopers with at least five years' experience, Red Cross First Aid certification, a thirty hour "intensive training course in paramedical procedures," and an additional ten days observing and assisting with patient care in a local emergency room, the program represented a level of training unusual for the typical ambulance service of the time.[57] Similar to the Pennsylvania program, the reviewers of Arizona's foray into police helicopter ambulance use discovered that medical evacuation alone was not cost-effective, and while the aircraft transferred over two hundred patients in its first nine months of operation (half of which were highway accidents), it flew five-hundred seventy other missions, including tracking and capturing a homicide suspect, locating a kidnapper in the desert scrub, and patrolling the highways.

In the end the more robust model of advanced helicopter medical service was the original: a hospital-centered operation, either with independent contractors servicing a consortium of institutions or, in the largest cities, an in-house flight crew. While the originals in this line were scaled in miniature at Santa Monica and Buffalo in the 1950s, the defining example was, and remains, the University of Maryland's Shock Trauma Center in Baltimore, entering the field in 1967, at a time when only twenty-nine states and the District of Columbia had operational ambulance heliports and the service was, still, a relative underperformer.[58] What would become arguably the leading civilian center for trauma medicine started with a disgruntled surgeon who couldn't figure out why he was leaving the hospital after a day of technically flawless open heart surgeries and coming in the next morning to watch his patients begin dying despite his brilliant technique and text-book closings. Sometimes it would take them weeks to "forget" that the operation was a success and die anyway, but again and again he watched surgery survivors succumb to the effects of shock, and he made it his business to find out why.[59]

The surgeon was R Adams Cowley, a man with a cliff-like brow over heavy features and a famous temper partly attributable to being condemned to go through life explaining that, no, he didn't use an initial—his first name was just the letter "R," short for nothing. (His bizarre christening came about through a wealthy uncle named Rufus who, for obvious reasons, preferred to use his middle name. When he learned Cowley's mother was pregnant, he asked her to name the child after him if it was a boy—sensing the possibility of a larger share of her brother's estate, she agreed, but since her brother always used an initial in lieu of his Christian name when signing something, she figured her son shouldn't have to use any more of his

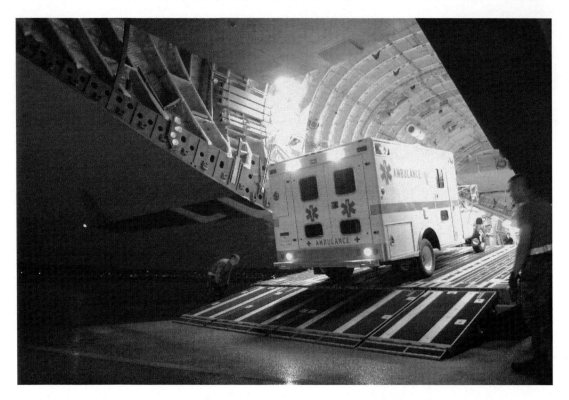

A literal take on the "air ambulance" as a C-17 Globemaster unloads its cargo at March Air Reserve Base in Augusta, Georgia (Sgt. Rick Sforza, June 2007. Courtesy DefenseLINK/DOD).

uncle's name than that, and so on his birth certificate Cowley's first name was reduced to a monogram.[60] Of course, why Rufus wanted his nephew saddled with a name he himself hated is a mystery equal to why a woman would name her child after a letter of the alphabet: in some ways one wishes that instead of being a cardiac surgeon Dr. Cowley had been a psychiatrist instead, since it appears the family needed one on retainer.)

In 1960 Cowley requested and received a $100,000 grant from the U.S. Army to study the relationship between shock and mortality, a question that obviously had tremendous application to military doctors contemplating the next war. The shock-trauma unit thus endowed grew larger as the brilliant surgeon attracted more and more able colleagues to assist him in what was becoming, year by year, a more important and well-funded branch of medicine. After Baltimore Hospital, where Crowley worked, built a helipad in 1967 the military started using their helicopters to ferry over their serious accident victims for acute care, and then in 1968 the Department of Transportation provided a grant to establish and study a "Helicopter Patrol," which resulted in a new heliport being built on an eight story parking garage next to Cowley's state of the art Trauma Center.[61] By April 1969, the "patrol" was operational, using a military surplus helicopter and operated by the State Police (in 1970 the department split off and began operating their own trauma medevac service, mostly handling traffic cases): at first, three quarters of the flights were simply patient transports from one hospital to another, but within two years the bulk of the missions were emergency transports, although the medical support available was at the level of advanced first aid, and the operation was little more than an airborne "you call, we haul." In 1971 the aircraft were retrofitted with mechanically operated suction and ventilation equipment and the crews were given advanced training in life-saving interventions, measures that had dramatic effect: by the end of the year the mortality rate for severe trauma cases arriving at the hospital had been halved.[62] The civilian helicopter ambulance had its first highly visible medical success story.

Hueys over Houston: The National Debut of Medevac

Even as civilian organizations, fueled in large part by DOT grants, experimented with helicopter ambulances in the mid–1960s, the military was field-testing its second generation of medevac choppers in the jungles of Vietnam. By now its Huey helicopters had sufficient space in the hold for medics to actually treat casualties in-flight, a departure from the pontoon transport of Korea, and the military deployed the larger machines to considerable effect. It was, therefore, foreseeable that tremendous benefits would be realized when Secretary of Defense Laird recommended, in March 1970, that military helicopter medevac units be deployed to civilian accident scenes: the military would benefit from the extra training and the crews would help abate "the nation-wide need for qualified rescuemen."[63] This proposal also coincided with a draw-down in our forces in Vietnam and repatriation of large numbers of trained medics to the States. From this coincidence of interests the Military Assistance to Safety and Traffic (MAST) program was inaugurated in July 1970, with the 507th Medical Company at Fort Sam Houston, Texas, using fifteen H-model Huey helicopters. The first "dust-off" came on July 17th, 1970, flying a man struck down by a truck in Dilley, Texas, to a hospital 75 miles away, and by August the program was in place at Mountain Home AFB, Idaho; Lake AFB, Arizona; and Forts Carson and Lewis, in Colorado and Washington, respectively.[64] As able as the flight medics were, they were still constrained by the same laws governing civilian ambulance crews, statutes narrowly prescribing the types of procedures that the non-physicians could perform in the majority of states. As one former navy corpsman volunteering for a ground-based rescue squad in Maryland put it:

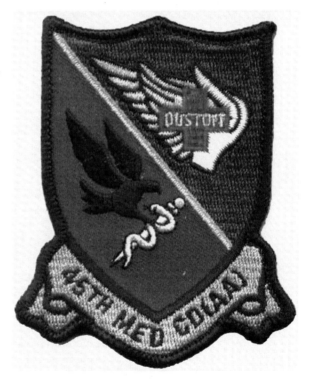

Military helicopter medical evacuation crews, like the 45th Medical Company, set the stage for a civilian revolution in air ambulance service.

> The Maryland medical practice laws are keeping us from saving lives. In one three week period, our squad transported two people who were DOA at the hospital. Using the skills I learned in the Navy I could have saved them both. One was an old man who had a head injury from a car crash, and the other a young woman who had some food lodged in her throat—neither could breathe. All it would have taken to save their lives was a simple trach[eotomy].... Even though I did more than 10 of those in Nam, the law still says no ... so they died.[65]

On the other hand, law or no law, the majority of MAST medics were apparently prepared to do whatever was necessary to save a life. A government spokes-

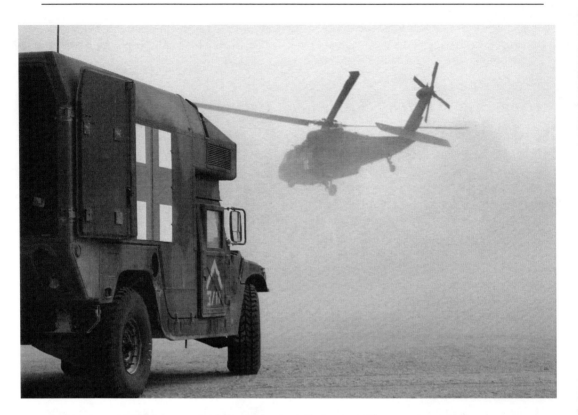

In Kuwait, an ambulance awaits the return of a UH-60 Black Hawk medevac helicopter en route to recover a wounded Marine in 2003 (Lcpl. Kevin Quihuis, Jr. Courtesy DefenseLINK/DOD).

man noted that ninety-five percent of Medevac crews had seen active service in Vietnam, where a year's tour gave them more trauma experience than most civilian ambulance crews saw in a lifetime—and many of these crewmembers were simply going ahead and starting tracheotomies en route if that's what it took.[66] When it worked, patients didn't complain, and if it failed families were often grateful that everything possible had been done. A Justice Department official, speaking on condition of anonymity, told a reporter

> We're holding our breath. I admit the [medevac] medics may be bending a few laws, but they're saving a hell of a lot of lives as they do it. I suppose sooner or later someone may try to bring a suit against the Army for their rescue efforts, but maybe the medical practice laws will be broadened before that happens.[67]

(Rule-bending or no, the program was successful, and continues nationwide to the present day, although not from Fort Sam Houston—after a force reduction in 1993 the 507th medevac unit transferred out after flying more than 5,000 rescue operations.)

As state laws on the practice of paramedics liberalized the inflight crews were given the authority to act in accordance with their training and the age of the air ambulance took on its recognizably modern contours, with increasing success: a North Carolina study found that after MAST flights went airborne with full paramedic services they decreased morbidity/mortality by 38 percent.[68] Today, helicopters and fixed wing aircraft are routinely staffed with specially trained flight-paramedics who each year provide care to nearly 650,000 patients in the United States alone.[69] From the first crude attempts to lash a stretcher to an airplane wing to the creation of specialized medical craft attended by the new profession of flight-paramedics, the aero-ambulance traveled an almost unimaginable distance in the space of

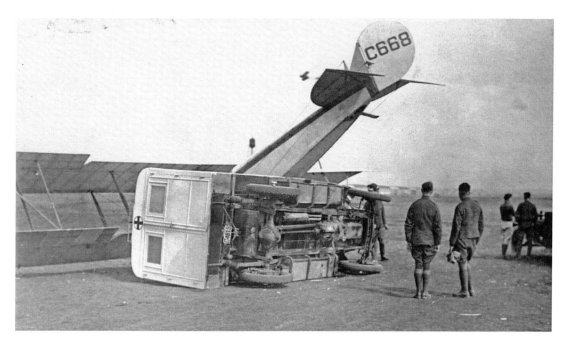

The marriage of airplane with ambulance was not always peaceful, as with this 1917 collision at Camp Borden, Ontario, Canada (courtesy Glenbow Archives, NA-3316-34).

two generations, a story that is one of the most exciting, and successful, in the annals of emergency medicine.

The Manufacturers

Of course, all of these improved ambulances, both terrestrial and airborne, were being built by someone, and before ending this chapter it would be wise to consider the artisans, the entrepreneurs, and the supporting cast of salesmen and advertisers who provided the working stock for the mobile medical services. The era began with the siring of the successful and widely imitated Bellevue ambulance service in 1869, an innovation promising an entirely new market for urban carriage makers, and among the first to benefit was the famous Abbot, Downing & Company (headquartered in Concord, New Hampshire, but with showrooms nationwide).

This renowned firm, the General Motors of the buggy trade, received the inaugural contract for the Bellevue ambulances, but, instead of nailing down a monopoly on the field, the partners concentrated on building the distinctive stagecoaches whose progeny can be seen kicking up sage dust in old Westerns and left the ambulance market comparatively open.[70] One entrepreneur quick to seize the reins was Manhattan's own Mr. Curley, a Broadway carriage maker. His skill was widely known, and when the internationally famous Massachusetts General Hospital went shopping for their first ambulance in 1873 they forsook the local craftsmen of Beantown to seek out Mr. Curley's shop. The trim, black beauty they took into service set the board back $700, a princely sum at the time.[71] Eight years later Mr. Curley's ambulances had achieved global reach, and in 1881 he proudly boasted to a visiting British physician that "I make the ambulances for nearly all the cities in the United States, and am now making three for Guatemala, Central America."[72] Volume, expertise, and possibly competition

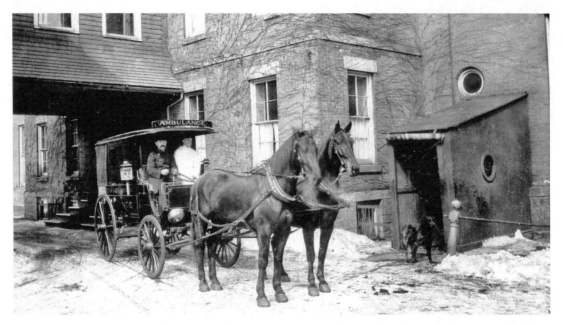

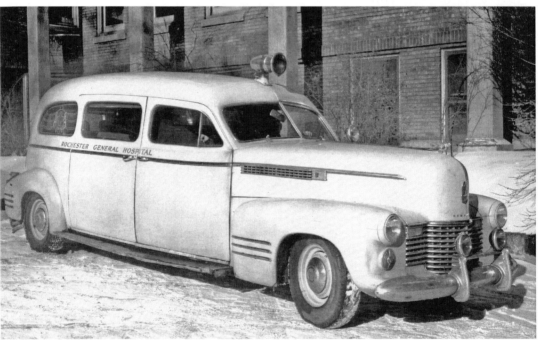

Less than fifty years separated the two ambulances seen here, both operated by the Rochester City/General Hospital, in upstate New York, but in manufacture and design they represent a titanic shift from reliance on locally constructed, hand-built ambulance wagons to centrally manufactured and nationally distributed automotive ambulances provided by a few large firms (courtesy Via-Health Archives Consortium, Rochester, N.Y.).

were reducing the cost, as he offered a one-horse ambulance for $550, and a two-horse model for $585.

As the horse gave way to the motorcar, carriage makers made a stab at fiscal survival by custom building ambulance cabs for automotive chassis, and down through the early 1900s most ambulance manufacture continued to be done on a local basis by the commercial descendants of Mr. Curley and his fellows. Even after Henry Ford irrevocably changed the industry with assembly line production, automakers like La Salle, Cadillac, Pierce Arrow, and Studebaker sold trainloads of chassis to the nation's ambulance builders so they could graft their own carriage work on top, although by now they were beginning to work in chrome instead of cherry, manganese steel instead of mahogany. By 1910 a perceptible shift was underway towards national advertising, and a comparatively small number of large firms began taking control of the ambulance market. Unquestionably the center of gravity for this second wave of ambulance manufacture was Ohio.

For mysterious reasons the Buckeye State had long been the center of the hearse and funeral car business, and its firms lost little time in taking the ambulance trade out of Mr. Curley's calloused hands. After all, both hearses and ambulances were designed to transport horizontal customers, and it was as easy to build one as the other. To streamline operations all the major hearse manufacturers duplicated as many design elements as possible when building ambulances. In fact, some companies used identical bodies for hearse and ambulance with the only difference being the color scheme or some small design detail, such as an elongated cab on the hearse model. During the early and middle 20th centuries Ohio was host to nearly all of the major ambulance firms—companies like Riddle Coach and Hearse Co. in Ravenna, The White Company in Cleveland, Meteor in Piqua, Superior in Lima, A.J. Miller Co. in Bellefontaine, and the venerable Hess and Eisenhardt in Cincinnati. Those were the names that appeared on the majority of American ambulances and whose ads filled trade magazines catering to funeral directors and hospitals alike. (In addition to building ambulances and hearses the companies also sold "combination" vehicles, designed to function as either. A detachable siren, removable casket brace, and a sliding floor plate that permitted an attendant to sit in the back were the only things required to transform a hearse into an ambulance, and these were popular sellers.)

By the 1950s many of the smaller firms had been bought out or had succumbed to more

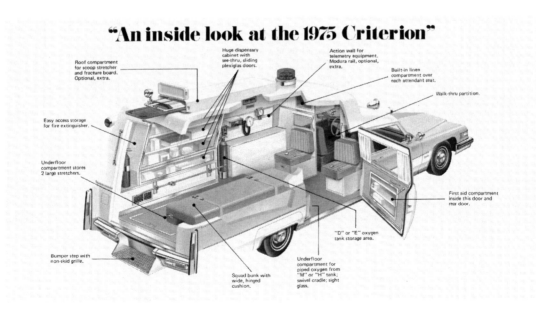

Miller-Meteor Inc., a merger of two venerable ambulance and hearse manufacturers, remained one of Ohio's leading ambulance firms through the late 1970s. This brochure page for their 1975 Criterion demonstrates the plentiful design features that made this vehicle one of the best selling ambulances of the year (courtesy Miller-Meteor/Accubuilt).

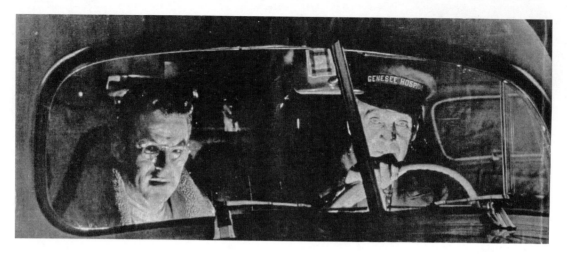

Limned by the dash lights, intern and driver appear tensely poised for flight in the Genesee Hospital ambulance in December, 1942 (courtesy ViaHealth Archives Consortium, Rochester, N.Y.).

aggressive rivals, but the major players, Hess and Eisenhardt, Meteor, A.J. Miller Co., and a few others, were still in the trade. Soon, however, their best customers, the funeral homes, began deserting the ambulance business, especially after 1965. Increases in the minimum wage and state regulations requiring new, and expensive, operating standards conspired to make an untenable extravagance out of a service that seldom turned a profit for the funeral home. Legislation in the 1970s required new ambulances to be built on the modern van/truck model, creations completely distinct from the "professional car" ambulances of old. The expense of re-tooling their production facilities was too much for companies that had spent decades creating ambulances and funeral cars that were virtually interchangeable in terms of frame and body work, and by 1977 the last hearse-style ambulances were rolling out of factories in Ohio and elsewhere. During this shift to specialty firms most of the hearse/ambulance carriage makers followed the lead of Superior and returned to the exclusive manufacture of funeral cars, while a few others looked for profits in new fields—the successor to Hess and Eisenhardt now specializes in armored cars and bulletproof limousines designed to keep its clients *out* of the ambulances and hearses it once sold by the train load. For nearly a century most American ambulances had been imitations of other cars—a hearse with a siren, a station wagon with a cot, a patrol van with a stretcher in the back. While the new manufacturers symbolized the fresh start for ambulance services, their more utilitarian designs have never captured the eye the way the mile-long profile of the old professional cars did, in all of their inefficient, impractical, and genuine beauty.

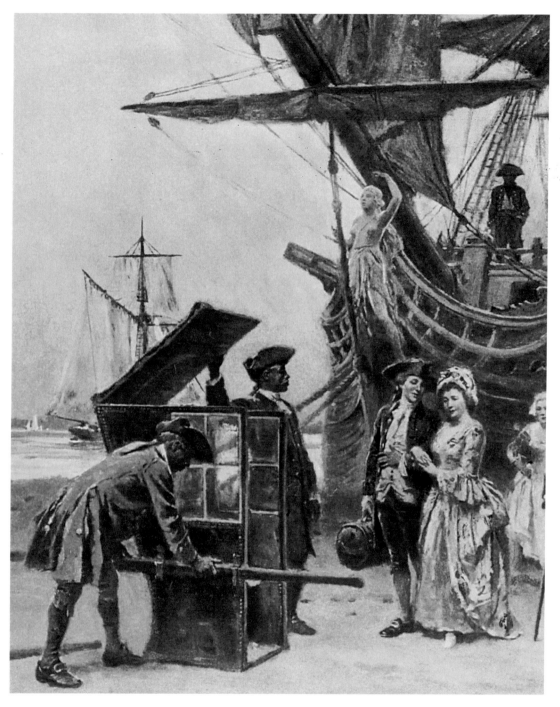

An 18th century "street chair" of the kind used by many hospitals of the day to bring in patients; the advantage of the chair was that it could be carried right to the bed or operating table. (J.L.G. Ferris, c. 1930. Library of Congress Prints and Photographs Division, LC-USZC4-9906)

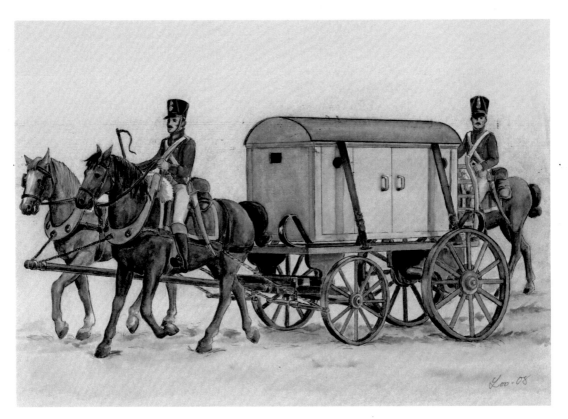

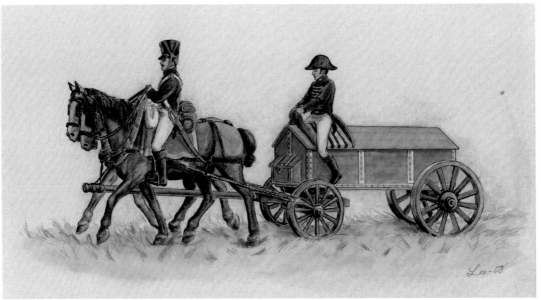

Top: Larrey's "ambulant volant" (inspired by similar carriages used by Napoleon's "flying artillery") redefined the ambulance with a combination of expert medical care at the scene, a special transport vehicle, and, of course, speed. *Above:* Baron Percy's wagon was designed principally to transport surgeons onto the battlefield, but the lightly wounded could be evacuated by riding astride the vehicle. The design was almost immediately superseded by Larrey's innovative ambulance. (Ann-Cathrine Loo)

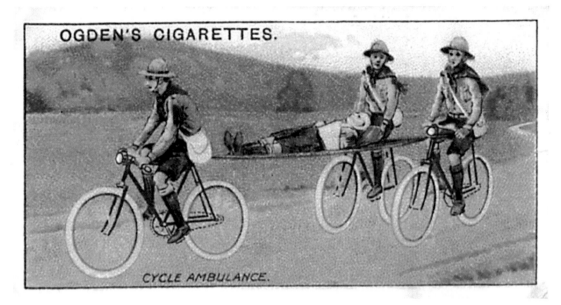

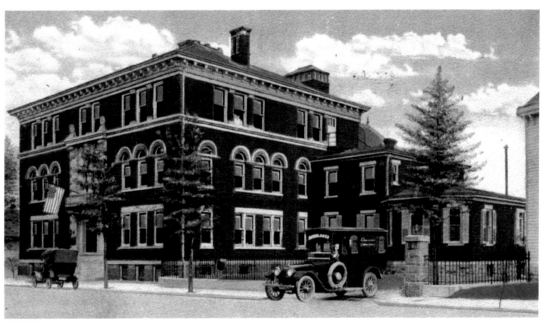

Top: Some ambulance innovations are born of necessity, as with this example from a turn of the century cigarette premium—apparently offered to encourage smoking among Boy Scouts. *Above:* In 1921 an ambulance was a symbol of a hospital's success and civic commitment, as with the aid car proudly displayed alongside the Easton Hospital in Pennsylvania. Thirty years later increasing costs and staffing problems made such hospital ambulances an unwelcome burden.

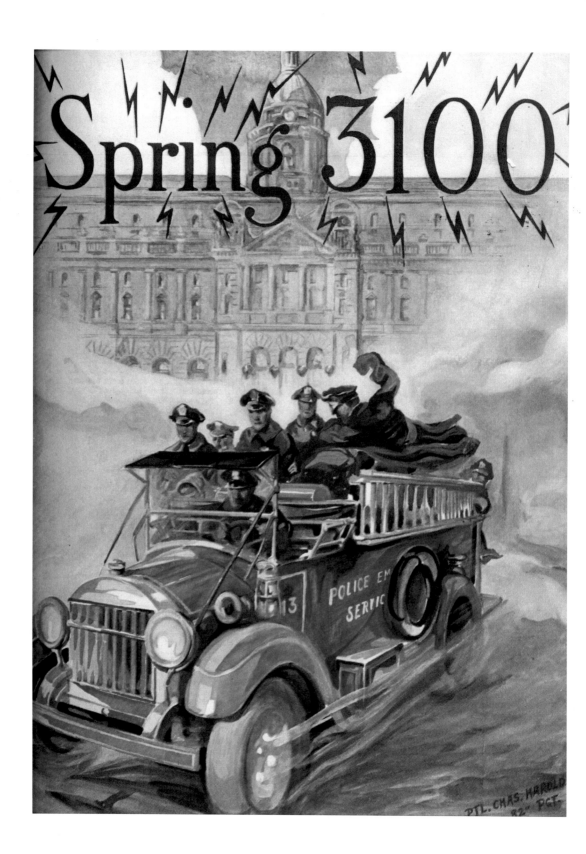

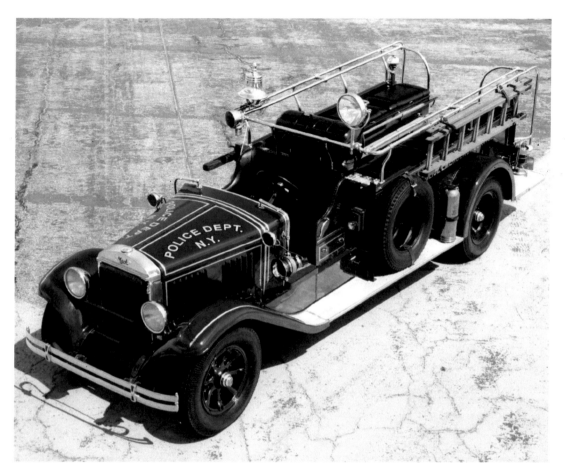

A restored Mack truck once used by the original New York City Police Emergency Service Squad. (Courtesy Kevin Reynolds. Copyright 2001, New York City Police Department, all rights reserved. Used with permission)

Opposite: This 1930 cover of the New York Police Department's house magazine featured a striking tribute to the newly re-organized Emergency Services Division, with their newly repainted Kelly-green squad trucks. (Spring-3100 was the telephone number of the old Centre Street police headquarters.) (Courtesy Kevin Reynolds. Copyright 2001, New York City Police Department, all rights reserved. Used with permission)

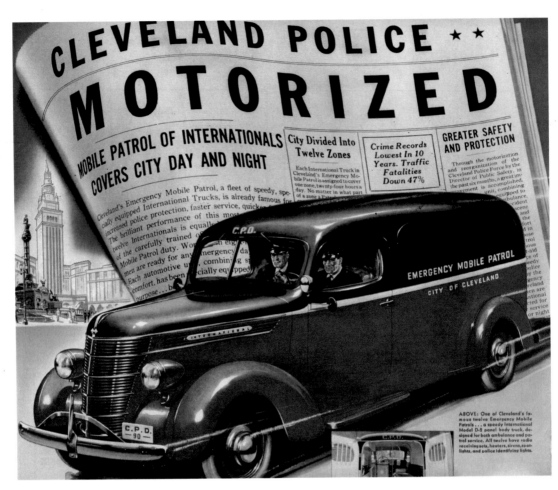

Eliot Ness, of "Untouchables" fame, was Cleveland's Public Safety Commissioner in 1938, when he created a Police Ambulance Corps with one dozen International D-2 panel trucks equipped with splints, first aid kits, respirators, stretchers and radio receivers. Staffed by unsworn departmental employees with first aid training, the fleet's organization, equipment, and radio control made it one of the most advanced civilian ambulance services of its time.

Opposite, top: The Jay W. Stevens Disaster Unit in all its Technicolor glory, in the early 1940s. With its dramatic flame-colored highlights and full panoply of emergency and rescue equipment, the "Coffee Wagon" was a stunning re-definition of the ambulance. (Courtesy Portland Fire and Rescue and the Portland Fire Museum Collection) *Opposite, bottom:* In 1974 the federal government adopted new design criteria for ambulances purchased with taxpayer funds, only accepting van or modular-style vehicles, such as those shown in this 1978 advertisement.

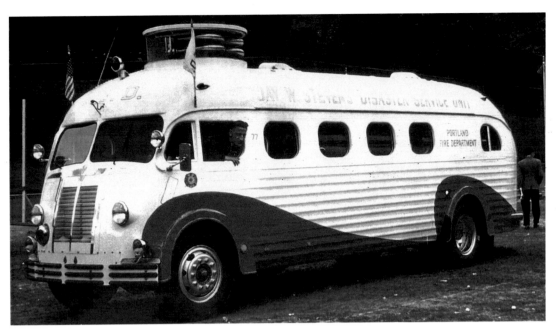

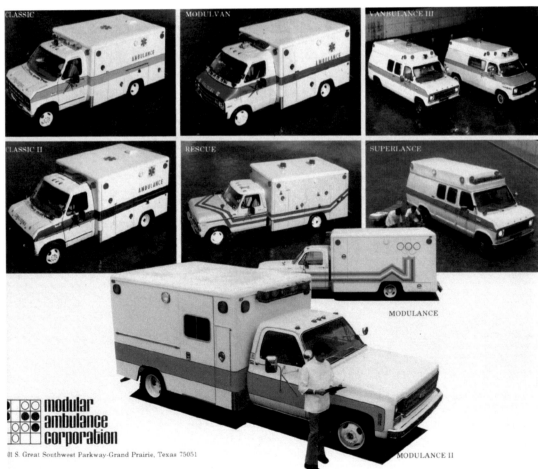

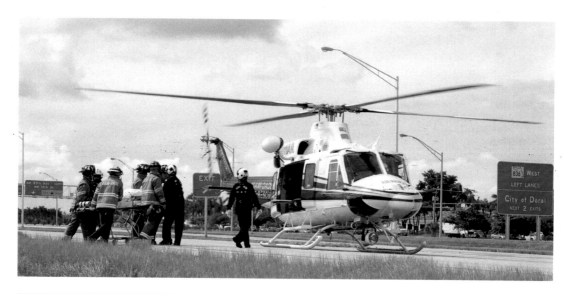

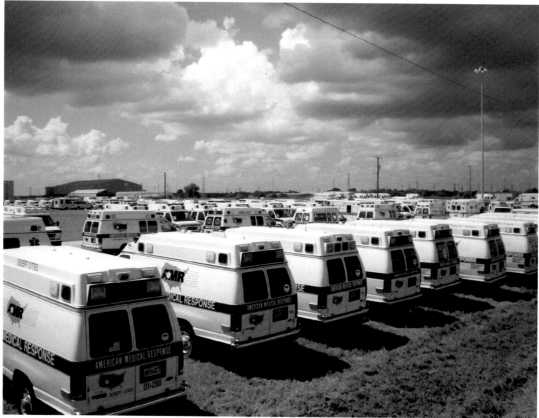

Top: A Miami-Dade Fire Rescue Department squad transferring a patient to a medevac helicopter. (Courtesy the Miami-Dade Fire Rescue Department) *Above:* Prior to Hurricane Dean nearly 700 ambulances were staged at San Antonio in August 2007—the largest civilian ambulance mobilization in United States history. (FEMA/Don Jacks)

• 10 •

Siren Call: The Lure of Speed

Almost from its inception the civilian ambulance service has been held to explain the difference between speed and recklessness, between medical necessity and merely feeding the human instinct for drama and action. Where to draw the line has bedeviled legislatures deciding to what extent emergency vehicles should be exempted from basic traffic laws, stymied administrators questioning the necessity of sirens, and perplexed physicians debating whether the excitement of a fast car ride was dangerous to the frail constitutions of the injured and ill. Time has brought experience but little wisdom, and the debate of a century ago continues. Here we consider the ways communities attempted to meet the need for ambulance regulation, from equine debates over when to trot and when to canter, through the Great Siren Controversy of the middle 20th century, and down to the modern era of black-boxes under ambulance dashboards and defensive driving.

Code Red and Traffic Codes

Shortly after New York City's ambulance service debuted in 1869, Albany gave the new vehicles a right of way over all carriages and wagons save the United States Mail, fire department rigs, and insurance patrols. (The latter, now happily extinct, were squads of men employed by underwriters to rescue movable property from fires, thus limiting the insurer's liability at the risk of their own lives.) A nearly identical provision was enacted in Brooklyn two years later, granting ambulances the right of way "against any person, carriage or incumbrance" who might interfere with their progress.[1] Similarly, in New Orleans the ambulance service of the Charity Hospital, from its origin in 1885, was given the right of way over everything on the road except, naturally, the omnipotent United States Mail. While seldom explicitly mentioned in the right of way ordinances, these ambulances appeared to enjoy immunity from prevailing speed limits as well, since they are invariably mentioned in the literature as "dashing," "flying," or "racing" along on their missions. (To the modern motorist, horses may seem laughably slow when flashing past an Amish buggy in your Chrysler, but speed limits were already old when the ambulance was new. Indeed, one of the earliest speed ordinances dates to 1635, when the maximum speed of a horse-carriage on the streets of London was set at three miles per hour, or a slow walk.[2] During the 19th century, most American cities followed similar limits, with the top speed in a business district usually ranging from three to six miles per hour.) The lesson that all should yield to the ambulance as a matter of morals as well as laws was inevitably put into uplifting verse by a civic minded Victorian, who reminded readers what to do when the ambulance came "Claiming its course with clang of gong / Forcing a way through the surging throng—/ That cross of red its right of way, / Let man nor beast its speed delay. / Open a way and let it pass!"[3]

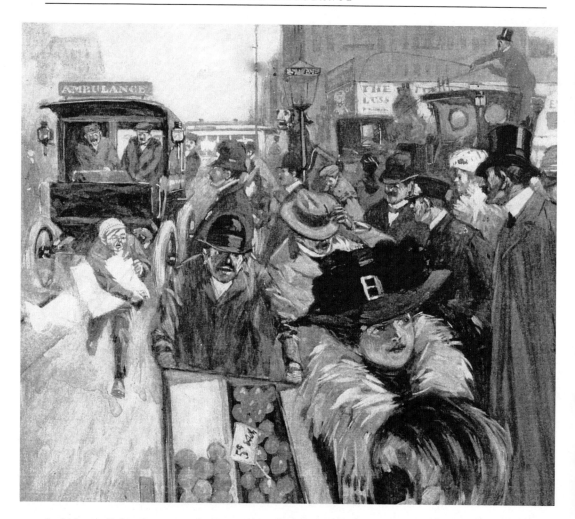

Ambulance right of way was freely awarded in New York, but not always observed. An electric ambulance, like this one, had the added disadvantage of running silently, necessitating the frequent use of the gong to alert the populace to its passage ("Clear the way for the ambulance!" Gordon Grant, *Leslie's Weekly*, December 12, 1901).

Tale of Two Cities

Not all communities were willing to grant the ambulance *carte blanche* on the boulevard, however, and those doing so were almost invariably municipalities with government run emergency services, as in New York, New Orleans, and Brooklyn. In comparison, where ambulance services started as a private business such exemptions were altogether rare. Portland, Oregon, and New York City represent object lessons in the argument that it mattered whether a municipal ambulance service was the first, or at least the dominant, emergency provider when predicting what exemptions to the traffic laws would apply and what level of oversight would evolve.

First New York, where the ambulance service began as a municipal enterprise and the state enjoyed a long history of regulating every aspect of citizen behavior coming to the attention of its legislature. As we have seen, Manhattan's city ambulance service started out well supervised, well regulated, and with a right of way on the city streets. Still, by 1909 the *New York*

Times had to observe that "the ambulance service of Greater New York has grown up in a haphazard way," and some social scientists argued that the competing interests of individual ambulance services would never spontaneously give rise to the "organization, control, and improvement" that could be expected from centralized command, since individual infirmaries would always be tempted to maximize their own profits at the expense of the community.[4] Indeed, some hospitals were ignoring an ordinance requiring ambulance calls to be forwarded to the central police station for assignment, preferring instead to simply snatch up whatever calls (and fees) came their way, regardless of whether another infirmary was actually closer to the caller. These cases were most common in neighborhoods with a surfeit of hospitals, but other areas, especially on the verges of the expanding city, had no local ambulance service whatsoever. Further, in the wake of the bank panic of 1907 decreased charitable giving caused some hospitals to scale back ambulance service, as when the Roosevelt Hospital terminated its ambulances in 1908. Apart from spotty service, reform-minded civic leaders were growing impatient with the variable quality of the services, attributed by many to a system that allowed the nearly forty hospitals sponsoring ambulances to make their own best guess as to how to train their surgeons and drivers.

To address these deficiencies the state legislature created the New York City Board of Ambulance Service, becoming operational in 1911. Presiding over the board was the police commissioner, seconded by the charities commissioner, with the remaining seats occupied by

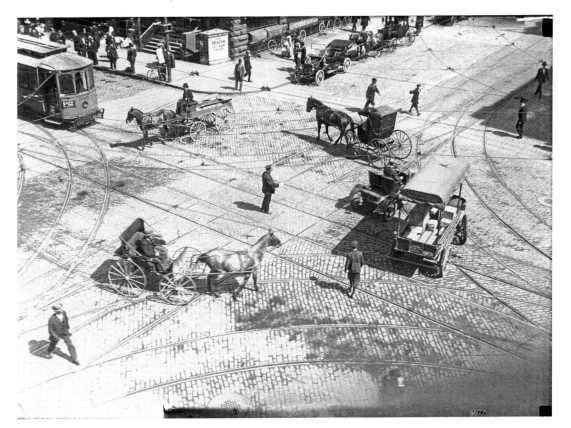

Traffic at Four Corners, Rochester, New York, in the early 1900s, as trolleys, pedestrians, wagons, carriages, and an automobile crowd a lone policeman directing traffic. Such chaotic scenes created dangerous environments for speeding ambulances and led to calls to slow the rigs down (from the Albert R. Stone Negative Collection, Rochester Museum & Science Center Rochester, N.Y.).

the president of the Bellevue and Allied Hospitals (representing the municipal infirmaries) and two members appointed by the mayor (representing whatever political interest had His Honor's ear at the moment). The board's jurisdiction only reached into those ambulance barns or garages whose rigs answered emergency calls, as opposed to services functioning solely as medical taxis to ferry patients to and from the hospital on a non-urgent basis.[5] (The city's proprietary interest in emergency medical services represented the durability of Mayor Wood's original decision, in 1855, to place all accident cases under the exclusive jurisdiction of the city police surgeons.) As a practical matter, the board had authority to inspect vehicles, collect monthly reports from every hospital providing emergency ambulance service (on the theory that such services were being provided on the city's behalf), investigate complaints, and could veto the appointment of any physician to ambulance duty (a draconian sanction it was willing to use, albeit sparingly, rejecting seventeen of the first three hundred candidates it reviewed).[6]

Each of these powers was identical to those the commissioner of charities had exercised over the pioneering Bellevue ambulance at its inception: the new Board of Ambulance Service simply extended this writ to the private emergency providers, on the principle that the city had an original obligation to provide emergency medical relief to its citizens, as first enunciated by Mayor Wood, and if it delegated some of this authority to private hospitals it retained a fiduciary duty to see that these services were provided in a satisfactory way. Private hospitals were motivated to accept this arrangement since all emergency ambulance dispatch was via the police department, and any infirmary wishing to receive their fair share of accident cases (with their attendant teaching value, potential for income, and the community standing an ambulance service brought with it), had no choice but to participate in this scheme. Thus the city of New York maintained close supervision over the ambulance services of the municipality and, by keeping a firm grip on ambulance dispatch via the central switchboard at police headquarters, could negotiate with private operators the same standards it set for municipal services. This pattern, an original and comprehensive city ambulance service setting terms for private ambulance operations to assume an accepted municipal function, was invariably associated with the most regulated, and best quality, ambulance services in the United States prior to the development of federal ambulance standards in the 1970s.

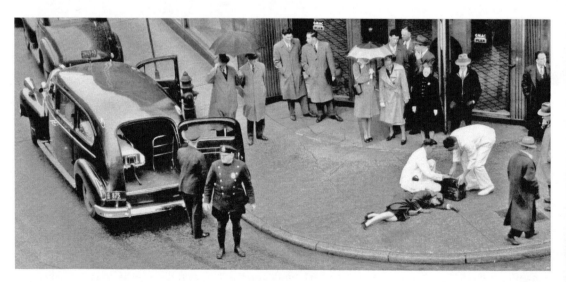

This scene staged for a Rochester film crew in the late 1920s illustrates the dilemma faced by ambulance crews: In the face of a sudden emergency, how fast was too fast when responding? (Courtesy ViaHealth Archives Consortium, Rochester, N.Y.)

Safety, by Order of the Board

The board's efforts at coordinating dispatch and becoming involved in training and equipment certainly benefited patients, but its writ also extended to ensuring the safety of the interns riding the rigs. While most cities who took the time to consider ambulance safety followed Brooklyn's lead in 1902 and limited themselves to enjoining ambulances from being "driven through the streets at such a speed as to endanger the lives or limbs of the public," the New York City Board of Ambulance Services started issuing detailed safety regulations in 1919 with its pocket-sized *Regulations Governing the Ambulance Service of All Hospitals in the City of New York*, which was updated and expanded a year later.[7] Still, even with speed limits and requirements to put on tire chains in wet weather the service remained an occasionally dangerous one. The apparently fearless Dr. Janet Travell left this account of her term on the New York Hospital ambulance in 1927, an electric model with a body like a delivery wagon:

> When the pavements were slick with rain or sleet, I developed a fatalistic attitude, no matter what kind of skid we made. I hooked my left arm through the looped strap, braced my back against one side of the bus and my feet against the other, with my legs stretched out on the cross-seat at the open end, and I fixed my eyes steadily on the book that I was reading.[8]

Not all of her fellows escaped unscathed, of course: during her term on the ambulance a classmate riding the Bellevue ambulance died when the rig slid into the Third Avenue elevated posts, and Travell herself had actually taken the place of an intern who was severely injured when his ambulance collided with a horse-cart and a wooden pole ripped through a side panel and struck him in the throat.[9]

Free to Drive Slow

While New York City's efforts were exemplary, much more typical of the nation as a whole was the *laissez faire* approach of Portland, Oregon, where ambulances came late and there was no comparable tradition of municipal control, however slight. In fact, municipal ambulance operations hadn't even begun until the fire bureau received its first ambulance, the George Baker Disaster Car, in 1933—a full fourteen years after private ambulance services made their debut in the business directories. By 1945 this bustling port city, with a population in excess of three hundred thousand, could yet claim only two publicly funded ambulances, both operated by the fire bureau. Unlike Manhattan, entrepreneurs had created the ambulance market in Portland, and these private concerns dominated the city streets.

On the other hand, Portland did share with New York an ordinance granting the right of way to emergency vehicles. Significantly, in Oregon that regulation was read as applying only to *municipal* apparatus, such as fire bureau rigs and police cars. Thus in 1945, when a car and a private ambulance collided while the latter was on a hurry-call, a municipal police judge held that a civilian auto had *no duty* to yield the right of way to a private ambulance, even one with siren blaring.[10] Paternity, not purpose, defined an emergency vehicle in Portland, and only municipal ambulances were legitimate. Naturally the city's private ambulance firms instructed their drivers to operate the machines in strict accord with all traffic laws, hewing scrupulously to the posted limits and patiently waiting out the lights. Then, only a few months after the court ruling, a terrible trailer fire killed three children outright and left two others seared with second and third degree burns. The local ambulance company was called, but under the new policy their response was so slow that one of the injured children was finally taken to the hospital by a frantic bystander in their own vehicle, while the other was transported in the fire bureau's late arriving J.W. Stevens disaster car. Both of the young victims later died of their injuries.

An editorial in the *Oregon Journal* addressing this grim outcome clearly struggled with the tension between private and public ambulances and the question of how to balance speed with the preservation of life, noting "Portland medical men hold that excessive speed and excitement may kill rather than save the lives of injured passengers, and ... the Stevens disaster car is [already designated] an 'emergency vehicle' and is as well equipped to save lives as a [private] ambulance."[11] While acknowledging that the disaster car could only be in one place at one time, the editor suggests "no lives would be lost if [private] ambulances, like fire engines, were 'emergency vehicles' going to an accident, but observed regular driving laws on the return trip." The editorial, exhausted by the seeming complexities of the case, trailed off with a rhetorical shrug: "no one will ever know whether the lives of the two small victims ... may or may not have been saved by quicker action ... if others like them are to live under similar circumstances, a lesson must be taken from this tragedy." But what was that lesson to be?

In 1959 the logic of the Portland police judge's 1945 ruling was extended to the entire state of Oregon: under Senate Bill 223 private ambulances were obligated to obey all traffic ordinances. Within days of the law taking effect in August an article appeared in the *Oregonian* under the headline "Death Heightens Controversy over Rein on Ambulance Operation."[12] In one case, an ambulance took thirty minutes to reach a residence, and when the patient subsequently died at the hospital his relatives charged that the delay in transportation contributed to the young man's ultimate death. Later that same day a teenager attempted suicide by hanging, and, as reported in the article, "the lad's mother, riding in the ambulance with the victim, pleaded with the driver to turn on his siren and speed through the red lights ... [but] the driver said he had to comply with the new state law, effective [that day] which requires ambulances to obey all traffic regulations like any other car." Behind the legislation were incidents like one cited by the bill's introducer, and quoted in the article, where an out of town ambulance ran a red light on Broadway and was involved in a wreck that injured seven, including the patient. It was widely believed that accidents like this were attributable to the generally poor quality of private ambulance drivers, a view endorsed by bill supporter Senator Grenfell:

> Personally, I think ambulance drivers should have the privileges of the drivers of police and fire emergency vehicles—if they were equally qualified.... But few of them are. They are not full-time, trained, professional drivers of emergency vehicles like our police and firemen. They get no special training. They are not required to pass special tests. Too often they are part-time drivers, students or hot-rodders.[13]

The solution proposed by the senator was not a race to the hospital, the excitement of which he felt might put the patient into shock: instead, Grenfell advocated equipping ambulances with interns who could provide medical care en route, eliminating the need for the high speed race to the emergency room. Warming to his theme, the senator added: "That's the kind of ambulance service offered in big cities. We handle our ambulance service like Podunk Center."[14]

What Senator Grenfell failed to appreciate was that, by 1959, the "big city" ambulance intern of his youth was already an anachronism, largely replaced by hospital orderlies and ambulance attendants. Instead, private ambulance services in municipalities like New York had long ago accepted city-imposed attendant training standards in exchange for operating subsidies and, almost incidentally, frequent exemption from traffic laws on emergency calls. As the ambulance marketplace evolved, administrative oversight had the opportunity to evolve with it, setting new standards and training requirements to keep pace with changes in medicine as well as traffic. On the other hand, while long usage had made these old firms docile under the municipal halter, this system was less appealing to firms just beginning their corporate career in the waning hours of the 20th century. After all, Portland's ambulance companies had little incentive to stand up and demand the right to spend more money on training in exchange for

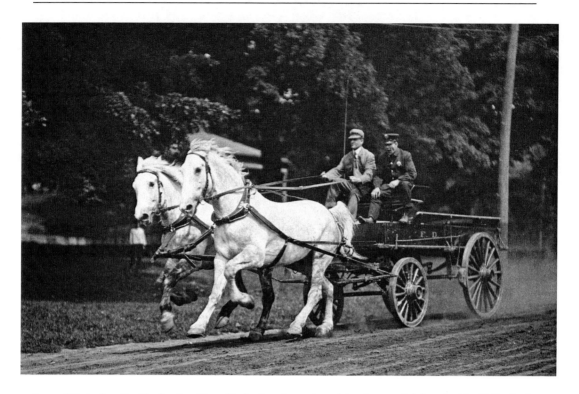

A candidate for the Rochester, New York, fire department is given a driving test in 1910. Such "defensive driving" training was part of the reason cities were more comfortable granting the right of way to police and fire ambulances as opposed to the unknowns handling commercial services (from the Albert R. Stone Negative Collection, Rochester Museum & Science Center Rochester, N.Y.).

the opportunity to speed and perchance to crash and pay higher insurance premiums. Indeed, many in the commercial ambulance field were desperately seeking ways to *slow down* their drivers, not encourage them to travel faster.

Siren Song

The problem for ambulance supervisors growing gray from worrying about crashes and insurance premiums was that in some difficult to determine number of cases speed *was* essential, while in others it was only a risk without a benefit—and how to predetermine which was which would tax any but the omniscient. The resulting temptation was to ignore the complexities, blame something small and comprehensible, and declare the matter solved—and so it came to be that the siren, which we now take for granted, was demonized as *the* evil mainspring driving the watch works of ambulance catastrophe. An early forum for the debate over sirens and their merits was *The Modern Hospital*, that monthly biopsy of the business of hospital operations. In a 1926 segment of its "Your Everyday Problems" column the editors raised the question "Should the Ambulance Be Supplied with a Gong or an Ordinary Warning Signal?"[15] (Sirens had yet to supplant rotary gongs as the preferred ambulance clarion, while the "ordinary warning signal" meant the standard horn.) The piece begins with an appeal to a shared irritation for the hardworking, dutiful overseers of modern temples of healing, where insurance rates had become as much a part of medicine as opiates and bedpans:

Most hospital administrators have had the experience of standing on the street corner and seeing an ambulance from their particular institution, with a clanging gong, dashing by at a speed too great for safety. Upon arrival at the hospital they were disgusted to find upon inquiry that the patient being transported on that particular ambulance call was one whose admission was in no way an urgent matter.

The editors note that, generally, the few minutes saved by dashing through the crowded streets are unnecessary—but in a fraction of instances, they become vital. Thus, they admit, the "gong is useful, if properly used." Alas, "the presence of a gong is a continuous invitation to unnecessary speed and to disregard of the traffic rules of the locality." After recommending care in the hiring of chauffeurs and mentioning the merits of a speedometer tape which records, for later review, the maximum speeds obtained by the ambulance, the editors advocate that the ambulance gong be abolished, with chauffeurs relying on their machine's horn to clear the way when extra speed is medically indicated.

The next year the editors were at it once again. Quoting *The Atlantic Medical Journal,* they agreed that too many ambulances were being driven as if every call were an emergency and the legal right of way was a magical shield protecting an ambulance from the careless and inattentive with whom they shared the crowded street. Even if an accident was avoided, there were other reasons to avoid speed while driving an ambulance: "[t]he peace of mind of the patient certainly should be taken into consideration. It must be a source of anxiety to a patient, who cannot see what is doing, to be shut up in an ambulance, lying flat on his back, and unnecessarily hurried along, turning corners on one wheel."[16] While older drivers were generally felt to be more reliable in these matters, many administrators echoed the despairing words of one

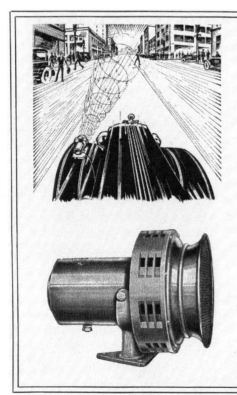
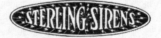

STERLING FREE ROLLING SIREN

the World's Greatest

Apparatus Siren

8 Reasons Why:

1: Greatest sound.
2: Free Rolling.
3: No clutches.
4: Beautiful design.
5: Marvelous motor.
6: Ball bearing throughout.
7: Greatest distance sender.
8: All STERLING made.

29 Years of Siren Experience

STERLING SIREN FIRE ALARM CO., INC.
61 ALLEN ST.   ROCHESTER, N. Y.

Siren advertisement, 1931. The use of sirens on ambulances was frequently a topic of concern for administrators, who feared they encouraged reckless driving (courtesy Sentry Siren, Inc.).

correspondent who, drawing on "many bitter experiences," averred that any "chauffeur with an excellent record, once placed in charge of an ambulance with a gong at his hand seems to pass from the sane to the dangerous."[17] By the late 1920s the issue was a live one for many hospitals, with directors trying a number of schemes to improve safety records. At the Jewish Hospital of Brooklyn, for example, executive director Dr. John E. Daugherty was actively seeking some mechanism that would shut down the power drive of his ambulances if they exceeded a predetermined maximum safe speed (what would happen to an ambulance that suddenly lost its motor in mid-careen was, apparently, a problem for the driver, not the administrator). His mechanical abilities falling below his ambitions, Dr. Daugherty found himself reduced to offering $50 bonuses to drivers who went six months without an accident, a policy not unknown at the time. While disappointingly pacifistic, he had to admit this gentle scheme "has been productive of some improvement."[18] (Not the kind of improvement you'd get from booby-trapping the accelerator, but no doubt he kept working on it.)

The question of whether sirens were appropriate for ambulances was answered in the negative not only by weary administrators, but occasionally by local governments as well. Typically representative of national trends, Rochester, New York banned sirens in the 1930s, only to have to ban them again in the 1950s. New York City experimented with abolishing ambulance sirens in the early 1950s and saw a 60 percent decrease in accidents involving ambulances, prompting Dr. MacLean of the New York City Hospital Council to note tartly that sirens in ambulances are "just spectacular stupidity."[19] Where ambulances were operated by fire or police departments, however, such bans were seemingly unknown—suggesting once again that, as with the right of way question above, the problem was not so much the siren, but the inadequate training of most drivers and attendants. With the wholesale revolution in professional-

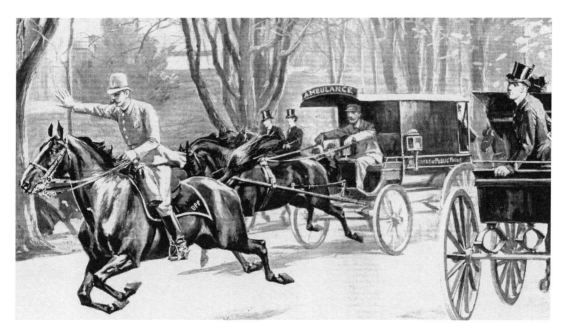

The problem of speeding ambulances predated the internal combustion engine, of course. In 1936 a sober and respectable Dr. George Goler of Rochester, New York, decried the reckless speed of automobile ambulances, but admitted that decades earlier he had clung "precariously to the back step of horse-drawn ambulance [and] enjoyed the thrill of having people turn in the street and follow his mad flight" (Henry W. Clune, "Seen and Heard," *Democrat and Chronicle*, January 28, 1936). (Courtesy the National Library of Medicine.)

ism that began in the late 1960s the demonization of the ambulance siren dissolved into the pattern of history and is scarcely remembered at this date.

While the siren debate and angst over whether private emergency vehicles deserved the right of way are no longer current, the issues which made them live are still a significant, if not well understood, problem. The former debate on speed was two pronged: first, that speed caused accidents, and second that it was psychologically damaging to the patient. This latter view survived into modern times, with Pennsylvania's 1965 *Ambulance Attendant Training Manual* helpfully pointing out "a high speed ride is often a traumatic experience for the patient and can do more psychological damage than is merited for possibly a few moments saved in transit."[20]

As we are now a nation that considers the fifty-five mile an hour speed limit a childish superstition, the psychological trauma of a fast car ride has disappeared from the debate. How many lives are lost due to high-speed ambulance driving versus how many are saved is, however, a calculation that continues to defy solution. A convincing, and relatively early, look into the necessity of speed occurred in 1957, when a Midwestern community hospital set out to calculate not only how much time was actually saved by speeding ambulances and rights of way, but whether the difference in time translated into lives saved.[21] First, hospital staff set out a 4.4 mile course through the city streets and timed their ambulance under varying conditions. With siren wailing and taking the right of way, but without driving in excess of thirty miles per hour, the ambulance reached the hospital in ten minutes or less. When it was driven in scrupulous

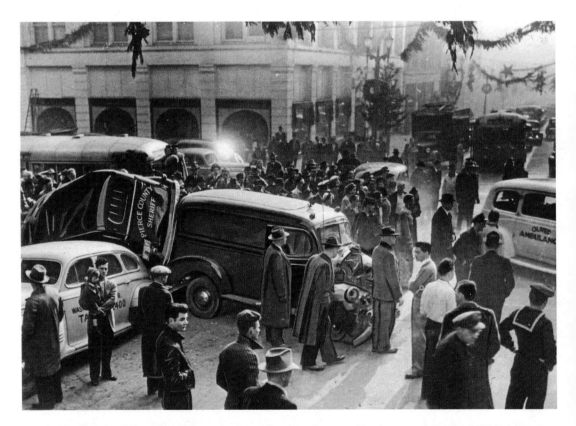

Professional public-safety drivers were not immune from accidents, as seen in this 1941 fatal accident involving a Tacoma, Washington, sheriff's car. A responding ambulance is seen to the right (courtesy the Seattle Museum of History and Industry).

accord with the traffic regulations, however, the trip took anywhere from thirteen minutes to just under half an hour.

Next, the authors collected data on the next 2,500 ambulance cases arriving at their emergency room. Of that number 2,455 had outcomes that would have been unaffected by arriving even ten minutes sooner—either their injuries were relatively mild, or they were so lethal that had they been struck down on the threshold of the operating theater they would still have been beyond earthly aid (such as the several patients with high, complete transection of the spinal cord). A mere 2 percent could have conceivably benefited from arriving ten to eighteen minutes earlier, and none of these would have received any medical benefit from the extra time saved by averaging sixty miles an hour rather than thirty en route to the hospital (assuming an average journey of 4.5 miles). Calculating the increased risk of crashes, in this study at least, the authors concluded that while the right-of-way was necessary, speeding was not. (A study conducted in California in 1964 was similar: the Department of Health evaluated 3,284 ambulance runs and concluded that speeding resulted in an average savings of about two minutes and forty seconds—a difference that was potentially significant in only 8 percent of the observed cases, mostly involving poisoning.)[22]

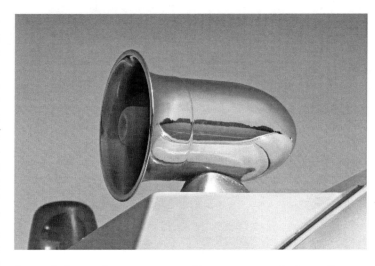

An ambulance siren announces its presence and clears the crowded street. How fast the ambulance should travel in the open lanes, however, is the subject of ongoing debate within the profession.

Modern numbers have added weight to the supposition that terrific speed is seldom vital, and invariably increases the risk of an accident. For example, the number of accidents involving ambulances is reckoned to be anywhere from sixty-five hundred to twelve thousand a year, and between 1991 and 2000 at least three hundred fifty-seven people died in ambulance crashes.[23] When compared to the millions of miles driven by ambulances each year these numbers may seem unimpressive, but looked at another way the estimated EMS worker job fatality rate is more than *double* that of the average worker: 12.7 per 100,000 EMS workers versus 5 per 100,000 for the general workforce.[24] (In comparison, police officers suffer 14.2 work related fatalities per 100,000 employees, and the fire-fighter rate is 16.5 per 100,000.) Small studies in various communities have estimated the average time saved by full-on lights and siren versus a silent run to be anywhere from 43.5 seconds to 3.02 minutes, an incremental difference that authorities generally agree could only benefit a small subset of patients: further, assuming that some significant percentage of ambulance accidents, and thus excess morbidity and mortality, could be avoided by driving at posted limits, there may not be *any* case, on a population basis, to justify aggressive driving.[25] Still, it is clear that more information is needed before definitive conclusions can be drawn. In the meantime, a number of products on the market discourage reckless driving and enforce company policies on ambulance operation: on-board "black box" computers with names like Road Safety and Silent Witness record speed, seat belt usage, use of emergency lights, acceleration and braking patterns, and even cornering, while some can be programmed to deliver a warning to the driver if pre-set thresholds have been crossed,

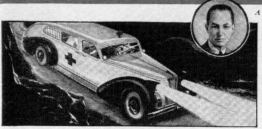
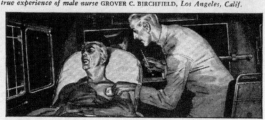
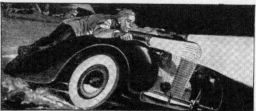

A 1941 ad for Eveready Batteries reminds us that, as with an evolving myocardial infarction, speed can be a critical factor. Of note, it was unusual at the time for a nurse on an ambulance rig to use cardioactive medication without physician supervision, an innovation prefiguring the paramedic movement of the late 1960s (copyright 1942 Eveready Battery Company, Inc., St. Louis, Missouri).

and all can be downloaded at the end of the shift for evaluation. Even lower tech products, like windshield-mounted video cameras, have demonstrated an ability to reduce accident rates. Illustrating the kinds of gains in safety that can be achieved by combining better training with electronic chaperones, LifeCare Ambulance, of Battle Creek, Michigan, stresses "low-force" driving, includes driver mentoring during the probation period, and puts a "black box" on every ambulance: in the program's first five years company drivers covered three million miles without a single serious injury.[26]

Much has changed in the world of emergency services since the Portland Police Bureau urged that ambulance horses not exceed a canter except in the direst emergencies, and the New York Hospital Council warned chauffeurs that driving the new automotive ambulances in excess of fifteen miles per hour was presumptively reckless.[27] While police and fire ambulances drew from traditions of formal and informal training in what we would now call "defensive" driving, the private sector had less incentive to incur more costs for additional schooling for its drivers, and lawmakers responded by denying such ambulances the immunity from traffic ordinances that would otherwise be their due. Now the young profession has matured to the point where most improvements and innovations are coming from its own self-policing and enlightened self-interest. Historically the incentive for our recent driver standards came from withholding federal highway dollars from states that did not enforce new, rigorous standards for ambulance service. With standards came professionalism, and Senator Grenfell's part-time

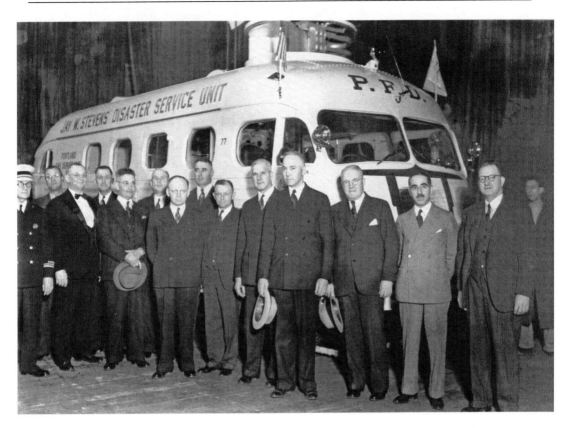

The Jay W. Stevens Disaster Unit, built in 1939 for the Fire Department of Portland, Oregon, was the first civilian mobile hospital/rescue response center of its kind. It was donated to the city by Aaron Frank, second from right (courtesy Portland Fire and Rescue and the Portland Fire Museum Collection).

hot-rodders followed Dr. Goler's impetuous wagon drivers onto an historical off-ramp. With them passed the former dichotomy between private and public ambulances relative to the traffic laws, as now ambulance pilots are trained to their jobs and share the privilege to speed with the other emergency first responders, the firefighters and police. The question of *when* speed and aggressive ambulance driving are appropriate, however, is still much with us, and it is unlikely that the debate will ever be gaveled closed. There will always be the need for rapid transport of the most critically ill, just as there will always be the temptation to star in a drama of one's design so long as human beings can thrill to speed—and dream of the glorious achievement of saving a human life by virtue of reflexes, nerve, and a responsive machine tearing down a boulevard on a sled of wailing siren screams.

• 11 •

Specialty Squads and Disaster Cars

The ambulance can be said to have been born twice: once as the creaking wagon of Queen Isabella's time, designed simply to collect the fallen and haul them off the battlefield, and again as Larrey's ideal of a miniature hospital providing medical care en route. In its various civilian incarnations the earliest ambulances oscillated between the two visions: most ambulances in most places for most of the time were "scoop and go" operations whose minimally trained attendants valued speed because that was all they had to offer, outside of a warm blanket and a reassuring word. Periodically there erupted on the scene stunning repudiations of these simple vehicles, elaborate "disaster cars" spilling out teams of specially trained medics or combining heavy-rescue with first-aid. While such pioneering vehicles and crews prefigured today's paramedic and rescue squad ambulances, they often labored in such obscurity that the ultimate success of their innovations depended more on reinvention than adoption. These proud ambulances were born in the smoking pits of collapsed mines and crawled up from the reeking trenches of World War I; they rolled out of police precincts, fire stations, and, in one notable case, the show-windows of a West Coast department store.

War Wagons and Mine Cars

As was so often the case, innovation in emergency medicine was the harvest of combat. The Great War was only a few months old when an article in the September 1914 *Scientific American* described a new French "Motor Hospital."[1] Built on a panel truck chassis, this specialty ambulance was outfitted with miniature operating theater complete with X-ray machine to localize shrapnel and a motorized trepanning instrument to quickly open the skull. It carried little water, intending (perhaps over-optimistically) to rely on an ultraviolet sterilizer to purify what would be drawn from streams and standing pools with an electric pump. Later, in 1917, the British Joint War Committee unveiled its latest take on the ambulance: a two patient aid car with sound-proof paneling and exhaust pipes carried under the beds to warm patients. These additional comforts made this vehicle "more like a ward on wheels than anything which has yet been attempted in a motor ambulance" according to enthusiastic reviewers.[2] In the United States perhaps the first vehicles dramatically altering the scope of care offered by an ambulance and crew were designed by the Bureau of Mines, a government agency facing a casualty problem the equal of many militaries. Indeed, when Congress created it in 1910 the bureau was faced with over two thousand mining deaths annually—a slaughter unchecked by feckless state governments incapable of challenging a lucrative industry presided over by mining lords like the Guggenheims and the Rockefellers who, in turn, seemed immune to the suffering of men whose lives were being snuffed out to feed their avarice. Without recourse in the law or any claim on the moral sense of their absentee landlords, miners were forced to strike

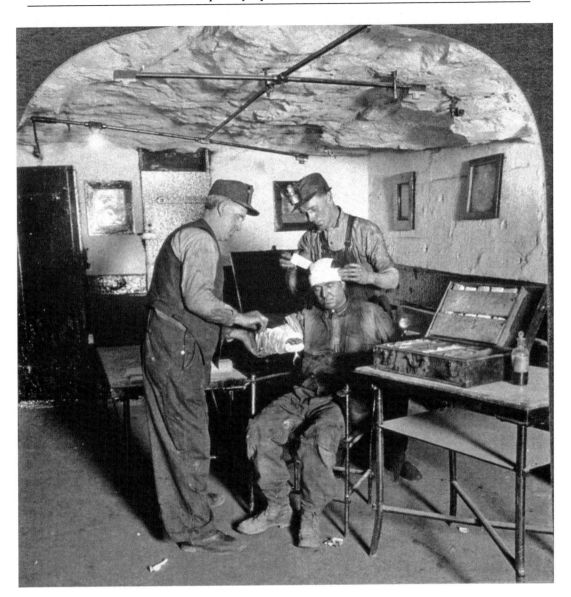

A small emergency hospital is carved into the rock in a Pennsylvania coal mine, circa 1915. In the early 20th century the dangers of mine work inspired medical innovations that significantly influenced ambulance development above ground (Keystone View Company; Library of Congress Prints and Photographs Division, LC-USZC2-6215).

for better conditions, leading to shutdowns, lost profits, and civil unrest. Such was the setting in which the bureau was given the job of improving safety practices, largely in hopes of placating the miners and making the industry peaceful as well as profitable. Even as the bureau set to work, however, the death toll kept rising, especially when the owners demonstrated a willingness to kill striking men above the ground as well as working men below it. Matters reached a head with 1914's "Ludlow Massacre," when a tent city of striking miners was raided by the Montana National Guard and twenty men, women, and children were shot and burned to death.

Shortly after the Ludlow incident the Bureau of Mines put on a very public display of the

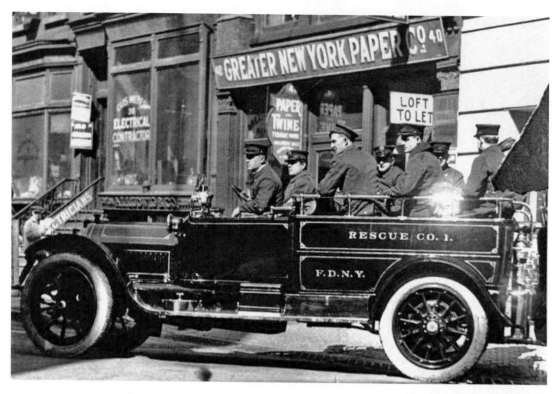

New York City's Rescue 1, formed in 1915, was an early example of how fire departments adopted advanced rescue and medical functions after the turn of the century (courtesy the Fire Department of New York City).

kind of improved ambulance it hoped would help appease the irate miners and bring a measure of calm to the industry. The setting was the Rescue Display at the 1915 Panama-Pacific Exposition, where the Palace of Mines and Minerals included a mini-excavation specifically designed to showcase a stunning new emergency ambulance and its equipment. Twice a day this government crafted "especially designed motor car" rushed across the exhibit grounds in response to an alarm from the mock mine site.[3] In photographs it appears as an oversized truck body on a heavy chassis, with curtained panels and tiered stretchers, and in addition to standard first-aid equipment the "disaster car" contained self-contained breathing apparatus with goggle masks and built in radio equipment.[4] These ingenious transmitters featured a throat microphone held tightly over the wearer's larynx to transmit speech, via a wire unspooled behind the crew, by the vibrations of the throat. The breathing apparatus was demonstrated to Exposition crowds by placing wearers inside a glass cubicle filled with smoke and toxic vapors, and also by projections from the depths of the artificial mine itself, beneath the floor. In time, these technologies would be exported far beyond the mines, most notably to fire department emergency squads who faced similarly dangerous fumes while battling blazes.

Fire Department Ambulances and Volunteer Rescue Squads

Ambulance creativity was not confined to the men who moiled for ore, as by the early 20th century independent "rescue squads" began appearing. Amongst the nation's occupations the fire-fighters found themselves most frequently deployed into the midst of dangerous and toxic environments: chemical manufacturing was becoming more prevalent (in one notorious instance, a dozen Milwaukee fire-fighters died in 1913 after inhaling arsenic fumes at a chemical works fire); growing cities were increasingly dependent on cold storage plants to keep perishable food stocks for their populace, plants that depended on dangerous refrigeration systems involving high pressure ammonia; and subway tunnels and building excavation sites were getting deeper as technology improved, making cave-ins and fires ever more lethal.[5] In each case the potential for disaster was omnipresent, and the city desk seldom had long to wait for some new horror filled headline to pump circulation. In response, fire departments across the country began considering how improved rescue techniques and better on-site medical care would improve a firefighter's chance of survival when confronted by deadly ammonia leaks, suffocating smoke, or the danger of a cave-in.

One of the first agencies to organize and deploy a rescue squad with special training and equipment for such emergencies was the New York City Fire Department. Called Rescue Squad 1, it was built around a particular piece of technology, the smoke helmet—literally a flameproof, self-contained breathing apparatus, a fiery counterpart to the aqualung popularized by Jacques Cousteau decades later. While smoke filters and breathing apparatus specifically for firemen had been patented since at least the mid–1880s, it wasn't until the early 1900s that they became reliable enough to be broadly adopted by European fire fighters, and New York City

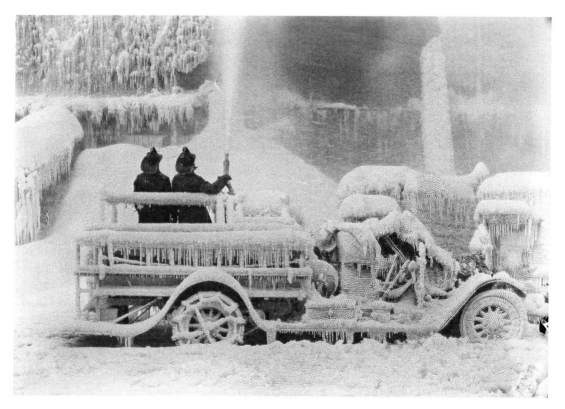

A 1927 fire at a cold storage plant in Rochester, New York, resulted in a deadly ammonia leak (the ice was created by the rapidly condensing fumes). Increasing numbers of industrial accidents made improved breathing apparatus, medical gear, and well-equipped ambulances necessary equipment for modern fire departments. (The rippled pattern is an artifact of the emulsion separating from the photographic plate.) (From the Albert R. Stone Negative Collection, Rochester Museum & Science Center Rochester, N.Y.)

Fire Commissioner Robert Admanson was sufficiently impressed with their performance overseas to commit, in 1914, to the creation of his own squad of "smoke eaters."[6] With final preparations complete by the end of the year, training for nine picked men started January 1915, and the new squad reported for duty to Engine 33 on Great Jones Street in March. The helmets the men relied on were similar to a diver's rig, with oxygen cylinders rated to provide eighty minutes of air at two liters per minute (sixty minutes on the dial, with an emergency reserve of twenty minutes for the tardy). In order to test the equipment's effectiveness the squad's captain, John J. McElligott, put himself in a concrete cell at the Firemen's College along with a smoldering pyre of excelsior, straw, old rope, rubbish, and plenty of sulfur.[7] The door was slammed shut and for sixty minutes he endured temperatures up to 280 degrees Fahrenheit, enveloping smoke, and toxic fumes that rotted his clothes till the rags sluiced off in the runnels of sweat pouring from his soot grimed skin. After an hour the door was pulled open: the helmet, and the captain, had passed their first test.

The squad started operations with a special motor car equipped with a Blaugas cutting torch, pulmotors to revive the nearly asphyxiated, stretchers, a life-gun, extinguishers, fire axes, asbestos gloves, and their elaborate Draeger smoke helmets.[8] The success of the program was immediate, as by September their unique apparatus had been instrumental in containing a factory fire poisoned with arsenic fumes, an explosion at a cooling plant that sent a toxic cloud of ammonia boiling into a city street, and a deadly leak of sulfuric chloride gas at a rubber company in midtown Manhattan, the oily yellow miasma spreading like ground fog throughout the building and sending the first firefighters on the scene reeling into the street gasping and clutching their throats.[9] While the Rescue 1 truck was not intended for ambulance use, the team foretold the future of fire department emergency squads with their combination of advanced equipment and basic medical training. The squad got a less hazardous chance to demonstrate their prowess at the Fire Department's Fiftieth Anniversary celebration in June 1915, as a large crowd watched a crew wade into the pall of smoke billowing from a mock tenement house, relaying their progress to the fire captain via an umbilical radio wire strung out behind them and ultimately carrying out a smoke inhalation "victim" on a stretcher and reviving him with a pulmotor.[10] As was often the case, the team was assisted at the scene by a departmental Fire Surgeon, but as their training and expertise increased over the years the attendance of such surgeons became increasingly rare, until they were ultimately supplanted by fire fighters cross-trained as emergency medical technicians.

A similar development was taking place in rural areas, with more immediate impact on the trajectory of ambulance services in America. Outside of the cities increasing numbers of volunteer rescue squads began appearing in the late 1920s, such teams frequently equipping themselves to retrieve the injured as well as transport them, since they might be the only emergency provider on the scene if the sole sheriff's deputy on duty was patrolling a distant area of the county or the volunteer fire department lacked a trained ambulance crew. The earliest of these volunteer rescue squads was the Belmar (New Jersey) Rescue and First Aid Squad, inaugurated in 1927 by a former army ambulance driver named Charles Measure.[11] His military experience, work as a volunteer fire-fighter, and training in first aid as part of a safety program at the power plant where he worked all combined in a scheme to train volunteers to provide top-flight emergency medical care—and to bring a measure of safety to the "lusty first aid game as practiced by willing but ignorant hands," in the words of an early news story.[12] (Some accounts suggest the original impetus behind Measure's idea was a local policeman who almost bled to death after breaking out a window to escape a burning building, a medical emergency the untrained volunteer fire crew struggled to manage until a passerby stepped in and properly bandaged the wound.)[13] Initially called the Firemen's First Aid and Safety Squad, the volunteer crew started first aid training sometime in 1927 under the guidance of Dr. Daniel Traverso, and

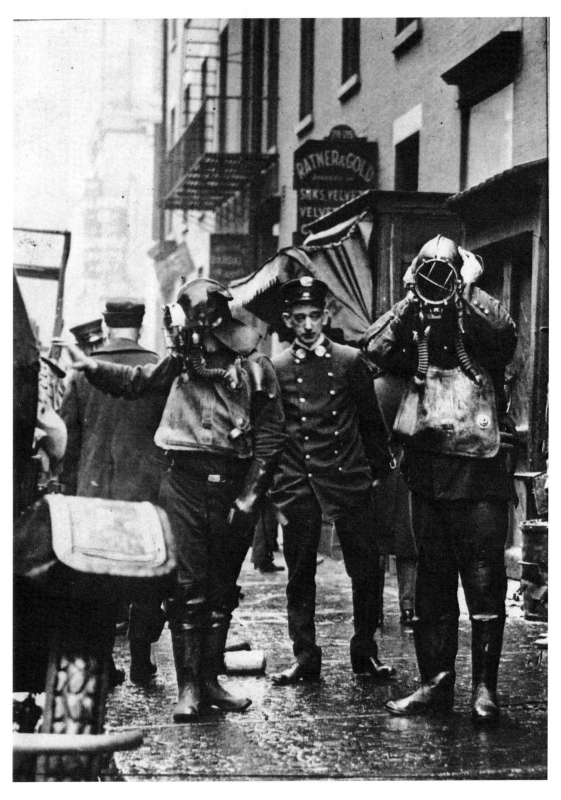

Steel helmeted salamanders: New York Fire Department Rescue 1 crew members in standard uniform and full rescue kit, including Draeger smoke helmets, in Manhattan around 1916 (courtesy the Fire Department of New York City).

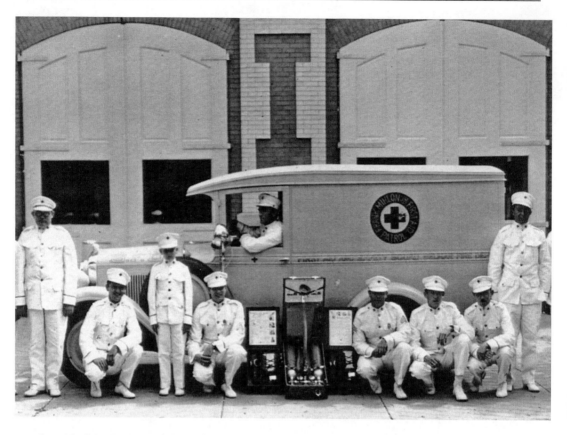

Several of the Belmar First Aid and Safety Squad members outside their old headquarters in 1928 show off their new dress uniforms. The young man in the center is Frank Mihon, Jr., who donated his birthday money towards the purchase of the squad's first ambulance (courtesy the Belmar First Aid Squad).

acquired its first ambulance prior to March 1928 with a donation from local businessman Frank Milhon, Sr. (whose thirteen year old son volunteered his birthday present money for the cause).[14] Within a few years the gold cross of the Belmar ambulances had been adopted by aid squads across New Jersey, leading to their affiliation as the New Jersey First Aid Council in 1929, with Measure as president, and by 1941 Gold Cross ambulances and rescue societies had been established from Minnesota to Rhode Island.[15]

Another profoundly influential organization was Virginia's Roanoke Life Saving and First Aid Crew, formed in 1928 by Julian Wise (although it is likely that the ex-lifeguard was supervising drills in water rescue in 1927).[16] When he was a boy, in 1909, Wise had watched helplessly as two men capsized their canoe on the Roanoke River. Bystanders ran to the water's edge and heaved tree branches towards the struggling figures, but after a few minutes the exhausted, panic-stricken men sank beneath the waters and were drowned.[17] This terrible sight haunted Julian Wise for the rest of his life, and the image of two men futilely fighting for their lives in open water, within sight but beyond help, was the inspiration for what would become his life's work. In 1927 he had just returned to Roanoke, Virginia, gotten married, and taken a job as a clerk for the Norfolk and Western Railroad, but amidst the welter and the work of establishing a new life the young newlywed felt the spell of the long ago drowning in the river that ran just outside the town, and he decided to put his plan into action. By 1928 he had formally organized nine other railroadmen into a "Life Saving Crew" (later the Roanoke Life Sav-

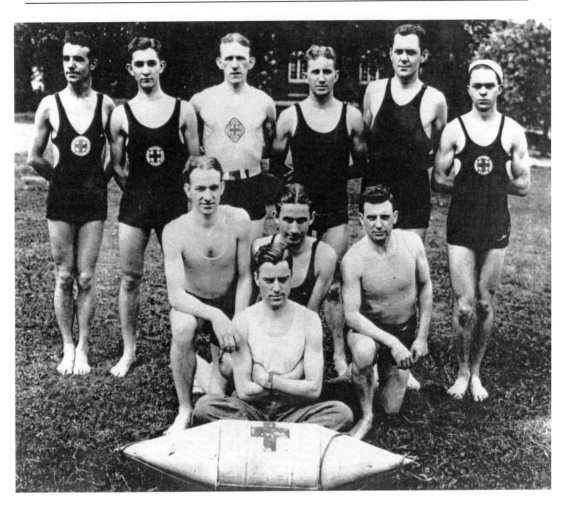

In keeping with the drowning deaths that inspired its creation, the Roanoke Life Saving Crew was well trained in water rescue. Here, Julian Wise (third from left) poses with early members of what was then called the "Life Saving Corps, R.N.C." Such lifeguard training apparently preceded the formal debut of his rescue squad by several months (courtesy "To The Rescue Museum," Roanoke, Virginia).

ing and First Aid Crew) and advertised their services to the town: anyone needing the squad telephoned the railroad's chief clerk, who rounded up available crew members and sent them flying in a Reo truck outfitted with a variety of rescue gear and the crew's official medical kit— a three dollar tackle box containing smelling salts, a poison ivy antidote, some topical bactericide, and an assortment of other basic supplies.[18] (Notably, the quantity of rescue materials packed into the rig prevented its use as an ambulance, and for some time the squad relied on local mortuaries to transport patients to the hospital.) Word was slow to get out (in the first year the squad was only dispatched six times), but it gradually built a name for itself, and by 1934 its first protégé appeared when the Lynchburg (Virginia) Volunteer Life Saving and First Aid Crew incorporated itself and accepted delivery of a second hand rig from the Roanoke crew as their first ambulance. Other squads soon followed, each successful imitator creating its own ripple effect, inspiring yet more neighboring communities to form their own combination rescue and first aid squads, usually with some attendant ambulance service as well.

The obvious question is *why* did so many small communities develop rescue squads in the

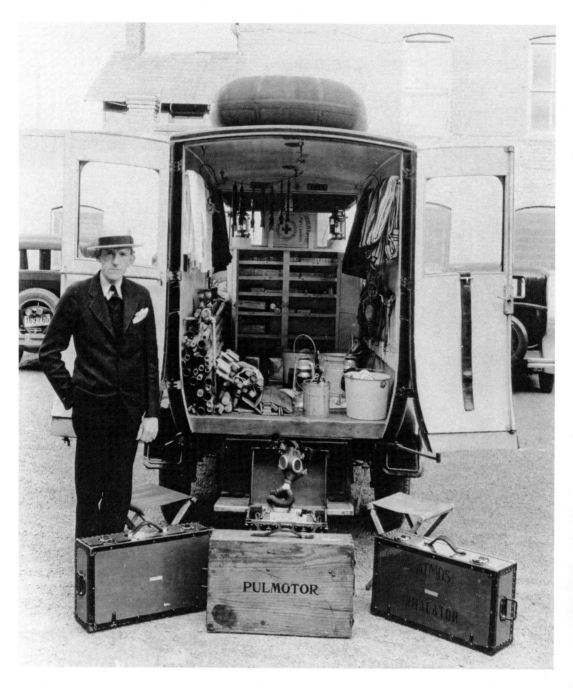

In a later photograph, Mr. Wise stands beside a well-equipped rescue van, complete with stretchers, grappling hooks, inhalators, and a variety of medical supplies. Mr. Wise went on to found the Virginia Association of Volunteer Rescue Squads in 1935 and helped establish the International First Aid and Rescue Association in 1948, later serving as its second president (courtesy "To The Rescue Museum," Roanoke, Virginia).

1920s? First, there was the evangelizing of the movement's pioneers, especially Julian Wise, who tirelessly promoted the idea of well-trained mobile rescue squads with lectures and personal visits from coast to coast, a campaign creating ever more successful models to propagate his cause by example. Secondly, the end of the First World War sent home many doughboys who had served on ambulance crews in France, and, as had happened to their grandfathers in the Civil War, many of these veterans saw a need to bring this military technology back to their towns and cities. In an early example of this process, eighteen members of Delaware's American Legion Post No. 14 in Smyrna formed an ambulance corps in 1924.[19] (Unlike later outfits forming in Belmar and Roanoke, this American Legion ambulance was not a rescue squad, but was designed to transfer the seriously ill to distant hospitals with speed and comfort, in lieu of the prevailing practice of taking them to the depot and waiting for the next available train to deliver them to a well equipped infirmary in Dover, twelve miles south, or Wilmington, thirty miles north, depending on both the severity of their condition and the direction of travel of the first train to stop.) Finally, this was simply the historical moment when second-hand ambulances began entering the retail market in sufficient numbers to guarantee low prices and easy availability. After all, the used "disaster car" market could only exist five to ten years after the first wave of mass-produced ambulances, which had occurred during the late teens and early twenties. Taken together these factors explain the timing with which volunteer and small ambulance services began appearing all around the country, from Virginia to Coney Island, from the Midwest to the Pacific coast.

In the larger cities the trend was slower to develop, most likely because by the 1920s the typical American metropolis was well-stocked with hospitals, police departments, and private concerns going fender to fender to provide ambulance services. Such operations were not always satisfactory, however, particularly since few ambulances of the era were routinely equipped with oxygen tanks or resuscitators and so were ill equipped to deal with the effects of smoke inhalation, by far the most common fire-associated injury. The natural response of many fire departments was to start fielding their own ambulances especially equipped for respiratory support, an effort supplementing the recovery-oriented rescue squads pioneered by New York's Rescue 1. (Practically speaking, fire bureaus had always had an incentive to guarantee effective medical care for their own crews, of course, with fire surgeons long a fixture of many departments, and ambulances appearing in fire department fleets from the late 19th century, but this augmentation took on new speed in the 1920s.)[20] The excellence and profession-

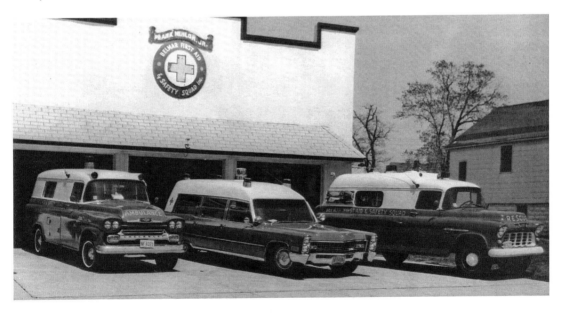

The Belmar First Aid Squad was started in 1927 as part of the local volunteer fire department. By the early 1970s their ambulance fleet included two Chevrolet panel trucks and a 1968 Cadillac hearse-style ambulance (courtesy the Belmar First Aid Squad).

alism of these fire department ambulances in general, and their particular expertise with pulmotors and other respiratory aids, frequently made them the provider of choice for local physicians or the police and often resulted in their services being made available community-wide. An astonishing example of how dependent physicians were on these lay providers is an event that occurred at Johns Hopkins in the early 1920s. Then, as now, Hopkins was synonymous with elite medical care, and its clinical staff would have been the first to tell you so. Nonetheless, a physician recalls being in the operating theater during a urological procedure when the anesthesiologist looked up and told the surgeon that the patient's pulse had stopped and their blood pressure was not palpable: the surgeon coolly peeled off his gloves, turned his back on the patient, walked over to the telephone, and proceeded to call the fire department.[21] After explaining the crisis he hung up the receiver and everyone—surgeon, attending physicians, nurses—stood around feeling gloomy for the next fifteen minutes until the firefighters burst through the doors lugging their resuscitation equipment and fell to work on the cooling body, pumping oxygen into the lungs with their pulmotor for several minutes before giving it up as hopeless. While today surgeons are now trained at least as well as firefighters in resuscitation methods, we are living with the natural evolution of these early rescue squads and the majority of calls made to fire departments are for EMS services.

Rose City Rescue

A particularly lustrous example of how a fire bureau augmented its historical mission by adding emergency medical service occurred in Portland, Oregon, during the height of the Depression, when a gift to the fire department ignited a statewide revolution in civilian emergency response. It started in 1933 when fourteen businessmen in "The Rose City" formed a committee to raise $8,000 by public subscription to buy and equip a modern disaster car, which they donated to the Portland Fire Bureau for the exclusive benefit of, in their words, "this group of public employees who are engaged in a very hazardous service."[22] Since 1924 the department's first aid apparatus had been a squad truck with some first aid equipment tucked in amidst the chemical fire retardants and rescue gear, but the committee invested its capital into a 1932 Lincoln sedan that was then re-engineered into what its sponsors believed was the finest emergency ambulance in the country, with its specially built trunk and interior cabinets bursting with a complete surgical kit and a miniature pharmacy of prescription medications (for use by any physicians who happened to be on hand), a full set of first aid materials, a combination inhalator and resuscitator, ambulance cot, chemical hot pads, canteens, grappling hooks, sledgehammers, crowbars, chisels, gas masks, tannic acid spray for burns, disinfectants, everything that could wished for to rescue, relieve, or revive.[23] The car was lacquered over in a brilliant red, souped up with a 100 horsepower engine promising a top speed of ninety miles an hour, and christened "The George Baker Emergency Car" in honor of the popular Portland mayor who was retiring that year after sixteen years in office. The new ambulance was officially given to the fire department at a gala celebration on Portland's Jantzen Beach, June 30, 1933, in a ceremony that included a demonstration of the crew's resuscitation skills with a staged rescue of a swimmer dragged out of the Columbia River and restored to life for the delight and edification of the assembled throngs.[24]

While the original intent may have to been provide first aid to firemen, the crew made itself immediately available to the general public, and by 1935 it averaged 350 cases a year—including, in the reckoning of the aid car's skipper, Captain Fred Roberts, heart attacks, pneumonia, infantile paralysis, drowning, electric shocks, carbon monoxide poisoning, "all types of suicides," auto accidents, and struggling newborns.[25] Had the Baker Emergency Car confined

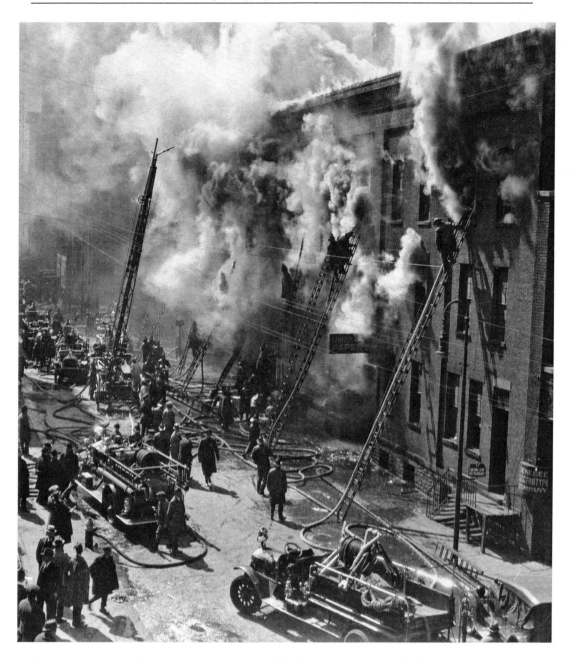

The perilous nature of fire-fighting, as with this 1924 blaze at the Lawless Paper Company, inspired departments to invest heavily in emergency medical equipment for the benefit of their crews (from the Albert R. Stone Negative Collection, Rochester Museum & Science Center Rochester, N.Y.).

itself to Portland it would have repaid the investment of its philanthropic patrons many times over, but just as the sight of Union Army ambulances darting through city streets in the 19th century had educated the public about the utility of ambulances, so the Baker Emergency Car achieved similar results by undertaking a summer barnstorming tour of Oregon in 1935. The tour was initiated by Governor Martin, who had just formed a state "First Aid Committee" to encourage duplication of the Baker Car in a minimum of fifteen Oregon towns and cities. The

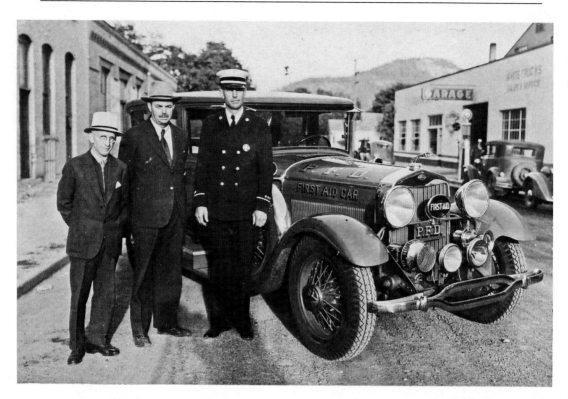

Captain Fred Roberts with town leaders in Grants Pass pose alongside the George Baker First Aid Car on its tour of Oregon cities in 1935 (courtesy Portland Fire and Rescue and the Portland Fire Museum Collection).

governor was not only impressed by the admirable record of the Portland squad, he was appalled to discover that in the entire state of Oregon there were only five inhalator units in use, and a single certified oxygen instructor—Captain Roberts. Meanwhile, Washington State had more than 200 such devices in operation and California boasted at least 400 of its own (and further claimed that this equipment could be delivered to any citizen in the state within twenty-minutes, something that Oregon couldn't begin to approach—even with the ninety-mile an hour Baker car to deliver the equipment).[26] Even allowing for differences in population size, it was clear that, outside of the Rose City, Oregon was making a poor showing relative to the neighbors when it came to providing emergency medical service for her citizens.

Accordingly, Captain Roberts was asked to drive the vermillion mercy car up, down, and across the state in an effort to inspire local townships to replicate its services. In a summer tour that took him from the sands of Seaside to the Grand Ronde valley in eastern Oregon, it was estimated that thirty thousand people had a chance to admire Portland's rescue car at over a hundred public appearances at fair grounds, skating rinks, library lawns, and fire stations: among the throngs meticulously recorded by the Fire Bureau's hard working public relations department were 508 doctors, 187 nurses, and over 500 Oregon firemen—as well as one newborn at Klamath Falls who was given four hours of oxygen resuscitation in an unplanned field trial.[27] In all, the Baker Car visited twenty-six towns, and within a month twenty-three of them were raising funds to acquire their own first aid cars—pulp and paper mill workers outside Salem agreed to donate fifty cents each towards their local campaign, the Baker Elks Lodge staged a circus to kick off their fund raising rally, and everywhere city councils looked hard at their budgets for the funds to purchase an inhalator or a used ambu-

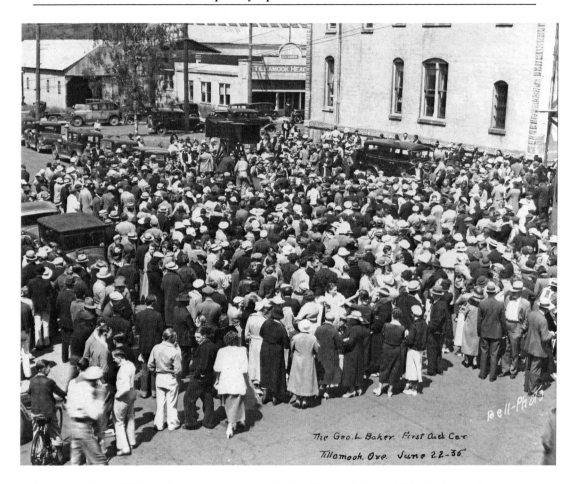

Crowds gather in Tillamook, Oregon, to see the Baker First Aid Car in 1935. In all, the demonstration tour reached twenty-six towns and cities, and twenty-three of them were inspired to acquire new ambulances as a result (courtesy Portland Fire and Rescue and the Portland Fire Museum Collection).

lance of their own.[28] Even as Portland's smaller rivals raced to keep up, however, the city was on the verge of taking an unprecedented stride over the very horizon of ambulance possibilities: in 1939 the Baker Emergency Car was going to be eclipsed by the debut of the Fire Bureau's massive "Coffee Wagon," an ambulance demonstrating the fantastic future of emergency response vehicles.

This successor to the Baker car was a bus-sized behemoth whose $30,000 cost (over $400,000 in 2007 dollars) was carried by mercantile king Aaron Frank, son of the co-founder of Meier and Frank, the Portland department store fixture. Mr. Frank, a gifted amateur mechanic, had been favorably impressed by the 1933 George Baker Emergency Car, but he envisioned a greater, even gargantuan, version of that ambulance — a colossus of mercy that could face down any emergency.[29] The result of his scheming was a modified bus christened the "Jay W. Stevens Disaster Service Unit" in honor of a friend and former fire-marshal. Nicknamed "the Coffee-Wagon" for its resemblance to a mobile diner, it was the first civilian all-in-one disaster unit of its kind, a radical expansion of the ambulance that has never been surpassed.[30] The colossus made its public debut on March 25, 1939, when the curtains of the Municipal Auditorium parted and the Disaster Service Unit was there on the stage for the assembled thousands to

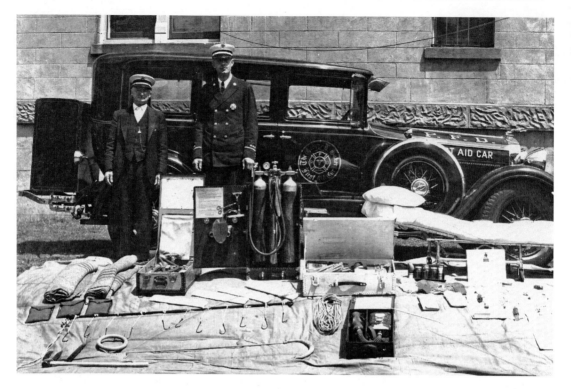

Captain Roberts and a town official in Tillamook, Oregon, pose next to some of the Baker First Aid Car's equipment. In addition to first aid and rescue supplies, it also carried a complete surgical kit and a medicine chest for use by physicians.

gape at. Among the crowd was a modest Aaron Frank, who wasn't interested in accolades or public applause—unfortunately for him, several enthusiastic members of the Portland Fire Department were nearby and, amidst cheers, they seized hold of Frank and carried him kicking and screaming into the spotlight on center stage.[31]

Without question, Frank and his Disaster Unit deserved all the applause they received that night. He had given the city a vehicle whose portable power plants could generate sufficient electricity to restore lighting to a good sized office building and which were hooked up to a range of electronic marvels, including floodlights burning enough candle-power to illuminate an entire village, a long-range public address system audible two miles away, and a miniature radio station that sent and received messages from the specially equipped gas and smoke helmets worn by its rescue and fire-fighting squads: in addition, it was equipped as a complete emergency hospital with resources for surgery and could transport seven patients at a time.[32] It had a predictably overwhelming effect on a city whose previous conception of an ambulance was a stock hearse or a comfortable looking sedan with a cot in the back and an oxygen tank. One awestruck local reporter who stepped inside the white bus with the red highlights over the wheel-wells found himself staring at a "multiplicity of mechanical miracles which [will] probably remind you of an artist's conception of a world of the future."[33]

In addition to its miniature surgery suite the Disaster Unit had a bevy of heavy rescue equipment and enough tackle to open a hardware store, and so, according to a brochure put out by the Portland Bureau of Fire, it was admirably equipped to handle "not only fire, but all such disasters as train wrecks, plane crashes, [the] collapse of tall buildings, bridges or elevators; shipwrecks, highway disasters, snow slides, earth slides, floods, jail breaks, riots, epi-

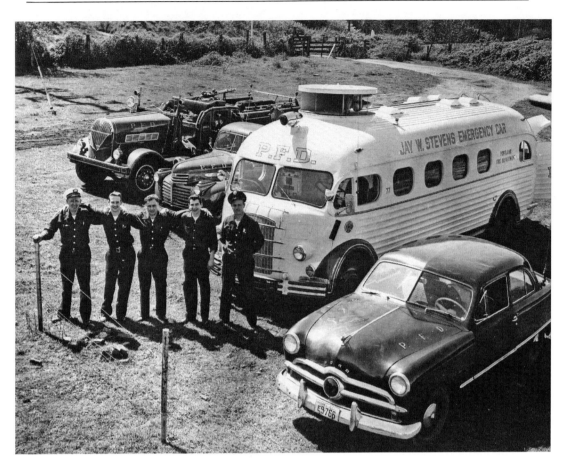

Roy Love, Jeff Morris, Jim Tyrell, Ron Raschio, and an unidentified firefighter pose with some of the Portland Fire Bureau's apparatus in the 1940s, after the Disaster Unit had been renamed the "Emergency Car" (courtesy Portland Fire and Rescue and the Portland Fire Museum Collection).

demics, explosions, mine or tunnel disasters, storms" or any other emergency that might make headlines in the Rose City.[34] Fortunately for the citizens of Portland the Stevens Disaster Car (as it was later called) was generally called out for less catastrophic emergencies, such as house fires and auto accidents. It was also sent out to major incidents occurring well outside the city limits when its special services were required, as with the time in 1952 when it responded to a collision between a Mercury sedan and a logging truck jack-knifed athwart a highway some thirty miles from Portland: the resulting fireball killed two men and injured three women, and, in a macabre detail, it was noted that a Thanksgiving turkey sitting in the back seat of the sedan had been burned black.[35] Aaron Frank died in 1968, but his "Coffee Wagon" stayed on duty, not being inventoried into a city warehouse for storage until May 9, 1972: by then it had been in operation for almost thirty-three years and had logged over 48,000 miles, certainly earning it a place in some Vehicular Valhalla.[36]

Widely discussed in the press of the day, the Stevens Disaster Unit had many imitators, especially in the post-war years when a rising economy and newly unfettered manufacturing plants fueled a flood of new products. In the Eisenhower era of huge cars and fascination with scientific progress, such hyper-technical, all-in-one disaster units were a compelling article, and both large cities and small-town rescue squads invested in them. Ultimately, however, they proved impractical for most services — for example, while it was true that a super-rig could

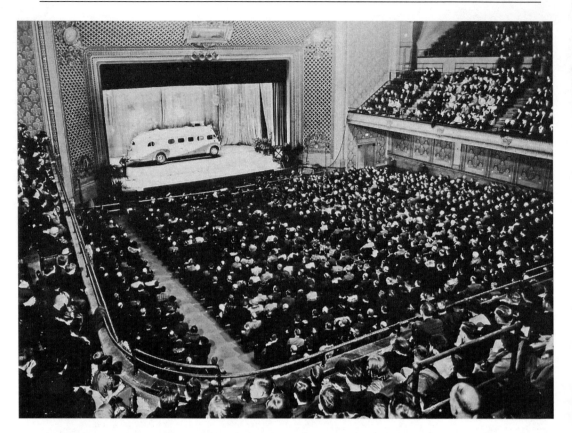

Thousands came to the Municipal Auditorium on Saturday night, March 25, 1939, to see a public demonstration of the new Jay W. Stevens Disaster Unit (courtesy Portland Fire and Rescue and the Portland Fire Museum Collection).

provide the tools to light up an accident scene and extricate victims from the tangled wreckage of a car crash, once the bodies were free the crew faced a dilemma: leave all the tools on the pavement and drive away with the patients, or let them wait in the back while all the gear was gathered up and stowed before taking off for the hospital. In addition, prior to the late 1960s there was no accepted curriculum to train non-physicians in advanced medical service, so often the mega-ambulances rolled out with a crew holding Red Cross First Aid Cards and sitting in the middle of a small surgical theater surrounded by specialized equipment they couldn't use (cost was also an issue, as replacement parts were more expensive for a vehicle the size of a bus than they would be for a sedan-sized ambulance). By the early 1960s few of the super-ambulances had survived, having given way to "modular" response squads consisting of separate vehicles for patient transport and heavy rescue.

Perhaps nowhere was this evolution realized in a more dramatic fashion than New York City, the metropolis that, fittingly, started our ambulance revolution in 1869. It was just two years after the "Coffee Wagon" made its first appearance that Manhattan caught up with Portland when Mayor La Guardia, after a visit to Oregon, enthusiastically welcomed his own "Super Truck" to the city police armamentarium in 1941.[37] Physically similar to the Jay W. Stevens Disaster Unit, the new rig likewise carried its own generator to power the obligatory floodlights and was fully equipped as an ambulance, field hospital, and disaster command center. A news photo showed a vehicle that was nearly a dead-ringer for Portland's Coffee-Wagon, although perhaps a foot or three shorter and without the flame-red highlights.[38] Impressive as

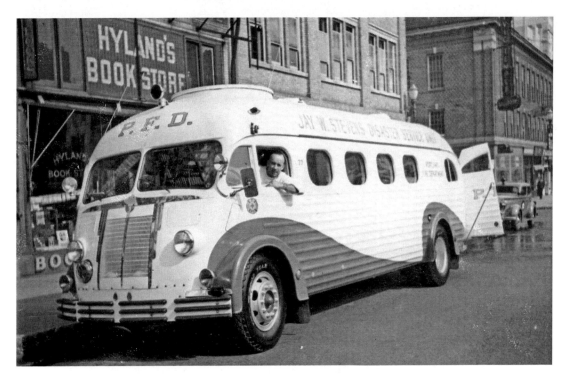

The first civilian ambulance of its kind, the Jay W. Stevens Disaster Unit was over twenty-nine feet long, almost ten feet high, and its locally designed roof-top loudspeaker could transmit intelligible speech two miles in all directions. Receiving national attention, the unit inspired many imitators, breaking ground for today's heavy-rescue response teams (courtesy Portland Fire and Rescue and the Portland Fire Museum Collection).

it was, this new disaster truck was only the latest member of a storied New York rescue squad whose scope of services foretold the heavy-rescue paramedic teams of the 1960s — and beat them to it by forty years. Its history follows the entire trajectory of the super-ambulances, while also prefiguring the revolution in training and equipment that marked the beginning of the age of the paramedic and the emergency medical technician. While almost anonymous today outside of New York City, this police rescue squad had its own television special a decade before Jack Webb's *Emergency!* introduced paramedic services to America, pioneered modern emergency response techniques at a time when horse drawn wagons were still seen on city streets, and after eighty years is still setting the pace for emergency services in the city where it all began.

Emergency Service Division: Going Like Gangbusters since 1925

"People always are getting into unusual situations. If the cop on the beat can't handle it, out we roll."
    — Deputy Chief Inspector McKenna, Emergency Service Division, 1949.[39]

From the first stretchers tossed into the back of a horse-drawn paddy wagon and the earliest first-aid courses taught by dedicated police surgeons, American law enforcement demon-

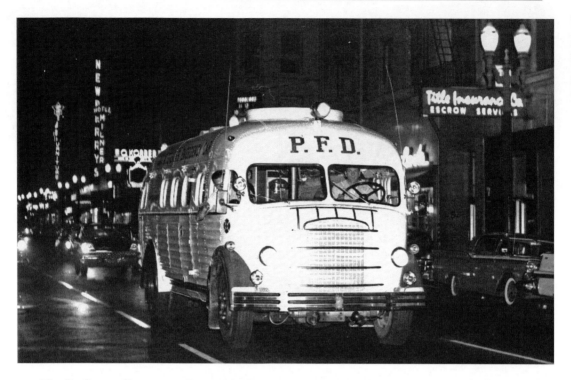

The Jay Stevens Emergency Car sprints through a sweltering summer night in Portland, sometime in the 1960s. The mega-ambulance was a reassuring presence until its retirement in 1972 (courtesy Portland Fire and Rescue and the Portland Fire Museum Collection).

strated a willingness not only to participate in local ambulance services, but to seize the wheel and take the lead. Nowhere did the police ambulance accelerate faster or transform itself more thoroughly than in New York City during the height of Prohibition, when a group of officers were brought to together to function as a rescue squad, pulmotor crew, and light infantry, operating out of open trucks designed to answer both as rolling armory and high-speed field hospital. The impetus behind this bold experiment was the realization that the NYPD was already the first responder to every imaginable form of mayhem that the modern city could devise, and by investing in additional training and equipment the police department could substantially enhance the services its officers provided while awaiting the arrival of the ambulance or the fire department.

Influenced by the appearance in 1915 of the Fire Department's Rescue 1 Squad, in 1925 the police department was ready to invest in its own rescue unit and so re-organized the Riot Squad into a Police Emergency Service Squad (in a nod to their predecessors, crewmen got their smoke-helmet training courtesy their counterparts at Rescue 1.)[40] Intended for deployment to major accidents, riots, and the occasional mad-dog killer holed up in a tenement house, the two squads were each budgeted approximately $6,000 worth of equipment, including complete surgical outfits, pulmotors, stretchers, one Thompson sub-machine gun apiece, life lines and rope cannons for water rescues, fire axes, hydraulic jacks, searchlights, firearms, gas helmets, blankets, and "many items of minor importance" (the importance of minor items soon became apparent: by 1949 the squad was using four-thousand thumb-sized corks a year to plug refrigerator coolant leaks).[41] To haul these armamentariums through the streets the city turned to the White Motor Truck Company (descendant of the White Company, a pioneer in steamer ambulances) and purchased two elongated, open topped rigs costing a hefty $14,000 apiece.[42]

Enameled in dark blue and lettered in gold, the emergency trucks could rocket along at up to sixty-miles an hour—"the average gait at which they are expected to travel," according to a reporter who broke the story for *The New York Times*.[43] (One wonders how many times this reporter had driven Manhattan's crowded streets with their pushcarts and the occasional horse wagon, where to maintain a speed of sixty-miles an hour your best bet would be to shove your Stutz-Bearcat roadster off the roof of the Chrysler Building.)

One truck was assigned to cover Manhattan and the Bronx, the other guarded Brooklyn and Queens. Nothing like this had ever been seen before, and their combination of rescue equipment, surgical and medical supplies, and advanced training prefigured modern paramedic rescue squads. Typical of the crewmembers was Walter Klotzback, a six foot, two-hundred pound former pipe-fitter who joined the Riot Squad in 1924 before enlisting with the Emergency Service in 1926.[44] Klotzback and his fellows on the Emergency Service Squad responded to riots, every fire of more than two alarms, and major accidents involving plane crashes, train derailments, or multiple automobiles. They also handled more mundane affairs—with cutting rings off pudgy fingers occupying a surprising amount of time: as then Inspector Klotzback recalled some years later, "Since the E.S.D. came into being we've cut an average of four rings a week off people's fingers. We've cut off thousands, and haven't lost or hurt a patient yet."[45] (Klotzback stayed with the Emergency Service for thirty years, becoming its Commander and earning the sobriquet "Mr. Emergency" before retiring with the rank of assistant chief inspector.)

The small squad was just three years old in December 1928 when New York Mayor Jimmy Walker pulled his old friend Grover Whalen out of the manager's office at Wanamaker's Depart-

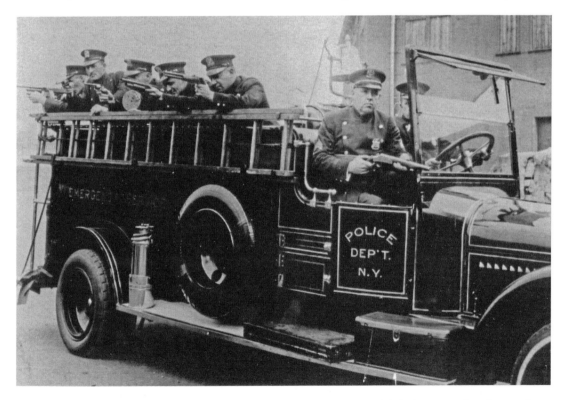

One of the original Emergency Service Trucks, with oxygen tanks and inhalators, various items of rescue equipment, and officers well armed with a Thompson submachine gun, a Remington shotgun, a Winchester rifle, and Smith and Wesson revolvers. (Courtesy Kevin Reynolds. Copyright 2001, New York City Police Department, all rights reserved. Used with permission.)

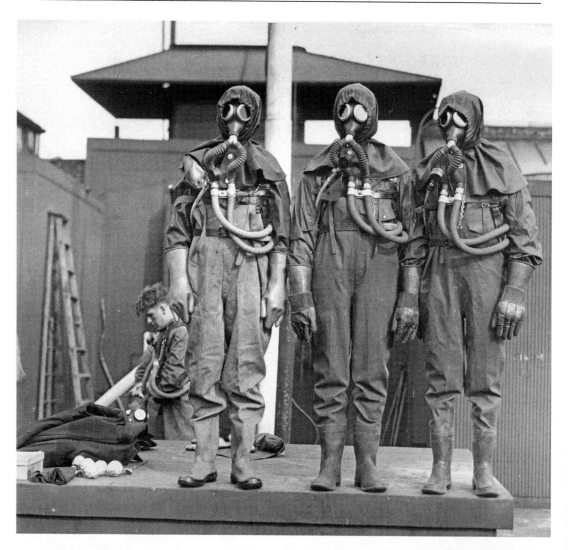

Emergency Division crewmembers Maurice Fitzgerald, John Farrell, and Edward McWilliams in 1932. Their breathing apparatus and protective suits are the sort of special gear that was once limited to fire department rescue squads. Indeed, when the Police Emergency crew was formed they received their initial hazardous atmosphere training from the Fire Department's Rescue 1, formed in 1915. (Copyright 2001, New York City Police Department, all rights reserved. Used with permission.)

ment Store and installed him as the new Police Commissioner. A successful businessman who had dipped in and out of the political scene for a decade, the impeccably dapper Whalen (whose carefully waxed moustache was as geometrically exact as his bespoke suits) would play a crucial role in expanding and promoting the Emergency Services Squad. Of course, Whalen had his work cut out convincing the city that he could manage a segue from supervising floorwalkers to bossing flatfoots, but he was up to it. First, he was savvy enough to tailor his message to his audience: when addressing the city's social and political elite at the dedication of his new police college he tuned his pitch to the key of Dale Carnegie, solemnly telling the tuxedo and mink set that "the police department is a business, having a commodity for sale. That commodity is service."[46] The demimonde got a different broadcast, advertised under his famous slogan "there is plenty of law at the end of a nightstick," a message he tried to deliver to every gangster in the city courtesy strong-arm squads made up of "blackjack wielding huskies," according to a police reporter with the *New York Times*.[47]

Not surprisingly in a man known for his sartorial exactness, he knew the importance of image, and in his first week in office he arranged for a complete remodeling of police headquarters, banishing the stained concrete floors under rich blue carpet and papering over drab walls.[48] Lest anyone mistake flair for frivolity, during his first month in his remodeled offices he made it clear incompetence and underperformance would be rewarded with dismissal, firing patrolmen walking a beat despite being in their sixties, abolishing the Homicide Bureau after discovering that it had made a paltry two arrests in twelve months of police work, and swinging his fountain pen like a fire-axe through the officer's list, discharging or demoting men he felt lacked the competence for their posts, be they a captain or a patrolman.[49] Amidst the remodeling, the Emergency Service Squad was almost certain to capture his attention, reflecting as it did his own solicitude to those in need of society's aid and willingness to use ruthless force against those who made society their prey. It was an innovative program that would interest a man determined to foster and reward innovation, and its service record was enviably productive. By every measure it was a successful operation, and like any sound businessman he set out to expand the franchise: with a single order from the commissioner's desk the two blue trucks of the Emergency Service Squad became a fleet of twenty shamrock green rigs under the banner of the newly created Emergency Services Division. He engineered a corresponding increase in staff by bringing in men from the recently dissolved Machine Gun Squad, a special task force that had cruised the city streets on motorcycles with armored side-cars, smashing breweries and hitting organized crime targets, and drafting men from the four-hundred strong Reserve Squad, whose members had often assisted the fire department at rescue jobs (the same tools that could cut through the steel doors of speakeasies could also extricate civilians trapped amidst the debris of train wrecks or a collapsed building).[50]

Divided into nineteen squads, the twenty trucks and crews of the re-organized Emergency Services Division went on active duty in April 1930: according to the end of the year police report the division was "dedicated to speedy and merciful service in the relief of distress, [and they] saved 533 human lives" in their first nine months of work, and in addition to saving human lives the crews were soon coming to the aid of distressed animals at the rate of two a week, whether it was a horse that had fallen into an excavation or pulling kittens out of trees.[51] Whalen was also keenly interested in improving police training (as with his re-invention of the Police College), and the Emergency Services Division was no exception: crewmembers were given advanced training in first aid and heavy rescue, and, because they were part of the police department during the bloody days of Prohibition, squad members were expected to handle Tommy-guns, lob tear gas bombs and grenades, and be crack-shots with their revolvers. In fact, with their fleet of twenty trucks they were expected to handle any emergency the metropolis could conceive of. Whalen's replacement, Police Commissioner Edward Mulrooney, put it this way in a 1931 letter to the Mayor:

> The ESD is a most important arm of the service. It consists of motor trucks with trained crews, with emergency and technical equipment for any condition that may occur.
> Where the main purpose is to transport members of the department to emergencies in a short period of time, such as fires, riots, and catastrophes, its activities are many and unusual, ranging from bombing the lairs of criminals, releasing by means of acetylene torches dead or injured from elevator pits, dispersing disorderly crowds and raising wrecks from the river beds, to applying inhalers to new born babies to start natural breathing....[52]

Even this impressive litany did not exhaust the brief handed to the Emergency Services Division. In the first few years of the newly reorganized squad's existence its members not only

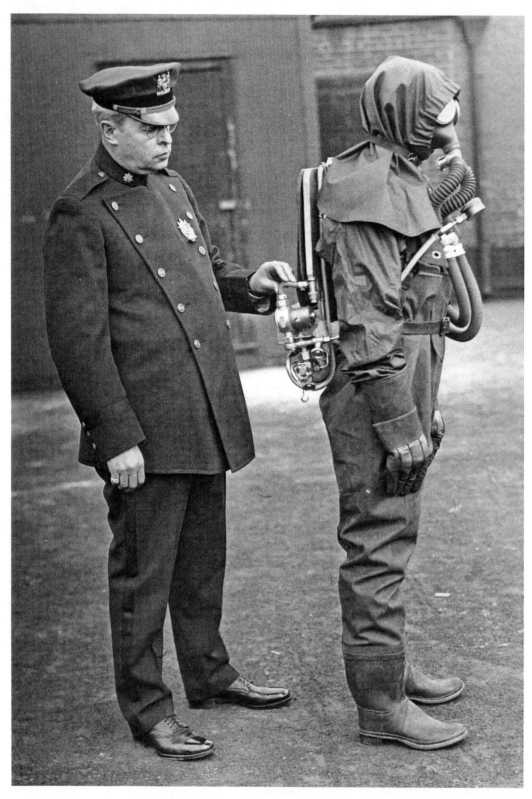

Inspector Daniel Kerr, chief of the Emergency Service Division, adjusts the breathing apparatus of crewmember Edward McWilliams during a 1932 trial of new hazardous atmosphere equipment. (Copyright 2001, New York City Police Department, all rights reserved. Used with permission.)

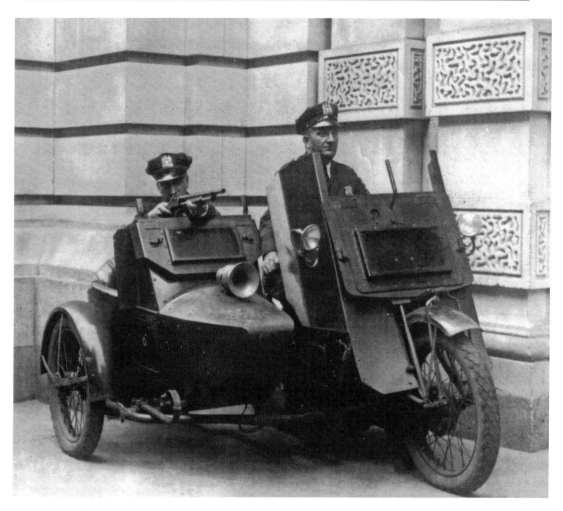

When the Machine Gun Squad was disbanded, many of its members were transferred to the newly reorganized and expanded Emergency Services Division. (Copyright 2001, New York City Police Department, all rights reserved. Used with permission.)

saved the imperiled from icy death in the city's rivers and rendered medical aid of every description, but frequently they had to "help subdue a desperate criminal brought to bay [and] often they must resort to gas bombs to force the surrender of an insane person armed and out do murder."[53] When not gassing homicidal maniacs, they might used their horse-belt to pull an animal out of the East River, use their inhalator to revive a cyanotic newborn, rush an accident victim to Bellevue in the back of their rig, or even hoist a six-hundred pound circus woman out of her apartment in order to deliver her to the hospital for her semi-annual check-up.[54] At this point the emerald green trucks were long and open-topped, with a chassis not unlike a hook-and-ladder rig, and each outfit carried no less than one-hundred and ninety-three pieces of equipment—"articles for the saving or destroying of life and for solving many of the difficult situations into which careless or unfortunate persons are sometimes thrown," in the words of one news story.[55] As the running boards groaned under the weight of oxygen and oxyacetylene tanks, inside they carried stretchers, boat hooks, medical equipment of every description, hydraulic jacks that could raise a trolley car, and, at the front, at least one Thompson submachine gun ready for the "battle against humanity run amok."[56]

While the rigs used by the Emergency Services Division were clearly designed more for delivery of equipment than the removal of patients, they could and did function as ambulances—in 1931, for example, they carried one hundred patients to the hospital, out of over four-thousand calls.[57] The Emergency Service Division was notable for its high quality of emergency medical care, with members trained in the best cardio-pulmonary resuscitation techniques of the day (which involved putting the victim on their stomach with an oxygen mask over the nose and mouth while an officer rhythmically pressed the ribs to mimic the usual action of respiration; the body was kept warm with hot pads and blankets and the effort was continued until the body was cold or the victim was pronounced dead by a physician.) In one notable instance a relay crew kept up continued artificial respiration for twenty hours on a woman overcome by gas fumes in her kitchen: she finally revived, only to die the following day.[58] By 1949 the Emergency Services Division was staffed by five-hundred and two handpicked specialists, and their original open-topped rigs had been replaced by "covered wagons," heavy-duty trucks with thick-windows in their side panels: that year the service answered 15,609 calls, successfully resuscitating a record thirty-eight hundred asphyxiation victims.[59] After experimenting with smaller prowl cars in the 1950s, the Division adopted combination patrol/ambulance cars in 1961 that featured a station wagon body bolted onto a truck chassis. Resembling the classic "professional car" ambulance used by many police ambulance services at the time, each rig was equipped with two stretchers and a stripped-down emergency medical kit sufficient to support a non-critically injured patient en route to the hospital, or to stabilize the more serious case at the scene pending the arrival of a fully equipped rescue truck.[60]

It is clear that, in its first forty years, the ESD pioneered much of the field equipment, training, and operations of modern rescue EMT and paramedic squads. While modern paramedics benefited considerably from the popularity of the classic television program *Emergency!*, once again the Emergency Services Division preceded its better known imitators—because ten years before Gage and Desoto drove Rescue 51 into the living rooms of America there had been the television premiere of *Police Emergency!*, a one-hour documentary airing February 18, 1962, on the old "DuPont Show of the Week." Narrated by Walter Matthau, it condensed three months of work by two Emergency Service Division patrolmen, Officers Walter Chadwick and Eugene Corcoran, into sixty gritty minutes showcasing their "dangerous, exciting, routine and sometimes ludicrous" work.[61] In keeping with the eclectic tradition of the service they dealt with a heart attack, an armed robbery at a Western Union office, and a high pressure steam leak trapping sixty people inside a building, each incident another of "the ugly strands of the tapestry that is New York," in the words of one reviewer.[62]

Thus, in small ways and large, the Emergency Services Division acted out on the New York stage a drama whose outlines would be recast forty years later, when the new paramedics took the country by storm. Unfortunately, it is impossible to dissect how many of the future leaders of the paramedic movement had been watching NBC the night *Police Emergency!* aired, or read Norman Lobsenz's 1958 history of the Emergency Service Division (*Emergency!*), or had any personal knowledge of the innovations pioneered by the officers of the original squads. It is likely that this service was more innovative than imitated, although its efforts were in the highest tradition of the ambulance services. Today the Emergency Service continues operations in New York City, although they have undergone yet another name change to become the Emergency Services Unit. A complete listing of its current activities is beyond the scope of this chapter, but they remain a vital component of the city's emergency response system. By the turn of the 21st century the ESU was handling more than one-hundred thousand calls a year—compared to somewhat over two-thousand calls during its inaugural year. Heavy trucks and smaller Radio Emergency Patrol Vehicles are deployed, in addition to specialty vehicles such as armored cars and Construction Accident Response Equipment. All officers are cross-

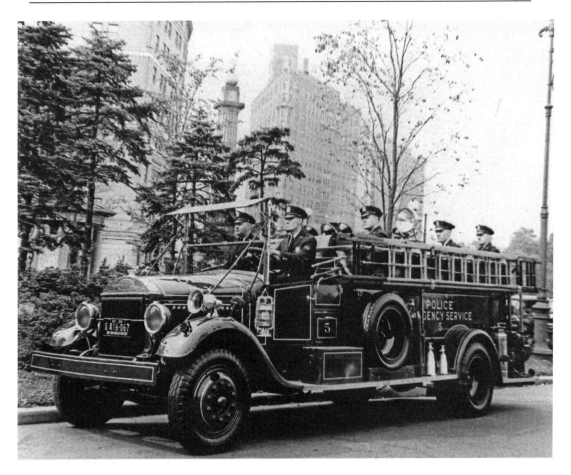

Emergency Services truck and crew from the early 1930s. (Copyright 2001, New York City Police Department, all rights reserved. Used with permission.)

trained as EMTs, with some staff receiving Advanced Life Support training: in addition, there is an effort to keep at least one M.D. in uniform in order to provide the required supervision for officers with Physician Assistant certification, allowing them to provide even more intensive field interventions. Kevin Reynolds, a former EMT instructor for the Unit, explained the importance of medical training for the squad:

> The training helps us to know what the next people down the line are going to do with the person — if we have someone injured inside a wrecked car, we know how quickly do we need to get them out, because we know how seriously they're hurt: that way we're not just grease monkeys with a tool, taking a car apart. We can even be an extra set of hands in the ambulance, so we don't need to tie up as many medical units at the scene.[63]

In addition to its special tactical medical teams, since 1942 the Division has operated regular ambulance services free for departmental personnel and their family members. (Funded entirely by employee contributions, this police ambulance service also oversees provision of in-home durable medical equipment such as oxygen and hospital beds.) The success of New York's original Emergency Service Squad is measured not only in its own proud history of service, but in the similar outfits it inspired in other major cities, where special police medical and rescue units supplement or replace traditional squads when an ongoing situation poses too great a risk for non-tactical medical personnel.[64] While the St. John Ambulance Association

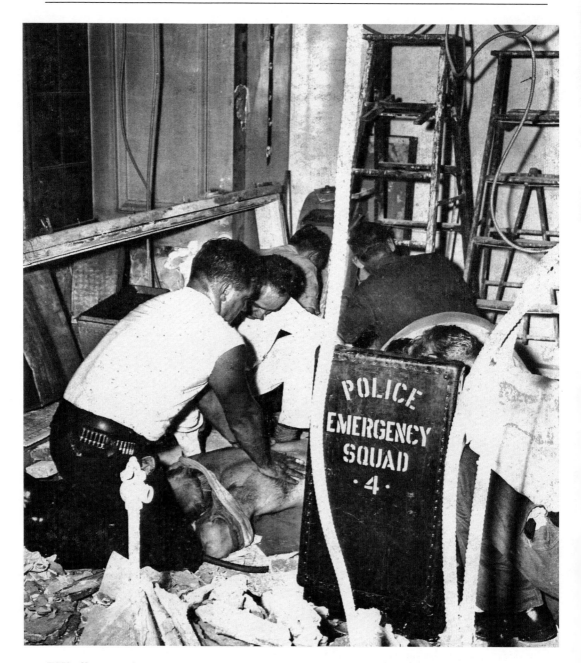

ESU officers perform an early form of artificial respiration. (Courtesy Kevin Reynolds. Copyright 2001, New York City Police Department, all rights reserved. Used with permission.)

began in the 19th century as a modern incarnation of the Hospitaller warrior monks, it is these modern tactical medical units whose operations most clearly evoke the proud lineage of an ancient order whose members also swore an oath to "serve and protect" and provided medical aid under cover of the sword.

Taken as a whole, all of these various pioneering ambulance services, from the Bureau of Mines disaster car to the "Coffee Wagon" and the daring crews of police Emergency Response Units, formed a preview of the paramedic rescue rigs that would dominate emergency serv-

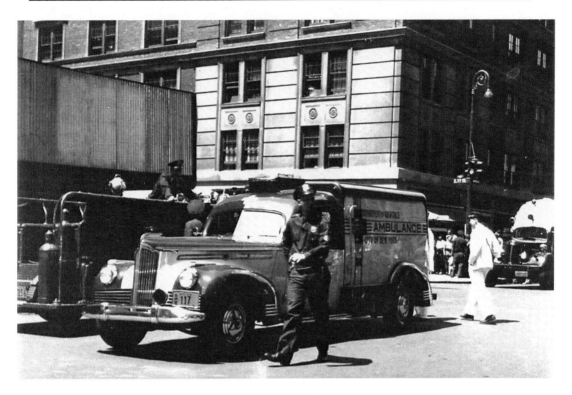

An original Emergency Services rig alongside a Bellevue Packard ambulance, with a new Emergency Services truck parked further down the street. (Courtesy Kevin Reynolds. Copyright 2001, New York City Police Department, all rights reserved. Used with permission.)

ices from the 1970s forward, with each of these earlier incarnations representing a distinct and important effort to re-imagine what an ambulance could be.

Ambulance Innovations

Of course, innovative responses to the problem of emergency medical needs had been part of ambulance history from the beginning, and a brief detour in the chronology of the ambulance will provide a context in which to understand the radical changes that came to the emergency medical services in the second half of the 20th century.

One of the signal moments in ambulance development came with the 1867 *Exposition Universelle* in Paris, a world's fair attended by forty-two nations vying to outshine one another with their innovations in the arts and technology. The festivities marked the public debut of the hydraulic elevator, reinforced concrete ... and new models of ambulance design. The French, who had pioneered the modern ambulance in 1792, did not fare too well: one commentator dismissed their prototype ambulance as "simply a bad omnibus" with stiff springs, poor ventilation, and not enough room for its passengers.[65] Considerably better received were those from the United States, of which a British observer declared "of those special conveyances exhibited, none possess the conditions desirable in ambulance conveyances to a greater degree than those used in America."[66] In a rare example of Anglo-French detente, the French agreed, awarding a *Grande Prixe* to the American Sanitary Commission for its military medical exhibit.[67] This Grand Prize was a notable achievement for a nation whose previous ambulances had been nicknamed "avalanches" by disgruntled survivors, although the models that crossed the Atlantic had the benefit of newly improved spring systems. Other nations received commendations for improvements in wheeled litters and stretchers, and the exposition marked the beginning of serious, concerted efforts to improve ambulance design.

Ultimately, the most significant innovation in 19th century emergency vehicle design was likely the adoption of the humble rubber tire, shielding the patient from the rude shocks transmitted by unyielding wooden wheels. A more unusual innovation in the late 19th century was a streetcar ambulance operated by the St. Louis Board of Health, the custom trolley making regular stops around town to collect patients and deposit them at the various municipal dispensaries, hospitals, and asylums and enjoying right of way over all other lines.[68] Making its maiden run on December 27, 1894, it was staffed by Health Department employees, had seating for eighteen inside its cherry, oak, and maple lined interior, and its amenities included surgical supplies, stretchers, heating, and two bathrooms with "earth closets" in lieu of plumbing.[69] For all its advantages, this elegant system couldn't survive the transition of street-cars to buses after the turn of the century.

While inherent limits on the size and weight of a vehicle drawn by a horse kept radical ambulance innovations at a minimum in the 19th century, these restrictions became superfluous as the automobile age dawned. As noted, the first motor ambulance appeared in 1899, an electric model owned by Chicago's Michael Reese Hospital, although it did not long endure the introduction of the gasoline ambulance with its superior range and economy. Heaters (originally using pipes warmed by the exhaust) were introduced on automobile ambulances as early as 1909 by the Cunningham Company of Rochester, New York, while the air-conditioned ambulance didn't debut until 1937, courtesy Cincinnati ambulance builder Sayers & Scovill.[70] By 1942 Buck Ambulance in Portland, Oregon was the first major ambulance provider to include

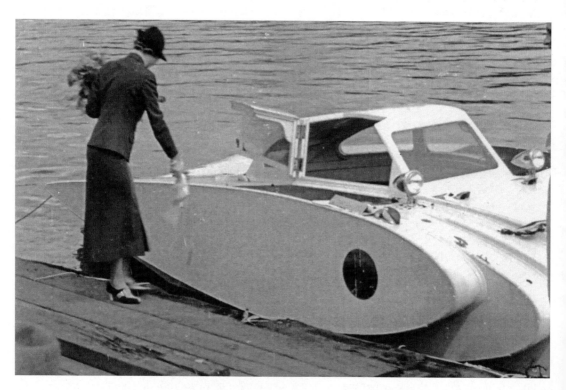

An experimental 1938 hydro-ambulance in Portland, Oregon.

oxygen tanks in all of its rigs, a response to the number of asphyxiation cases coming from the city's shipyards, where builders were often overcome by gas fumes while working in poorly ventilated compartments.

A less practical innovation were the two Cunningham ambulances built for the Memphis funeral home and ambulance firm, J.T. Hinton & Son in 1927. At the time mob-ravaged Memphis was popularly known as "The Murder Capital of the World," and Hinton's $13,000 ambulances were armored with boiler-plating and fitted with bulletproof glass in order to prevent conscientious hit-men from getting a second chance as a wounded victim made the dash to the hospital.[71]

By the 1950s the earliest boxy automobile ambulances, which had resembled the delivery-wagon bodies of their horse-drawn predecessors, had been replaced by the hearse or station-wagon "professional car" design. Long, lean, and dramatic looking, they sought to distinguish themselves from competitors with design innovations, such as side doors with hinges facing the front (making them less likely to be pried open by the whipping wind of a fast run), or saucier fins over the taillights.

Whereas ambulances had once been limited by what a horse could pull, now the limiting factor was what the ambulance provider could charge: with most such bills being paid out of pocket, there was simply no way for the average ambulance provider to finance radical departures from these relatively simple "scoop and go" rigs. In 1960, however, Baltimore's fire depart-

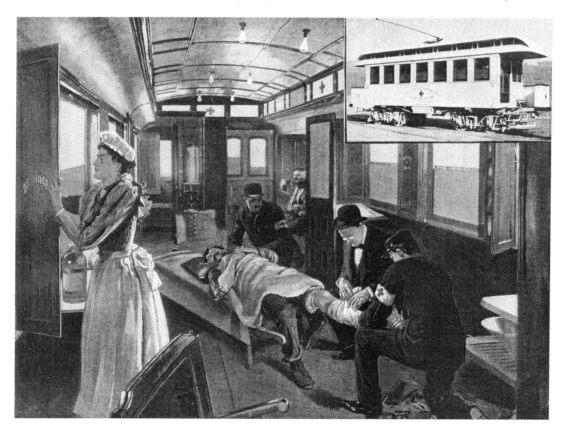

The St. Louis ambulance street car included "earth closets" in lieu of indoor plumbing and contained all the equipment necessary for simple surgery en route to any one of the city's sixteen infirmaries. A similar vehicle went into use in Brazil at around the same time (*Harper's Weekly*, March 23, 1895).

ment began a collaboration with a small wagon builder in Pennsylvania that sparked the most important ambulance innovation of modern times.

The Baltimore Fire Department had been in the ambulance business since 1927, when it had volunteered to take over the job from the police (citizens had complained that the combination patrol wagon/ambulance rigs were less than ideal in configuration and, equally important, it looked unseemly to have a paddy wagon parked in your driveway whenever you developed appendicitis).[72] By 1959, however, Baltimore Ambulance Chief Martin McMahon was a man with a problem: his department was using the same hearse-style ambulances as the rest of America, and the hard usage was shaking them to pieces. As he told a mechanic at the time, "hell, the transmissions are on the bench more than they're on the road!"[73]

His solution was to customize one-ton Chevrolet panel trucks for ambulance duty, trusting that their substantially more rugged construction would give his mechanics more free time and his spare-parts budget a rest, and the work was contracted to Pennsylvania's century-old Swab Wagon Company. One of the mechanics on the job was Mike Margerum, a great-grandson of the company's founder, and he recalled how, in 1960, the company turned a ten-foot panel truck into an acceptable ambulance by putting in a cot holder, laying in cabinet work and linoleum flooring, rigging up suction equipment, cutting in a side-door, and building up a proper step in the back.[74] The entire job, including the basic medical equipment inside, ran half the cost of a traditional ambulance and marked the beginning of modern civilian ambulance design.

In 1963 Chevrolet discontinued its one-ton panel truck in favor of a smaller ¾ ton rig, and Chief McMahon faced a dilemma: either convert his fleet to the smaller configuration, writing off his stockpile of replacement parts and adjusting to a smaller working space for his crews, or ask the Swab Company to build an entirely custom job on bare one-ton chassis. He opted for the latter.

Once more the job fell to Margerum to come up with something suitable, and he sat down one day and started sketching. "I knew we could build a body for him," he recalled, "so I made a little drawing for him ... it was a couple inches shorter than the panel-truck, but it was a little wider and a little higher, using a one-ton chassis with a body behind the cab, not a panel.... We didn't copy 'em from anybody else, but this wasn't rocket-science, just a box behind a cab."[75] This modest description belied a vehicle that revolutionized ambulance design, and Margerum recalls the Chief shouting "This is IT!" after being shown the original sketch. McMahon ordered four rigs without waiting to see a prototype, at a per unit cost (including most equipment) of approximately $6,500. ("You couldn't buy the paint job for that, today," Margerum observes drily.)

The work area was separate from the cab, with no walk-through, and "the box" was originally fifty-four inches high, not tall enough for a crewmember to stand upright. This low ceiling was a specific request of the Chief since some Baltimore hospital ambulance bays weren't high enough to clear a taller truck, and he also wanted his men to be able to brace their backs against the roof for stability when bending over patients during a ride.[76] While Chief McMahon was delighted with the new ambulances and ordered more each year, the rest of the nation was a slightly tougher sell. Margerum recalls taking his ambulance to trade-shows around the country and drawing stares instead of orders: "People are hard to convince to change, you know, and they just looked at it, being a truck, and said it would ride too rough." Chief McMahon, however, proved the most able salesman the Swab Company ever had: he was rapidly achieving national prominence as a brilliant innovator in emergency services, and he seldom missed an opportunity to plug the Swab ambulances he was deploying in Baltimore. "He'd tell people 'You call Swab and tell 'em to build you an ambulance: They're the best damn ambulances I've ever had,'" Margerum remembers. "Pretty soon people were calling me and ask-

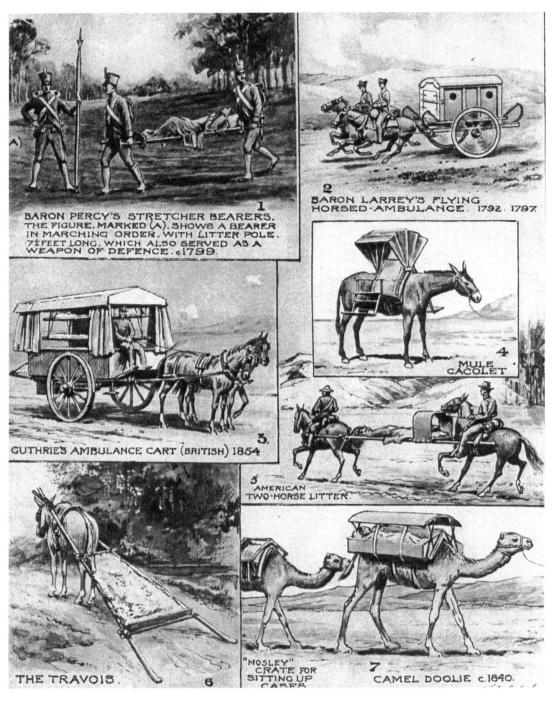

Military exigencies have always been a catalyst for ambulance innovation, as seen in this retrospective prepared for a British journal during World War I (*Illustrated War News* [London], February 2, 1917).

ing us to build 'em an ambulance—that's the best kind of sales work there is, when they call *you* up."

By 1968 the Baltimore Fire Department was running fourteen Swab ambulances, and their modular capability meant the "box" could be lifted off and switched onto a new chassis as needed—much cheaper than buying a new rig, of course.[77]

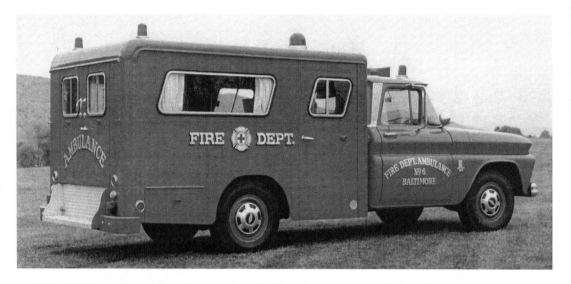

Eagle 110

THE "ORIGINAL" BALTIMORE UNIT — NOW WITH INCREASED INTERIOR BODY AND COMPARTMENT DIMENSIONS.

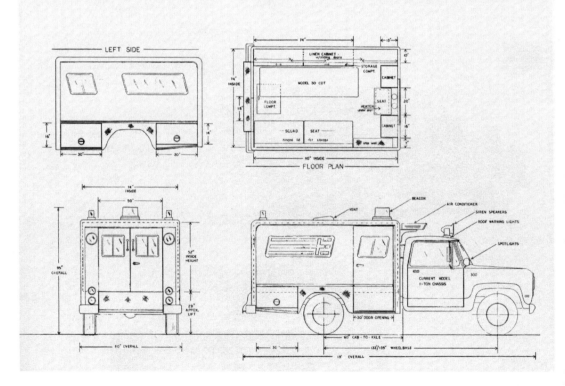

Top: The 1963 Swab ambulance built for the Baltimore Fire Department. This was the first "Type 1" squad ambulance ever built, revolutionizing ambulance design (courtesy the Swab Wagon Company). *Bottom:* Schematic of an early variation of the Swab's original Type 1 ambulance, circa 1966. After federal regulations made ambulance testing too expensive for the small company Swab had to give up its patient transport vehicles, although it remains a leader in rescue and fire rigs (courtesy the Swab Wagon Company).

The rig wasn't the only advancement in ambulance technology, either. A comparison between the medical equipment found on the Bellevue ambulance of 1869 and a Swab wagon (which in 1968 represented one of the top services in the country), is instructive. In the 19th century a New York intern went to the scene in a horse drawn wagon equipped with the medications and equipment that could fit into a black leather handbag, a pocket surgical kit, a

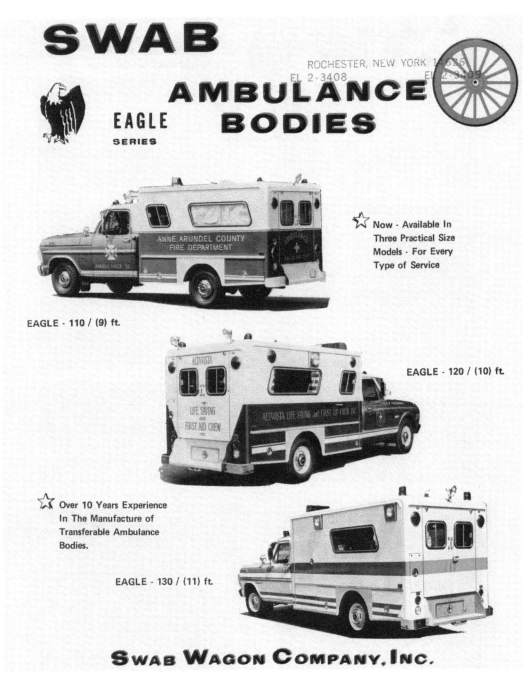

A Swab catalogue from the early 1970s showing some of its various makes and models (courtesy the Swab Wagon Company).

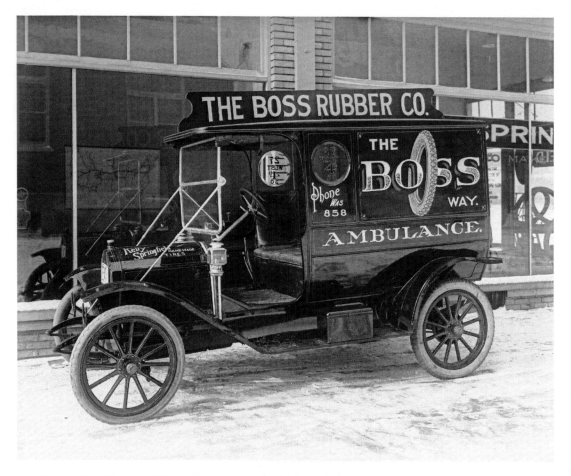

Unquestionably one of the most important ambulance innovations of the early 20th century was the use of pneumatic tires, first on some wagons, later on all automotive aid cars. Rubber tires provided a dramatically smoother ride for patients, reducing the re-injury rate en route to the hospital (William Shipler, photographer; used by permission, Utah State Historical Society, all rights reserved).

tourniquet, wadding, splints, bandages, a flask of brandy, and a bottle of persulphate of iron to help stanch bleeding in minor wounds. In the late 1960s a Baltimore fireman with a Red Cross Advanced First Aid certificate and additional physician training in resuscitation, childbirth, and fracture stabilization, among other topics, climbed into an air-conditioned Swab modular ambulance with the following gear[78]:

> *Front coach*: leg and arm air splints; two light blankets and one heavy; two mortuary sheets; bag resuscitator; emesis basin; vacuum pump; two oxygen bottles; gauze; ammonia inhalants; triangular bandages; resuscitator; three airways (with one child face piece); flashlight; second alarm keys for call box.
> *Coach*: seven-way adjustable litter; combination litter/wheelchair; two folding chairs; infant medical kit; aspirator; Westinghouse "Iron Heart" (an mechanical device that clamped onto a patient's body and squeezed the chest to maintain cardiac output); carbon dioxide fire extinguisher.
> *Side compartment*: orthopedic stretcher; five restraint straps; Kelley-Blake splint; jack handle; wood splints; oxygen bottle, first aid bag.
> *Rear floor compartment*: jack; oxygen bottle; first aid bag.

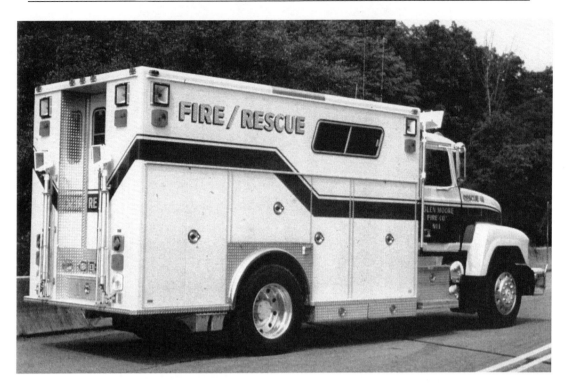

In addition to heavy duty rescue rigs like this one, Swab also manufactures smaller "squad" rigs suitable for transporting medical and rescue equipment to emergency scenes and has become the industry's leading innovator in animal control trucks (courtesy the Swab Wagon Company).

After a slow start, the Swab ambulance became popular throughout the country and its modular design became an industry standard but, in the end, the success of the Swab ambulance was its downfall. The improved work-area, smooth ride, and durability of the Swab design made it the logical starting point for the new federal ambulance specifications adopted in the late 1960s. To meet federal standards, however, manufacturers had to pay for crash-testing and other costly capital investments, which amounted to an outlay the small Swab Wagon Company couldn't afford.

Today they specialize in rescue vehicles designed to transfer equipment rather than patients and are industry leaders in fire-equipment and animal transport vehicles. Sadly, a fire in 1978 destroyed most of the company's old records and artifacts, including Margerum's original sketches, correspondence, and the bills of lading that would have tracked their ambulance sales around the country. Still, the innovative ambulance that started it all can be seen at the Baltimore Fire Museum, a gleaming monument to a small firm in Elizabethville, Pennsylvania, where the most influential ambulance innovation of the 20th century was born on a draftsman's pad and reared by hand in the Swab factory shop.

Innovation in ambulance design has continued apace, although over the last twenty years the appearance of the rigs has solidified into a few basic patterns. Neonatal ambulance units enjoyed a brief vogue in the 1970s, although current standard models can easily be equipped as needed to transport such tiny, fragile patients. Aircraft ambulances, both fixed wing and helicopter units, finally came into their own in the 1960s, after formally debuting in the 1920s, and are now staples of trauma services across the nation. Currently the newest specialty ambulance is the "bariatric unit," designed for the increasing number of morbidly obese Americans.

Equipped with its own winch, this ambulance can accommodate patients up to one-thousand pounds, according to its creators, American Medical Response in Portland, Oregon.[79] As with all of medicine, innovations in ambulance design continue to reflect the unpredictable interactions between technology, economics, and evolving patterns of disease and injury in the population.

• 12 •

The 1950s: Losing the Battle

"It may be an irrational public conception, but a hospital without an ambulance is, in the public mind, like a doctor without a head-mirror, and, of course, no doctor is ever without his head mirror.... To turn over the ambulance to the police, the firemen, or private agencies is to deprive the hospital of valuable glamour, public recognition and public praise."
—John Nicklas, "Don't Overlook the Ambulance as a Public Relations Tool," *The Modern Hospital*, Vol. 75, No. 3; September 1950

For the first eighty years of the civilian ambulance's existence it enjoyed significant growth: in rural areas this was largely driven by volunteer squads and the contributions of funeral homes, while in most of the major metropolitan areas emergency transport was usually split between police departments and the larger hospitals. Infirmary ambulance services were generally the most advanced, delivering a spiffily dressed intern to the more serious cases. Even in cities where the police or the funeral homes handled the bulk of the ambulance fleets, municipally owned hospitals would usually dispatch an intern to the scene if requested. By the beginning of the 1950s, however, the old scheme was unraveling, as a crippling intern shortage forced more and more teaching hospitals to abandon the practice of sending interns out on ambulance calls. Complicating matters was a dramatic shift in modern medicine, one that would have a profound impact on how ambulance services were provided around the world.

Under Pressure

Formerly hospitals had been the resort of those too poor to provide a suitable environment for treatment and recuperation at home: now the entire community expected to be treated in a hospital. Reflecting this, United States hospital admissions increased from 7.2 million in 1934 to almost 17 million in 1949: to make room for this influx the average length of stay reached an all time low of eight days, as patients were discharged to finish convalescing at home.[1] Eighty years before, when the ambulance debuted, the average length of stay had been measured in *weeks* and those now remaining in the hospital were, on average, sicker and in need of more acute attention. Such changes in case complexity and patient numbers made sending interns or orderlies out on ambulance calls an expense and a disruption that hospitals were ill inclined to tolerate. Meanwhile, police departments continued to provide a significant percentage of ambulance services nationally, but the increase in post-war crime and the expense of continually updating medical equipment made the ambulance an increasingly peripheral and unwelcome expense. In rural areas, far from major hospitals, volunteer fire and rescue companies played an ever larger role, continuing a trend from the late 1920s, and a significant spike in the number of ambulances owned by such units accompanied the sudden rush of used vehi-

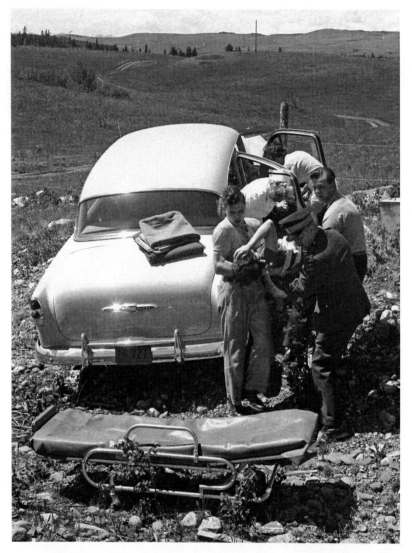

While many North American ambulance services declined in the 1950s, local exceptions could be found. In Canada, Ernest Starrs, veteran of the Royal Medical Corps and St. John Ambulance Society member, operated a well-regarded service in Alberta. Here, a Starr's Ambulance crewman and a nurse prepare to transport an accident victim after a highway blowout in 1954 (Jack De Lorme, courtesy Glenbow Archives, NA-5600-7520g).

cles into the market after civilian automakers resumed new production after World War II.[2] The discharge of thousands of medical corpsmen likely also played a role, echoing the effect of demobilization after the Civil War. Wherever police, private, and volunteer services were inadequate or absent, funeral homes took up much of the slack, ultimately dominating the South and holding other, isolated markets such as Chicago.

A truly up-to-date ambulance service was increasingly expensive with innovations in emergency medicine. Inevitably, the gap between what was *possible* and what was *seen* grew wider. Hospitals were squeezed by an intern shortage and rising expenses, police departments often lacked the resources or the will to continually upgrade their ambulance services, and an absence of state or national legislation setting ambulance standards allowed many providers to get away with offering little more than a station wagon with a cot in the back.

Simultaneously, innovations in trauma care produced by two world wars convinced the medical profession that there were real gains in life saving to be made—when and if those lessons were transferred to the civilian ambulance services. In the meantime, a 1954 report from the Trauma Committee of the American College of Surgeons reported that data from twenty-nine states indicated that only 15 percent of the injured were covered by "excellent" emergency transportation, while 28 percent were exposed to services that could only be classified as "fair to poor."[3] According to their report it made little difference whether the injury occurred in a large city or a small town, for by this date

> [m]orticians are responsible for most of the ambulances in this country with the remainder in charge of the police and fire departments, industry, volunteers and hospitals—in about that order. Whether effective, life-saving first-aid care and transportation are rendered depends largely on how much responsibility is accepted by the public, particularly the medical profession, to demand them....

Despite some efforts to drag the ambulance back into the medical mainstream, a majority of hospitals had decided that aid cars were too burdensome to deal with and ambulance service was increasingly relegated to whoever was willing to try and turn a profit with them. National surveys in 1955 and 1957 found just 16 percent of hospitals providing ambulance services for their communities, a new nadir in the steady decline that had started in the early 1900s.[4] Since the majority of providers who replaced the hospital ambulances couldn't match the level of equipment and medical expertise provided by an institutional service (and the profession had limited success in lobbying for legislation to extend hospital standards to all ambulances), the evaporation of traditional infirmary ambulances during the 1950s created an actual threat to public health.

Replacing the Hospital Services

The ambulance services filling the gaps created by departing hospitals were similar to ones providing services in those regions where hospital ambulance services had never been signifi-

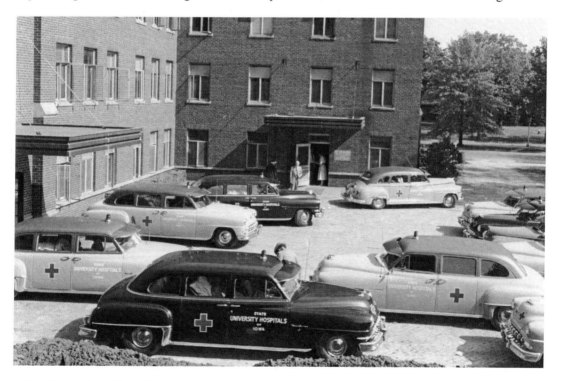

The University of Iowa Hospital's ambulance fleet in 1955 was an unusually large operation running counter to the national trend for hospitals to divest themselves of such services (Charlotte Brooks, *Look* Magazine Photograph Collection, Library of Congress, Prints and Photographs Division, Job 5-3979).

cant contributors: that is to say, they ran the gamut from the ultra-deluxe, such as Portland's "Coffee-Wagon," to simpler vehicles operated by mortuaries in America's small towns. Consider the representative Moss Funeral Home, in Breese, Illinois, which opened for business— and began providing ambulance services—in 1953: Moss' ambulance was just the company hearse with a cot in back and a flashing light on the roof. "We basically just sat back there and held their hand until we got to the hospital," a family member recalled in a newspaper interview fifty years later.[5] Still, such operations provided the best they could muster in places where no alternative existed. At the same time, the 1950s witnessed a second wave of urban fire departments providing ambulance services. Whereas in the 1920s and 1930s this had been, overwhelmingly, a phenomenon of rural areas and smaller towns, now firehouses in larger communities began revamping their operation to include emergency services in an effort to ensure that their firefighters received optimal medical care if injured on the job. In the event, this trend simply added another shard to the sloppy mosaic of American ambulance services, as demonstrated in a 1955 survey of forty-six cities by the American Municipal Association. According to the Association, in a third of the communities ambulance services were solely managed by private concerns (including for-profit ambulance companies, morticians, and private hospitals); in another third the ambulances were operated by municipal agencies, including police, fire and health departments, while the final third depended on some combination of these.[6] As the editors noted sourly, "in one place the Owl Cab Co. may send the ambulance; in another it may be Friendly Funeral System, the Good Will Fire Co., or Samaritan Ambulances, Inc.," and in this instance variety guaranteed inconsistency, with an inevitable surtax of death and suffering. (Responsibility for dispatching these rigs was less variable: police had exclusive

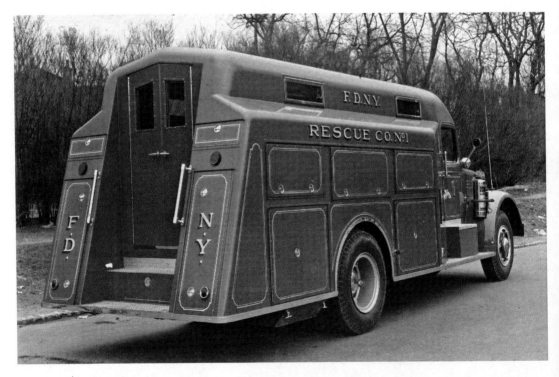

While Chicago's ambulance services suffered from poor coordination, inter-service rivalry, and inadequate funding, a few cities like New York were expanding their city-operated emergency medical services. By 1948 the FDNY Rescue 1 squad was operating this well-equipped rescue truck, one of several city-owned rigs (courtesy the Fire Department of New York).

control in more than half, and were at least partially responsible in a significant number of the rest.)

Among representative cities, in Cleveland police ambulances reigned supreme and alone, having displaced the mortuary ambulances that had ruled the thoroughfares since 1879, while in San Francisco the Health Department was still running a model system out of its five emergency hospitals. In New York City both municipal and private hospitals received annual stipends to defray their ambulance costs and handled all emergency cases between them; Boston relied on its police ambulances as well as those sent out by the City Hospital; Philadelphia depended on city morticians to supplement its fire-station ambulances, while in Dallas morticians contracted with the municipality to provide all the ambulance services needed. Overall some of these operations were superb, some were merely tolerable, a few were abysmal, but "nowhere," it was said, "is the possibility of being transported from the scene of an accident in a first-class ambulance much more remote than it is in Chicago."[7]

Chicago's Tale

While extreme, Chicago's experience with ambulance services illustrates broad themes that conspired nationally to impede uniform quality emergency services. Because it was Chicago, no bad decision was without its hint of graft, but even away from the fun-house mirror morality of the Windy City deficiencies in ambulance services were perpetuated by lapses in legislative oversight and inefficiencies in the market. (It's just that profitable mistakes get made more often, and resist rectification more successfully, than merely honest ones.) The Chicago Police Department had once dominated the local ambulance service, but they abandoned the field in 1922 after meddling citizens persisted in hauling off the injured before the police could arrive. Control of the ambulance service then passed to private outfits and the city's hospitals, all operating with minimal oversight (or interference, if you like) from the city or state. Then, in 1933, the city council passed one of the nation's first "splint ordinances," requiring all ambulances to carry, and their attendants be trained to use, first aid kits and splint appliances. Enforcement was left, for no discernible reason, to the Contagious Diseases Division of the Board of Health, who registered their disapproval by ignoring the statute completely. As the Depression ground on and funding streams dried up in the Dust Bowl wind, beleaguered Chicago hospitals sold off their ambulances and either did without or signed inexpensive service contracts with funeral homes and private firms, a decision whose tangible economic benefits had to be balanced against the practical decline in quality.[8] (Such desperate measures were not limited to Chicago. In Seattle financial necessity forced the county hospital to cancel its $700 a month ambulance contract in 1933, and similar economies were imposed on cash-poor infirmaries across the nation.[9]) In 1936 the Fire Department redressed some of Chicago's losses by acquiring five high quality International Harvester ambulances (similar to those used by Eliot Ness' police patrols in Cleveland a few years later), but overall city emergency services continued to erode.[10]

The war pre-empted further ambulance debate, but in 1949 the unreliability of the private firms resulted in police squadrols being given stretchers and blankets and ordered to collect the injured in addition to carting the drunk and disorderly back to the cells. (By court order these squadrols were exempted from the "splint ordinance" that applied, in name, to the private ambulances.) In 1954 there were eighty such police wagons on the streets, equipped with two-way radios, rubber sheets, blankets, stretchers, and two policemen with first aid training. They were still primarily used as "paddy wagons," functioning as crude ambulances if there was room in the back. Supplementing them were seventeen converted station wagons operated

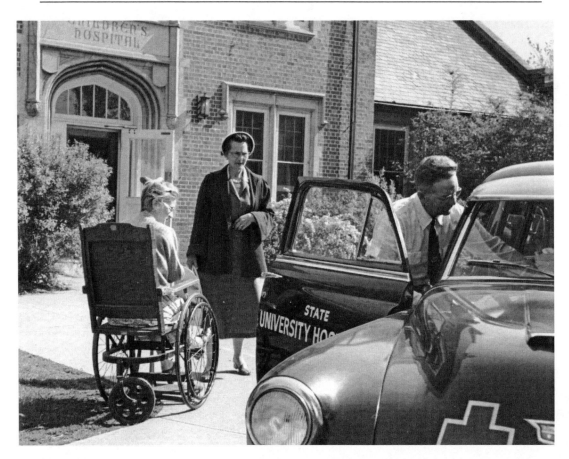

A University of Iowa ambulance takes a patient in a wheelchair to a clinic appointment in 1955. Many emergency ambulance services depended on such relatively lucrative work to subsidize their operations. Successful private ambulance operators often focused exclusively on these jobs, depriving their medically minded rivals of crucial funding. (Charlotte Brooks, photographer. Library of Congress, Prints & Photographs Division, *Look* Magazine Photograph Collection, Job 5-3979.)

by the independent Chicago Park District Police, which were marginally more effective as ambulances by virtue of being dedicated more or less exclusively to the work. Meanwhile, the fire department was operating a fleet of recently upgraded ambulances, vastly superior to the makeshift squadrols, but police dispatchers refused to send them to any accident on the public streets, relying on an old ordinance giving jurisdiction over such cases to the police.[11] Since citizens reflexively dialed the operator when calling an ambulance, they usually got a squadrol for their trouble. Attempting to bypass the police by calling the fire department direct could even be hazardous, as a reporter found out:

> The police, legally in charge of street accidents, sometimes discourage [calling a fire ambulance]. For example, a doctor chanced upon a window washer who had just fallen to the sidewalk from an apartment building. The man was badly hurt. The doctor asked a passerby to call Fire 7–1313 for an ambulance. A policeman showed up and the following exchange took place:
> "We have a fire department ambulance on the way," the doctor smiled.
> "Who gave you permission to call the fire department?" demanded the cop.
> "I don't need permission when I see a man lying on the street in need of an ambulance," retorted the doctor.
> "How would you like me to run you in for interfering with a policeman in the performance of his duty?" suggested the public protector.[12]

(In 1970 a Pulitzer prize winning series of articles in the *Chicago Tribune* discovered that police officers were calling private ambulance firms to transport the injured in exchange for $10 bribes, rather than taking patients to the hospital in their squadrols: it is tempting to speculate that such a scheme was extant in the 1950s, which might explain the patrol officer's reluctance to call the fire department.) The result of this bureaucratic inefficiency was that the twelve fire department ambulances averaged one call apiece per eight-hour shift in 1954, at $30 per trip considering the fixed expenses involved. (In New York City, ambulances averaged ten calls a day at a pro-rated cost of $5.50 a trip.[13]) That year a blue-ribbon committee recommended putting ambulance services under uniform regulation and reimbursing private ambulances for emergency services to the indigent, and Mayor Kennelly duly referred the matter to the city council, which referred the matter to a committee that referred the matter to a *sub*-committee that, as of a year later, didn't know a thing about it.[14] As to who profited from this morass, it was commonly believed that it was the operators of the city's forty-three private ambulances, mostly mortician firms. While loath to provide emergency services, which were inconvenient and offered limited opportunity to secure payment in advance, they had ensconced themselves in a lucrative niche of making private calls at $14 apiece, plus mileage, and apparently were concerned that this business would be impinged by a large scale, efficient municipal service. So, despite twenty years of committees and recommendations, nothing had changed in February 1954 when a mayoral committee surveyed eleven hospitals to see how Chicagoans were finding their way to Mercy's Receiving Dock. Of 2,582 emergency cases tabulated less than 6 percent arrived by ambulance, half came by private car, and another quarter were conveyed on a cot in the back of a squadrol: the rest walked.[15] At this date Chicago was the second largest city in America, with a population of four million, and the self-reliance that infuriated police surgeons in the 1920s, when they rolled up to find the injured had been whisked away while the police ponies were en route, was still getting a workout. Clearly, the Chicago ambulance "system" was a model in failure, but the problems it faced (lack of co-ordination, inadequate funding for municipal services, no safety-net of minimum requirements) were representative of the nation as a whole, even if their impact was unusually severe.

The View from Gotham

While Chicago was a metaphor for what could go wrong with ambulance services, Manhattan was emblematic of the difficulties facing even comparatively well-organized operations. By the early 1950s New York City's hospitals were operating one-hundred and twenty-four ambulances (in addition to the free-standing private services). The hospital fleet alone made 334,000 calls in 1954, down from 503,000 in 1941, a decrease attributed to the absence of ambulance surgeons after the war, removing the incentive to call an ambulance as a free substitute for a house call by the local doctor.[16] As for the Manhattan hospitals themselves, in 1955 a Hospital Council spokesman observed that modern infirmaries had no incentive to provide ambulance services since such operations inevitably lost money and "there is no penalty or stigma attached to not operating an emergency ambulance service."[17]

In fact, the Hospital Council of Greater New York had published a 1950 report alleging that the best solution to the ambulance problem was turning over the entire operation to a single municipal agency, preferably the Police Department. The NYPD was uniquely qualified since it was already the first to receive such calls, had the radio equipment to stay in contact with a fleet of ambulances, and its dispatchers had demonstrated over long years their skills in making reasonable judgments about whether or not to request a physician to ride along when

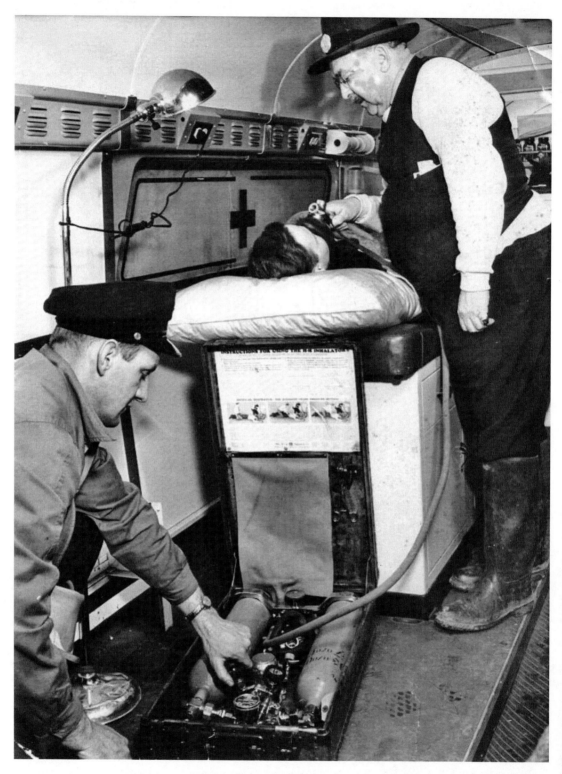

In 1950 the "Second Alarmers Rescue Squad" of Montgomery County, Pennsylvania, acquired an advanced rescue unit that, in addition to transporting ten patients, was equipped for medical services including transfusions and pulmonary resuscitation. Unfortunately, few ambulance services of the 1950s approached this level of service (courtesy Second Alarmers Association and Rescue Squad, Montgomery County, PA).

relaying ambulance calls.[18] Still, the report acknowledged that some of the city's hospitals persisted in providing ambulance service, noting:

> These hospitals believe that ambulances cruising in the neighborhood are visible evidence of a service being rendered to the community ... a bond with the outside world that sustains and supports the hospital. It may serve as means of attracting workmen's compensation and city patients as well as a means of selecting desired types of clinical material for the hospital's training program.[19]

(The use of the ambulance to bring in teaching cases, to solicit support, and to advertise the hospital's existence, were identical to arguments raised in the 19th century ... and the argument that they might conceivably be operated at a profit, even by indirectly increasing "workmen's compensation" and "city patients," is an argument that would reappear fifty years later, when a 2001 New York City Comptroller's report revealed hospital ambulances were ten times more likely to take patients to their home infirmaries than they were to deliver them to the hospital closest to the pick-up point ... a dangerous and illegal discrepancy not observed with ambulances operated by the city fire department, which lacked the financial incentive to bypass the nearest hospital in favor of their own.[20])

The financial burdens of an ambulance service were not inconsiderable, especially since it was often difficult to collect payment, and by 1948 only three New York City non-profit hospitals ran self-sustaining ambulance services, while close to thirty others were taking losses ranging from $2000 to $25,000 per year.[21] To help staunch the green hemorrhage the city paid an annual "subvention" to each non-profit hospital operating an ambulance service—between 1943 and 1945 this sum was $5800 per vehicle, but as these private hospitals posted ever larger losses in the post-war years (largely due to limited success in collecting payments) this prop was increased to $11,500 per ambulance by 1952.[22] Despite the largesse, Brooklyn emergency services took a triple hit when Beth El, Brooklyn Jewish, and Methodist hospitals all abandoned their ambulance services by 1954, saying that even with the city subsidy they could no longer afford to operate their aid cars.[23] Faced with the defections the city promptly increased the ambulance subsidy to $18,500: the disappointing return on their investment was a single ambulance added to the newly opened Long Island Jewish Hospital in Queens.

The case against hospital ambulance services was neatly summed up in an article entitled "Don't Overlook the Ambulance as a Public Relations Tool," appearing in *The Modern Hospital* in September, 1950. As the author noted: "Mention the word 'ambulance' to a hospital administrator, and his reaction will likely be a pained look of resignation, a triumphant grin, or a vacuous stare, depending on whether he has an ambulance in operation, has delegated the function to some outside agency, or has never operated an ambulance." Ambulances were, he continued, expensive, they scared away interns who were increasingly unwilling to work on them, and they entailed perpetual staffing problems since few good drivers were willing to cover long overnight shifts.[24] On the other hand, an ambulance advertised the hospital and generated good will that might translate into something tangible at an annual fund drive or a public vote on a city subsidy for capital improvements. Nonetheless, the 1950s saw a steady trend of hospitals quitting the ambulance business and more and more of these duties passing to independent providers. (*The Modern Hospital,* that revealing look into the in-basket of the mid-century hospital operator, gave an accurate reading of the trend. Starting in 1942 it sharply decreased the number of articles and advertisements dedicated to ambulance service, coincident with the intern shortage of World War II and its impact on hospital ambulance services, until by the mid 1950s the ambulance virtually vanished as either an editorial or commercial subject between its covers. These editorial changes paralleled the withdrawal of hospitals from ambulance service, just as the same pages reflected other historical trends ... for example, during the same time its dietary pages jettisoned sample patient menus featuring cream of onion soup and prune

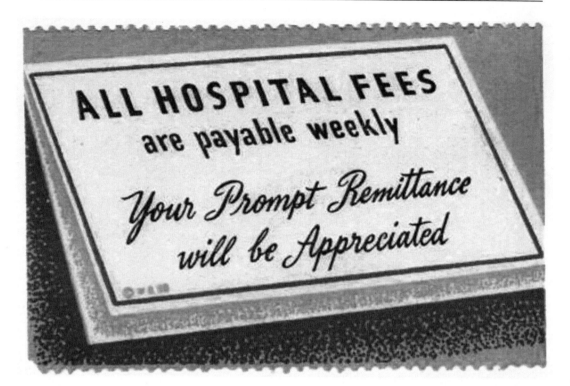

Well into the 1960s the majority of insurance companies imposed ambulance service deductibles that were much higher than the typical bill. As a result, ambulance fees were an out of pocket expense to patients, and hospitals and other providers frequently wrote off the bill as uncollectable.

shakes in favor of articles exploring the use of pre-frozen meals and vending machines to deliver calories to the inpatients.) Meanwhile, as administrators debated whether the PR value of ambulances outweighed their burdens and municipalities bribed providers to stay in business, a new and terrible argument for expanding and improving ambulance services was taking shape: the Cold War.

Duck and Cover

Ever since the U.S.S.R. detonated a nuclear bomb in August 1949 the government of the United States had been planning for "the unthinkable:" minimizing, to the extent possible, the civilian casualties of an atomic war. Medical preparedness was integral to this strategy, and Congress was quick to send Civil Defense dollars to protect the voting districts back home. These funds were eagerly received by a medical establishment beset with a host of problems in the early 1950s. As *The New York Times* reported in 1951, America's hospitals faced a crisis as they struggled with supply and staff shortages related to the "police action" in Korea and simultaneously assumed the burden of coping with threats of "atom bomb and bacteriological injuries, and also in training the thousands of volunteers that are being asked to serve in the civilian health corps."[25] Add to this the increasing numbers of hospitalized patients discussed earlier and it becomes clear why ambulances were getting short-shrift from the hospitals.

As hospitals started mothballing their ambulances, many concerned municipalities began upgrading their city emergency services: lending haste to their preparations were covers of *The*

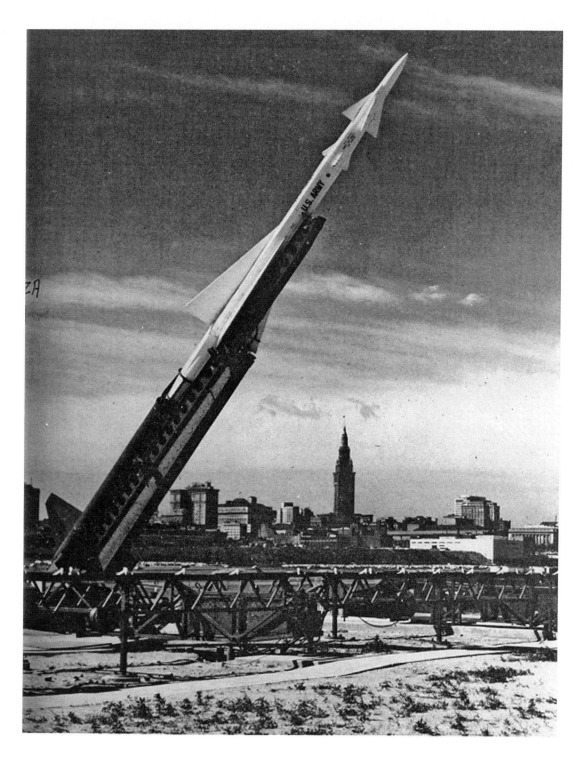

The new symbol of the age, a Nike missile battery guards Cleveland against Soviet bombers in 1954. The threat of atomic warfare was a critical element inspiring municipal ambulance reform across the country (United States Army Archives).

Bulletin of Atomic Scientists where, by 1953, the Doomsday Clock stood poised at two minutes to midnight. In this climate the emergency medical service was increasingly seen as a utility too important to leave wholly to the private marketplace. (Of course there were communities where this ethos had always been upheld: New York City made accident cases the province of the police in the 1850s and had explicitly reserved the right to regulate emergency ambulance services under the 1909 Board of Ambulances statute, and communities as disparate as Los Angeles and Yakima, Washington had been providing free or subsidized ambulance services for years.) Typical of many American cities was Rochester, New York, which in 1952 took several steps to reassert some municipal control over the crucial area of emergency response. It approved $10,000 for the acquisition of a new rescue vehicle to be deployed to major emergencies and disaster scenes and, on the recommendation of the Board of Fire Underwriters, purchased breathing apparatus, floodlights, oxy-acetylene torches, and construction grade cutting tools for placement in the cars of the fire department's Battalion Chiefs.[26] Significantly, 1952 also marked the first time that fire-fighting equipment, including city ambulances operated by the bureau, was cross-referenced with "Civil Defense" in the index of the City Council proceedings—proof that the government thought of emergency medical systems not as a simple product, like taxis, but as an element of the newly vital civil defense system.

Meanwhile, in 1954 the Mississippi Hospital Association rolled out its first "mobile disaster hospital unit," a grand title dwarfing its owner—a four-door sedan with emergency-lights and siren synchronized to its flashing red bumper lights.[27] A pale shadow of Portland's "Coffee Wagon," the MDHU carried a "heavy-duty" first-aid kit, high-pressure fire extinguisher, spotlight, flares, and, eventually, a PA system. It also sported a three-way radio to stay in communication with both the state police and the Civil Defense Council in case the Cubans invaded Biloxi, and its Highway Patrol designation number was painted on the roof for the benefit of spotter aircraft. While it could transfer the injured if absolutely necessary, its principle function was to carry medical specialists, such as neurosurgeons and specialty nurses, to disaster areas, or to take administrators and medical equipment to impromptu hospital sites when regular facilities were destroyed by natural disaster or enemy attack.

Perhaps the apogee of integrating ambulance services into the Civil Defense occurred in Chicago in 1955, when authorities experimented with using semi-truck trailers as massive, impromptu ambulances to carry hospital patients to the presumed safety of the suburbs ahead of threatened attack. Few contemporary commentators were persuaded that such efforts had any hope of success. Walter Trohan, chief of *The Chicago Tribune's* Washington bureau, had this to say about such schemes:

> ... few would be able to flee even if the roads were clear and few of these could be expected to survive if they could flee, and fewer still could be expected to reproduce their kind without mutations. It is a terrible thing to contemplate, yet the civil defense administration goes blithely on its useless way making ridiculous and unrealistic plans.[28]

Still, attention to civil defense co-ordination revealed a prevailing weakness in U.S. ambulance services: a frequent absence of central dispatch that caused chaos in the face of such quotidian disasters as a train derailment in Los Angeles in 1956 when ambulance teams crowded and jostled one another at the scene even as victims were being evacuated in private vehicles.[29] If competing, conflicting ambulance operations couldn't effectively handle a train derailment, how would they cope with atomic war? Additionally, the prospect of nuclear attack prompted civic officials to make thoughtful lists of what medical equipment would be needed—and more attentive leaders wondered if it wasn't time to make sure similar gear was available on the civilian ambulances their communities relied on every day. After all, if municipal ambulances being kitted out to respond to a theoretical attack by hydrogen bombs or germ warfare were up to the state of the art, why should the ambulances actually responding to the daily mayhem of

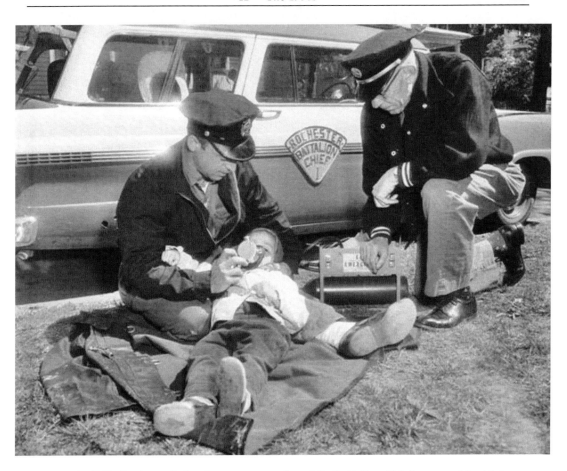

In the early 1950s Rochester's fire department equipped its Battalion Chief cars as aid vehicles on the recommendation of the Board of Insurance Underwriters. Similar changes were incorporated in Civil Defense planning nationwide and preceded the adoption of fully equipped paramedic rigs (from the Collection of the Rochester Municipal Archives).

city and suburban life be sub par and unregulated? Of course, one limiting factor in ambulance modernization was that during the 1950s ambulance expenses were borne by the patients themselves, since most insurance plans covered hospitalization only, not outpatient care, and the public safety-net programs like Medicare were still a decade away. (For example, even as late as 1969 the national average for an ambulance call was under $45, but major medical plans like Blue Cross/Blue Shield typically imposed a $100 deductible for ambulance services, meaning that most consumers continued to envision ambulance service as a household expense and, when choice was possible, selected accordingly.[30]) Ambulance providers, limited to out-of-pocket reimbursement, were faced with real financial restrictions on how much capital improvement could be poured into their vehicles.

On the other hand, portions of the medical community were becoming restive when it came to the quality of emergency response in the United States. Expanded interstate highways, built to facilitate the transfer of troops and material in the event of war, opened throughout the 1950s, and these wide, smooth concrete avenues allowed faster speeds which translated into more fatalities after the inevitable wrecks. Federal Highway Safety meetings had taken place since 1946, but they assumed new importance as the annual death toll for road accidents crashed through the 40,000 barrier in the late 1950s. Miles driven almost doubled between 1945 and 1949, and

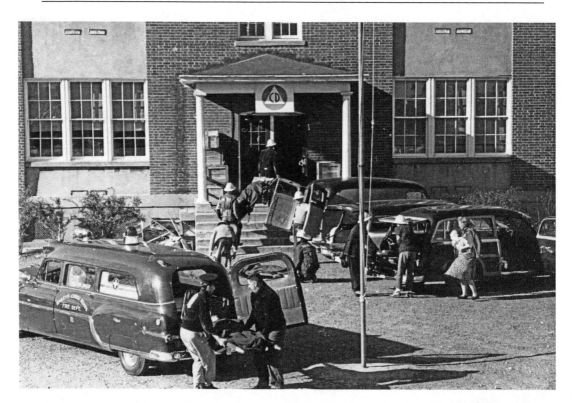

Ambulances assemble at a fall-out shelter during this Civil Defense drill in 1955 (Frank Bauman, Library of Congress, Prints & Photographs Division, *Look* Magazine Photograph Collection, Job 55-6354).

experts extrapolated ever-increasing death rates for the foreseeable future. The need for new safety initiatives was clearly a necessity, starting with more rigorous licensing standards. (President Truman told a 1949 Highway Safety Conference "Why, a man can go down to a drugstore from an insane asylum and spend a quarter and get a license to drive on any road in [Missouri], if he wants to."[31]) Other measures included widely distributed driver's education films, and in the name of highway safety American adolescents were treated to such 16mm treasures as "The Bottle and the Throttle" and "The Last Prom." Whether graphic footage of highway carnage actually made teenagers safer drivers is debatable, but there was one point upon which all parties soon agreed—although accidents were inevitable, the percentage of *fatal* accidents could be reduced if the quality of ambulance services improved.

An Era of Change Begins

Doctors saw the same headlines as the politicians, of course, and many also found themselves on the receiving end of shoddy ambulance services when bare-boned vehicles dropped off their cargo of misery at the hospital's back-door. Consequently, some physicians started looking for ways to stay involved with the shape and practice of emergency medical care, now that they were fast disappearing from actual ambulances. An early leader in this movement was the American College of Surgeons, which had actually entered the debate back in 1922 after forming their first committee on fractures, and by the 1950s this working group's transportation sub-committee was a strong voice for central ambulance dispatch, comprehensive

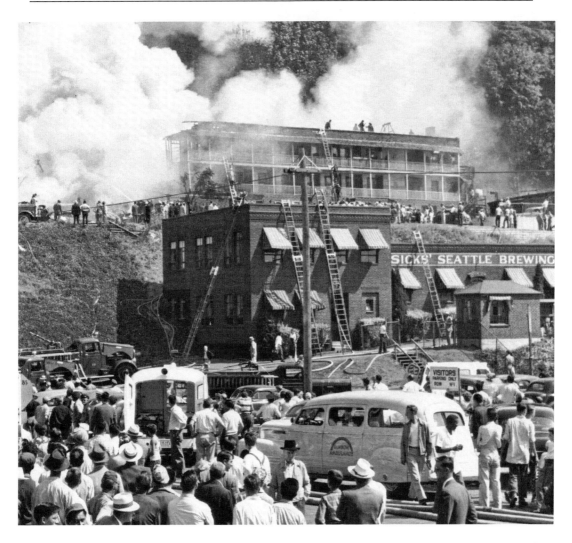

A Rainbow Ambulance Company crew responds to an apartment fire in Seattle, sometime in the early 1950s. Disaster responses such as this one were increasingly seen as integral to Civil Defense needs, leading to more government attention to the equipment and staffing of private ambulances during the 1950s (Seattle Museum of History and Industry).

oversight, modern equipment, and training to include at least a Red Cross Advanced First Aid Certificate. Specialty professional groups also began to form and take an interest in the debate, such as the American Association for the Advancement of Automotive Medicine (founded in 1957 by six physicians with a passion for race cars and an interest in what happened to their drivers when they crashed). In 1958 delegates from the American College of Surgeons, the American Association for the Surgery of Trauma, and the National Safety Council came together to form a Joint Action Program to raise the standards of immediate medical intervention in cases of traumatic injury, particularly through improved ambulance services. Lending impetus to the debate were trauma surgeons returning from the Korean theater where new medical techniques—including rapid response by skilled corpsman and swift transportation of the injured to well-equipped mobile surgical hospitals—had resulted in significantly improved survival rates, and the often dramatic contrast to conditions in many civilian hospitals was inevitably a source of frustration. Physicians were not the only group growing impatient with the inadequacies of most ambulance services in the country. As the Cold War progressed cities and states began critically examining their civil defense capabilities, an exercise invariably revealing a gulf between what they wanted for their municipal rescue vehicles and what was actually available to their citizens. Likewise, the public was beginning to appreciate the discrepancy between what was theoretically possible in terms of medical expertise and what was routinely available at the scene of the accident or the acute illness. A disparate, and largely inchoate, resistance to the emergency service status quo was building, and it was no longer a question of "if" they would see their reforms put into place, but when.

• 13 •

The 1960s: Changing Tactics

By the end of the 1950s the U.S. interstate highway system was unmistakably both an engineering triumph and a public safety problem. Not only did more people own cars thanks to the post-war prosperity, but the novel expressways beckoned them to drive further and faster than had previously been possible: inevitably, the traffic fatality rates that had grabbed Truman's attention in the late 1940s continued their relentless climb, and the problem was increasingly framed as one requiring a solution on the same scale as the roadway system itself. At the same time, emergency medical care, to the extent it engaged the federal government at all, was relegated to seldom visited bureaucratic cul-de-sacs. Throughout the 1960s the diligent might have tracked down one of these minor entities, the Department of Emergency Medical Services, buried within the massive enterprise that was the old Department of Health, Education, and Welfare. The EMS section was little more than a rounding error in the HEW budget, a cluster of filing cabinets and desks subject to having its name changed during periodic reorganization schemes and apparently able to do little more than correspond with the various private and non-profit organizations attempting to reform America's fractured system of ambulance care in the early 1960s.[1]

Meanwhile, in 1956 the United States Public Health Service had created a small and lightly staffed "accidental injury section," which even after being upgraded to the Division of Accident Prevention in 1960 continued to operate under conditions only slightly more generous than those prevailing for the EMS department at HEW. It focused on the prevention of domestic injuries by teaching people to be safer (poison control was an early area), and its involvement with post-accident care was limited to the occasional small research grant. This model—that resources were best spent on avoiding accidents rather than mitigating their consequences—was certainly logical in a "stitch in time saves nine" sort of way, but its application was hindered by an assumption that the best way to reduce injuries was to change human behavior, not product design, apparently assuming that it was easier to develop perfection in human being as opposed to safer stair risers, automobile glass, or lawnmowers. (For example, seatbelts only become necessary when you get in an accident, so rather than impose mandates on manufacturers to include them in all cars, the model would recommend teaching people to be safer drivers, thus making seatbelts unnecessary.[2]) While its oversimplification is easy to criticize, in the 1950s this model was an accepted truism among many academics and policy makers—as well as among industrial firms providing research grants and campaign contributions, and who were sympathetic to any theory that shifted liability from product to consumer. It was also a perception that paid little attention to the issue of what needed to be done to temporize the harm after an accident had already occurred.

Of all the federal services, the military had the largest interest in emergency medicine, but its research seldom reached the civilian world, although returning veterans from Korea and, eventually, Viet Nam, became more influential over time. Ultimately, the nexus for federal

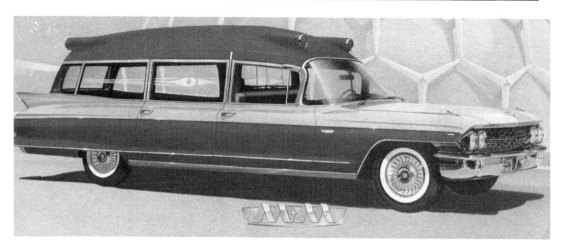

A 1963 Miller-Meteor "Volunteer" ambulance, one of the mid-range models marketed to the increasing number of voluntary emergency service providers stepping in to replace the ever fewer hospital and mortuary ambulance services (courtesy Miller-Meteor/Accubuilt).

attention to the question of how to improve civilian emergency medical service in the late 1950s and early 1960s rested in those portions of the government involved with the highways department. While apparently natural that those federal agencies busy constructing the freeways would take some interest in preserving the lives of those using them, this interest was actually pushed by a few government researchers who had become proponents of a then countercultural approach to injury prevention—the pre-accident, accident, and post-accident model of emergency medicine, giving equal weight to educating people on safe behavior, making industrial designs less harmful in the event of failure or misuse, and improving the quality of emergency service responding to an accident. By the early 1960s proponents of this theory had infiltrated the industrial, academic, and governmental fields in sufficient numbers to actually influence policy. This new emphasis on post-accident, pre-hospital care was reflected in the first widely distributed federal critique of ambulance and emergency medical services, *Health, Medical Care and Transportation of the Injured,* published by the President's Commission on Highway Safety in 1965.

The Commission looked at the widely variable emergency medical services in the country, from highly regarded rescue squads in New York and Baltimore to the minimalist station wagons and hearses operating out of gas stations and funeral parlors from Nebraska to Mississippi, and recommended that all ambulance crews be licensed and required to attend "complete and practical paramedical courses," ideally taught by physicians with expertise in trauma.[3] Acknowledging the dearth of research on what an optimal ambulance design might be, the Commission suggested that a reasonable minimum would include: seatbelts, heat and air conditioning, a way for an attendant in back to communicate with the driver (and thus, by implication, a minimum of two crew members), room for two litters in back, lighting enough to examine a patient, soundproofing, and a two way radio. They also urged that ambulances and rescue squads carry the "minimal equipment list" published in 1961 by the American College of Surgeons: bandages, tape, tourniquet, tongue blades, shears, safety pins, slings, padded boards for fractures, pillows, oxygen and a mask, oropharyngeal airways, and both adult and pediatric mouth-to-mouth airways. (For the ambitious, the Commission suggested that if the crew could be properly trained the ambulance might include mechanical suction gear, a bag and mask resuscitator, restraints, and IV fluids.)

The commission's modest recommendations were politely received by those who chanced

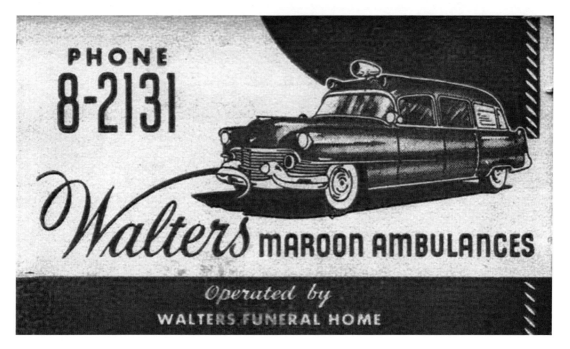

In McCormick, South Carolina, population 2,000, as late as 1973 only a red light on the roof separated the town ambulance from the town hearse. One resident said, "When the red light is on, you know it's an ambulance.... When it's off, it's a hearse. And if they switch it off halfway to the hospital, you know what happened" ("Ambulance Aid Deficient," *New York Times*, Aug. 19, 1973).

to read them, but the report was not widely distributed outside of Washington and the level of federal involvement in the local issue of ambulance operation remained negligible. The principal actors in ambulance reform continued to be motivated community members and national professional organizations, such as the American College of Surgeons and the Academy of Orthopaedic Surgeons. Their success was, unfortunately, largely at the margins: a 1965 survey discovered that only 22 percent of municipalities regulated ambulance services, and a mere 8 percent—seventy two communities out of nine-hundred—went so far as to require the Red Cross Advanced First Aid course for ambulance duty.[4] While there were certainly individual ambulance services who did not require legislation to improve training or equipment, there is no question that the overwhelming number of emergency medical providers were undertrained and underequipped, and when this was combined with ever increasing highway use, it becomes less than startling that in that same year, 1965, over 49,000 Americans died in automobile accidents, planting a new and grisly milestone along the ever expanding interstate road system. Also in 1965 Ralph Nader's *Unsafe At Any Speed* was published, a best-seller revealing how automotive manufacturers were retailing vehicles with designs they knew increased the likelihood of death or injury in a crash, but which they felt were justified because they made the cars more appealing to customers and, again, if people would just drive safely it wouldn't matter that the rigid steering column could crush their chests like a paper bag in a collision or that the chrome-heavy dashboard was gleaming buzzsaw at face level in a sixty-mile an hour crash. The combination of Nader's book and the new fatality record seized the attention of the public, and of Congress, and in an effort to get out ahead of the issue President Johnson used a line in his 1966 State of the Union Address to ask Congress to adopt legislation to reduce the traffic fatality rate.[5] While the public's attention was largely focused on dangerous car designs, the professional interest in improving after-accident emergency medical care also gained impetus from the national attention to highway safety. Ultimately, while the President's Commission on Traffic Safety may have made little impression with their 1965 report on deficiencies in the ambulance service, their motivations struck a chord with an increasing number of like minded individuals within the government, and their philosophy of combining safer industrial products with improved pre-hospital care would be reflected in the reforms to come.

On September 9, 1966, in good part due to Nader's book, the Highway Safety Act was passed, creating a National Highway Traffic Safety Administration (originally in the Department of Commerce, but soon reassigned to the new Department of Transportation, created in October). While the Safety Administration was given the broad task of overseeing government policies aimed at reducing morbidity and mortality due to traffic mishaps, the statute itself left the actual details to the Secretary to sort out later. Among the laundry list of actionable areas mentioned in the statute, the last one listed was the catchall "emergency services," an addendum finally putting ambulance regulation within the ambit of the Great Society.[6] This reference to the emergency services, while nearly an afterthought in the long litany of highway safety measures preceding it in the statute (licensing, roadway surfaces, pedestrian education, and so on), coincided with two critically important events influencing the manner in which the broad grant of authority in the 1966 Act was translated into actual change for ambulance services. The first was the collapse of the funeral home ambulance business in the United States, and the second was the publication of *Accidental Death and Disability*, a government report which became a template for ambulance reform for the rest of the decade.

Mortuary Ambulances

At the time the Highway Safety Act was passed the National Academy of Sciences estimated twelve thousand morticians collectively provided more than half of the nation's ambulances.[7] Their services were not distributed evenly, however. As far back as 1958 the country's largest mortuary association polled its members on ambulance service and found that medical transportation provided by funeral homes was directly linked to community size: in towns with populations of 20,000 or less mortuary ambulances provided at least 60 percent of the services, dwindling to a mere 6 percent in cities of 250,000 or more.[8] (The same study noted that private ambulance companies began to provide stiff competition once a community exceeded 20,000, with municipal services not becoming a significant challenger until the average city achieved a census in excess of 100,000.)

In addition to this population dependent distribution, funeral home ambulance services also showed strong geographical bias. South of the Mason-Dixon line mortuaries had long been nearly synonymous with ambulance service, and by 1965 morticians operated at least three quarters of all ambulances in Arkansas, Georgia, Kentucky, Mississippi, North Carolina, Oklahoma, Tennessee, Texas, and West Virginia, and enjoyed strong pluralities in all other southern states except Virginia.[9] (It was in the "Old Dominion" that Julian Wise had started his influential volunteer life-saving crew in 1928, and forty years later the Roanoke Rescue Squad and its successful imitators had made the funeral home ambulance nearly superfluous.)

Elsewhere, however, the various states and regions defied categorization. Some followed the South, trusting the living as well as the dead to the mortician, and funeral home ambulances dominated otherwise disparate jurisdictions like Iowa, Vermont, Kansas, and New Mexico. Similarly, the 1961–62 edition of the National Ambulance Directory listed sixty funeral homes providing ambulance service in Pennsylvania—alongside a mere five hospitals and ten free-standing ambulance services like *Russo's Convalett Service*, the *Snow Shoe Ambulance*

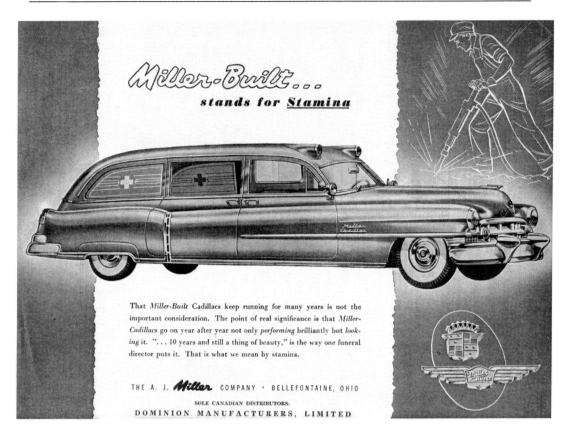

This 1951 Miller ambulance advertisement ran in the trade journal *Canadian Funeral Home*, since sales to mortuaries represented an enormous share of the post-war ambulance market (courtesy Miller-Meteor/Accubuilt).

Club, and the *Penn Alto Garage* in Altoona.[10] In Oregon, Utah, and Colorado the police and fire departments claimed a plurality. States with large numbers of volunteer ambulance services could be big and rural (Idaho, Montana, Nevada, Nebraska, and North Dakota, averaging fifty percent), or small and densely populated (Connecticut and Delaware, with sixty and eighty-five percent respectively), while only in California did commercial firms dominate emergency services, operating 53 percent of ambulances by the late 1960s.[11] Still, the truth was that for most Americans the only difference between an ambulance and a hearse was whether there was a cot or a casket in the back.

Despite their general dominance of the national market, when the end came for the funeral home ambulances it came quickly, under the guillotine of a falling profit margin. In 1965 the Labor Department issued a ruling that all ambulance providers were involved in "interstate commerce" as a matter of law, suddenly requiring those firms with gross receipts of $1,000,000 a year to pay employees the federal minimum wage—$1.25 an hour, with time and a half for anything over forty hours a week. This was an especial shock in the humid climes, as in the southern states a typical hourly wage for a mortuary ambulance attendant stood between seventy and eighty cents an hour. Further, crews routinely worked twenty-four-hour shifts and it was not uncommon for them to work sixty hour weeks with no overtime pay.[12] A year later the Minimum Wage Act was extended to businesses with gross volumes of $500,000, significantly increasing the number of ambulance firms affected by the mandatory increase in wages: for the typical ambulance provider, salaries made up 75 percent of their operating budget, so a

Southern operator paying the prevailing wage of seventy-five cents an hour faced roughly a 50 percent increase in overhead.[13] In Texas, where funeral parlors dominated the ambulance market, the reaction was swift and decisive, and by July 1967 fifteen Texas cities found themselves abruptly stripped of ambulance services when mortuary owners asserted poverty and abandoned the emergency service trade.[14] From Houston to El Paso one funeral home after another dropped their ambulance services, blaming the increase in the minimum wage, until a 1969 survey reported that emergency medical services had completely disappeared from five percent of Texas counties and the rest were underserved.[15] At the same time, the director of the Texas Division of Disaster Health and Medical Services reported that a fifth of all recent traffic fatalities could have been saved if adequate emergency aid and transport had been available.[16]

While undeniably dramatic, this financial pain was not confined to the Lone Star State or even to mortuaries. For example, a Washington State Hospital Association survey found that between late 1966 and early 1967 no fewer than nineteen local hospitals discontinued or cut back their ambulance services in response to the change in the minimum wage, while in nine Washington cities the change in the law had driven out every one of their ambulance providers.[17] As similar reports came in from around the country it was clear that a national ambulance crisis was under

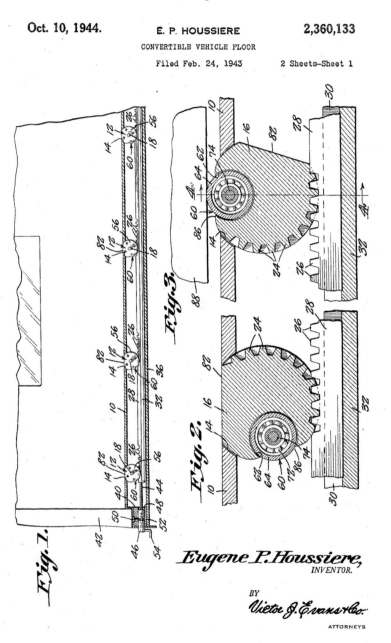

The retractable casket brace shown here made the conversion of hearse to ambulance simpler and safer, helping to create the market for "conversion professional cars" that were popular sellers through the early 1970s (U.S. Patent Office, No. 2,360,133).

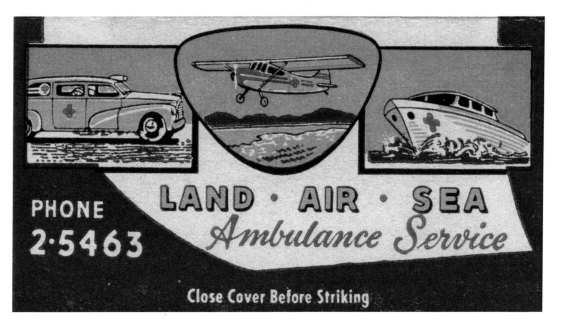

Details from a matchbook cover advertising the range of ambulance services offered by a northeastern mortuary in the 1940s.

way, a crisis coinciding with a federal mandate for the new Department of Transportation to set standards for emergency medical services that could be implemented at the state level. Guidance for the shape these standards would take came in the form of a report released contemporaneously with the Safety Act itself.

Accidental Death and Disability

As Congress was literally voting on the Safety Act, the Government Printing Office was finishing its run of a slim, twenty-three page pamphlet called *Accidental Death and Disability: The Neglected Disease of Modern Society*. Not much larger than a brochure, it was released in September, 1966, and within its economic maxims was concealed a critical mass of outrage that would dynamite the way clear for the second ambulance revolution. The report had started with the National Research Council, which had been the target of periodic lobbying by a number of medical professionals who felt the status of emergency medical care was under-researched. Finally, in 1963, the NRC put together a collaborative project to investigate the status of accidental death and injury as a national public health issue, significantly outpacing earlier efforts by the under-resourced Accident Prevention Division and its poor sisters throughout the bureaucracy. The task was assigned to the NRC committees on Shock, Trauma, and Anesthesia, with instructions to not only quantify the burden of accidental injury and death, but to pay particular attention to the status of initial care, an area long neglected in academic studies of the problem. The result was *Accidental Death and Disability*, a document destined to be quoted thousands of times in the ensuing debate over how to improve ambulance services.

Among the headline findings of the committees were that accidents were the leading cause of death for those under 37 years of age and were the fourth leading cause of death, overall. The Council report provided specifics, including some "salient factors which require early solutions," as follows:

1. The general public is insensitive to the magnitude of the problem of accidental death and injury.

2. Every ambulance and rescue squad crewmember, police officer, firefighter, "paramedical," and employee in a high risk industry, should be trained in the techniques of cardiopulmonary resuscitation, childbirth, and other lifesaving measures.

3. Local political authorities have neglected their responsibility to provide optimal emergency medical services.

4. Research on trauma has not been supported or identified at the National Institutes of Health on a level consistent with its importance as the fourth leading cause of death and the primary cause of disability.

5. Potentials of the U.S. Public Health Service programs in accident prevention and emergency medical services have not been fully exploited.

6. Data are lacking on which to determine the number of individuals whose lives are lost or injuries are compounded by misguided attempts at rescue or first aid, absence of physicians at the scene of injury, unsuitable ambulances with inadequate equipment and untrained attendants, lack of traffic control, or the lack of voice communication facilities.

7. Helicopter ambulances have not been adapted to civilian peacetime needs.

8. Emergency departments of hospitals are overcrowded, some are archaic, and there are no systematic surveys on which to base requirements for space, equipment, or staffing for present, let alone future, needs.

The report drew considerable attention, and its most famous statistic—that a solider shot in the Viet Nam jungle had a better chance of surviving than a housewife seriously injured in an accident on an American highway—was exactly the kind of memorable sound bite that wins political debates. The conjunction of the 1966 Highway Safety Act and the publication of *Death and Disability* guaranteed that the federal government would take an active part in the reform of ambulance services, and it was no surprise that when the Department of Transportation unveiled its new Emergency Medical Service Standards in mid–1967 they owed much to the themes sketched out in *Death and Disability*. Among other things, DOT made all federal highway funds contingent on a state assembling a program to ensure that victims of highway accidents received "prompt emergency care," creating training and licensing standards for ambulance and rescue vehicle operators, drivers, crew members, and dispatchers; setting vehicle and equipment standards for ambulances; establishing criteria to guarantee two-way radio communication between emergency vehicles and their base of operations; and instituting global policies to ensure that emergency medical services were coordinated between ambulances and receiving facilities: it was also required that the state periodically review its progress and report its findings to the DOT.[18] (Just in time for the new state standards, the American College of Surgeons published a revised "Minimal Equipment List for Ambulances" and saw it swiftly adopted by Virginia and North Carolina.[19])

From the beginning failure to achieve these goals by a set date would result in loss of highway funds—a threat that was never actually carried out, despite widespread failure to comply. Nonetheless, for the first time an attempt was being made to create universal minimum standards for ambulance services, standards that if implemented would represent a significant improvement in the prevailing standard of care. What was still missing were generally recognized specifics for ambulance design and crewmember training: the training standard remained the Red Cross Advanced First Aid course, but many physicians felt this was inadequate—in large measure because at this date the Red Cross considered external cardiac compression too dangerous to be taught to lay people, despite a growing consensus among emergency medicine physicians that the technique *could* be taught safely and was of vital importance in heart attack cases (the only alternative was a mechanical chest compressor like the Westinghouse "Iron Heart," a relatively expensive and cumbersome piece of machinery that encircled the patient's chest and then went to work like a trip hammer).

"Death in a Ditch" and Standardized Training

Critical to any progress in ambulance services would be training, and given its new mandate to oversee and promote improved emergency medical services as part of a national strategy to reduce traffic fatalities, the federal government needed a curriculum to distribute. In retrospect this was a pivotal moment, for the intensity and scope of the training given to the country's ambulance crews would directly influence the configuration and equipage of the vehicles they would be riding in. As it happened this critical history was built around a compelling unifying theme: Dr. Joseph "Deke" Farrington, the son of a Baptist minister who inherited his father's passionate certainty about the fundamental truths—as revealed to himself. (How this moral certainty played in the field is captured by a quote from a friend of Farrington's who recalls watching the great reformer arguing a point with a fellow surgeon: "I have a picture of Deke arguing with Cuthbert Owens in the middle of a ballroom in Washington in which he was apparently trying to do a thoracotomy on Owens with the index finger of his right hand while driving home a point.")[20]

Early in life he picked up the nickname "Deacon" in honor of his evangelical zeal, and

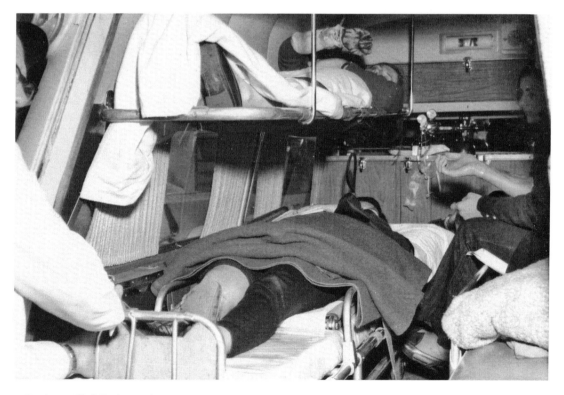

During a Civil Defense disaster drill in the 1960s a private ambulance firm provides transportation services in upstate New York. Use of realistic make-up was used to desensitize trainees and prepare them for the serious injuries they would encounter in the field (ViaHealth Archives Consortium, Rochester, N.Y.).

after graduating from medical school in 1933 he opened a private practice in orthopedics (where for the remainder of his life he treated clergy and their families free of charge, remembering his own family's poverty as they followed his father from one small southern church to another).[21] Tall, balding, and with a bushy goatee, "Deke" grew into a natural teacher and charismatic personality in his own right, and he was soon active in the Chicago branch of the Committee on Trauma of the American College of Surgeons. It was through their office that, in 1963, he and fellow physician Sam Banks taught a four day "Advanced Practical Course in Emergency Aid and Transportation of the Critically Ill and Injured" to the Chicago Fire Department's ambulance division.[22] The course became a yearly event, and was supplemented with semi-annual refresher courses, supervised by Farrington, where the crews toured the Cook County Trauma Center and watched educational films such as "The Four B's: Bleeding, Breathing, Broken Bones, and Burns."

In 1966 Farrington, after thirty-three years in Chicago, opted for a slightly quieter existence as a staff surgeon at Lakeland Memorial Hospital in the resort community of Minocqua, Wisconsin. The pleasant little community saw its population explode during the summer months, with vacationers hell-bent on having a good time: not surprisingly, a significant number of them wound up a night of high-living by barreling back to their lakeside cabins along unlit, unfamiliar roads, drunk behind the wheel of big cars with no seatbelts. Even less surprisingly, a good percentage of them wound up mangled in a ditch, and the route between the ditch and Dr. Farrington's operating theatre was traveled by the little community's volunteer ambulance service and rescue squad: a single converted hearse whose crew was equipped with basic first aid training, some gauze, and not much else.

In the words of a fellow surgeon, Farrington saw no choice but to "set about rectifying this hair whitening situation."[23] To do this he cast back to the short training course he had developed for the Chicago Fire Department several years earlier and expanded and adapted it for the local needs of an all-volunteer, all-purpose ambulance and rescue squad. The result was a twenty-one week evening course in basic trauma and emergency medical care, each class lasting three hours: memorable advice from one his teaching charts includes "Bring in severed parts" and "Do not reinsert intestines" (instead, he recommended wrapping the eviscerated torso loosely with tinfoil).[24] Among the most important aspects of his training course was the attention to careful extrication from a vehicle, particularly the use of back-boards and splinting to minimize the risk of aggravating orthopedic injuries—especially spinal injuries where improper movement could easily kill or paralyze a victim. (His methods for safely extricating and transporting patients with possible spinal fractures were detailed in a richly illustrated article called "Death in a Ditch," published in 1967: the piece was an instant sensation, with 10,000 reprints distributed within a year, and it became arguably the first nationally distributed ambulance training document to have a significant impact on field operations.[25])

The course Farrington assembled was superbly designed to deliver a high degree of technical skill to a lay audience in a minimum amount of time. As he had done with the Chicago firefighters, he relied heavily on creative and interactive teaching tools: students worked on manikins, watched 8mm films, went to the High School automotive workshop to practice vehicle extrications, and used copious amounts of fake blood (liquid starch and food coloring) to vividly mimic ghastly injuries and estimate blood loss by sight. A pre-requisite for enrollment was holding a Red Cross Advanced First Aid card, and the sixty-three hour curriculum that built on this basic training was as follows:

> **Session One:** Orientation (all classes three hours long)
> **Two and Three:** Physiology and Anatomy
> **Four:** Airway management and breathing problems

Five: Cardiac arrest
Six: Bleeding/Shock
Seven: Basic fractures
Eight: Wounds (including burns, electric, radiation, and animal)
Nine and Ten: Acute medical problems (epilepsy, stroke, poisoning, exposure, delirium tremens, etc.)
Eleven: Obstetrics and head/eye/abdominal and genital injuries
Twelve: Legal, public relations, and hospitals
Thirteen: Defensive driving
Fourteen: Practice session with manikins
Fifteen: Spinal fractures
Sixteen: Use of the spine board
Seventeen: Bandaging
Eighteen: Lifts and carries
Nineteen and Twenty: Splints and dressings in situ, and vehicle extrication
Twenty-one: Review[26]

A year after issuing "Death in a Ditch" the National Academy of Sciences/National Research Council published *Training of Ambulance Personnel and Others Responsible for Emergency Care of the Sick and Injured at the Scene and During Transport*—with Farrington the chairman of the College of Surgeons taskforce that actually composed the text. The report summarized many of the various schemes for advanced ambulance crew training then extant in the United States, analyzing seventy short "paramedical" training courses lasting from hours to three days, and evaluating twenty textbooks for ambulance and rescue crewmembers. They concluded that none of these materials was sufficiently complete, and while they failed in a variety of ways commensurate with their sheer numbers, the most prevalent deficiencies were in communications, safe driving, medico-legal issues, rescue techniques, and procedures to safely secure an accident scene.

The following year, 1969, the Department of Health, Education, and Welfare's Public Health Service, Division of Emergency Health Services formally contracted with the American College of Surgeons to develop a training course that would address the needs, and remedy the deficiencies, discussed in *Training of Ambulance Personnel*. (The Department of Transportation and HEW were on the verge of a bureaucratic turf war over who would take the lead on the suddenly vital topic of emergency medical services, although the training materials would eventually become a shared property.) Given Farrington's role in preparing the first report it was small surprise that the resulting *A Curriculum for Training Emergency Medical Technicians* was an almost verbatim reincarnation of his 1966 training course for the Minocqua Rescue Squad. The new course was twenty-four sessions long, adding an extra orientation session, two more review sessions, an expanded CPR section, and an examination at the end. To make room, the separate defensive driving and legal and public relations sessions were eliminated, while the back-board class was integrated into other relevant sessions. The result was a seventy-two hour course (still assuming pre-certification in Red Cross Advanced First Aid), augmented by four hospital training sessions of indeterminate length, exposing students to emergency room and the intensive care units.[27] In addition to the curriculum, the proposal included detailed lists of suitable training films and textbooks, as well as advice on how to successfully present the topics—tips taken from Farrington's own experience in Minocqua, right down to the recipe for artificial blood and a recommendation that instructors bring in rolls of tinfoil to demonstrate how to cover sucking chest wounds and disembowelment, or to wrap up a preemie infant like a baked potato when an incubator was unavailable. The Emergency Serv-

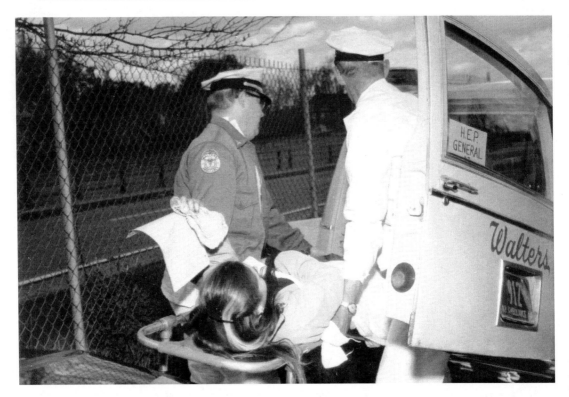

Crew members from Walters Ambulance in Rochester, New York, load a mock patient during a 1960s Civil Defense drill. By the late 1960s intensive and realistic training, as with this mass casualty exercise, was becoming more common (ViaHealth Archives Consortium, Rochester, N.Y.).

ices Division was pleased with the result and, with a few modifications, turned it over to the venerable Dunlop and Associates (government contractors who had been involved in traffic safety research since the 1940s) to create a formal teaching set with slides, manuals, and training films that could be used as a national standard for ambulance crew training.

Paramedics

While Farrington was developing what would become the modern "Basic Life Support" certification for emergency medical technicians, others were attempting to make a quantum leap from Red Cross First Aid training to ultra-skilled "physician extenders" qualified to render advanced medical care in the field. Unlike Farrington's work for the HEW, these early paramedic efforts were undertaken strictly as local experiments, without federal support or even acknowledgment. For the majority of these programs the inspiration was the Belfast Royal Victoria Hospital's Mobile Cardiac Care Unit (popularly known as the "Heart Mobile"), a high intensity ambulance service with physician staffing that began operations January 1, 1966.[28] The brainchild of cardiologist Frank Pantridge, the MCCU relied on a portable defibrillator unit to reverse life-threatening cardiac arrhythmias outside the hospital, at a time when large numbers of heart attack victims were arriving at the emergency room dead on arrival. While designed exclusively for cardiac interventions, its success helped break a psychological logjam that had become the received wisdom about the limits of out-of-hospital care and led to widespread imitation by a number of American and European services.

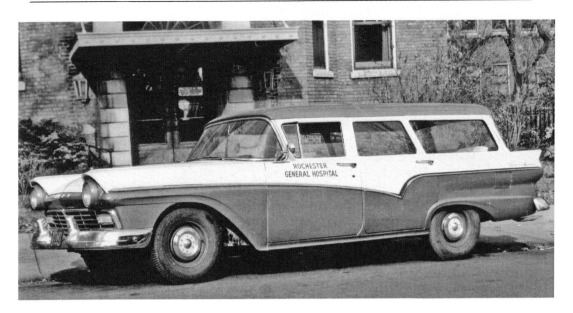

This 1960s station-wagon style ambulance, operated by Rochester (N.Y) General Hospital, was the kind of vehicle that reformers hoped to replace with elaborate models capable of supporting new, more intensive medical services by paramedics (ViaHealth Archives Consortium, Rochester, N.Y.).

In the United States a number of similar programs were operational by the end of 1969, including services that would eventually expand beyond cardiac care and become synonymous with full paramedic service in the early 1970s—Los Angeles, Seattle, and Miami, among them. Before these better known programs, however, there was another—the first true full spectrum paramedic training program, one that took no inspiration from Belfast but which was the brainchild of a civil rights activist in Pittsburgh, a city far removed from the major media markets that later became synonymous with the type of service it pioneered. Formed out of an alliance between a maverick anesthesiologist and a group of unemployed African Americans from an impoverished corner of the Hill District, it began as an experiment to prove that the poorest and least educated citizens in the country could be taught to save lives and operate the finest ambulance service in the world, and ended with that audacious idea triumphant—and the service destroyed.

"We Were the Best": Freedom House Ambulance Service

The story of Pittsburgh's path-breaking ambulance service had its origin in upstate New York, where the man who originated the idea of training the chronically unemployed to staff a top-of-the-line ambulance service had his own introduction to the realities of mid-century emergency care. In 1952 Phil Hallen, a doctoral student in English at Syracuse, learned the cold truth that while the surest way to starve is to try and make a living writing poetry, a close second is writing about *other* people's poetry, and he had been supplementing his income with a variety of jobs at Syracuse's Crouse-Irving Hospital. When he learned that the hospital gave its ambulance drivers rent-free lodgings above the garage, Hallen polished off his driver's license and applied. By this date, medical interns only went outdoors for the most urgent calls, forcing drivers to study enough first aid to handle a variety of simple, and not so simple, cases. To make matters worse, the doctors rotated out each year, so veteran drivers soon knew more emergency medicine than the young physicians they picked up, almost literally, at the steps of the medical school each summer. As Hallen recalled, "Every July first the new interns would show up, and they didn't know [anything]: pretty untrained, but with an M.D. after their name. So, all the drivers would joke with them and tell 'em to stand back and look like you know what you're doing while WE handle it."[29]

A few years piloting Crouse-Irving's beige, hearse-style ambulance gave Hallen a pavement-level look at how what happened in the hospital was limited by what did, or didn't, happen in the field. He drew the logical conclusion that better care in the ambulance saved lives, and a subsequent turn at Yale's prestigious School of Public Health gave him the training and the credentials to do something about it—someday. In 1960, after graduating from Yale and holding administrative posts at several Boston hospitals, he joined Pittsburgh's Hospital Planning Association and found a racially divided city depending on mortuary rigs for routine transfer while medical emergencies were covered by a police ambulance service with well-intentioned officers crippled by poor training and inadequate equipment. Years later Hallen recalled, "I came to Pittsburgh and saw things that were twenty-five years behind the times. They were using police vans and canvas stretchers ... and the white-owned funeral homes didn't want to go near what we used to call 'the ghetto.'"[30] By then Pittsburgh's hospitals had long since abandoned their ambulance services and the Hospital Planning Association provided Hallen no leverage to shift the status quo. A few years later, however, he was named the president of Pittsburgh's Maurice Falk Medical Fund, a foundation with a reservoir of community program dollars. At last Hallen had resources to commit to health care reform, and circumstances soon inspired him to look, once more, at the dismal condition of local emergency services. The opportunity came when David Lawrence, a former Pennsylvania governor and Pittsburgh's mayor between 1946 and 1959, paid the ultimate price for his city's failure to provide adequate ambulances. After years during which private citizens slipped into death and

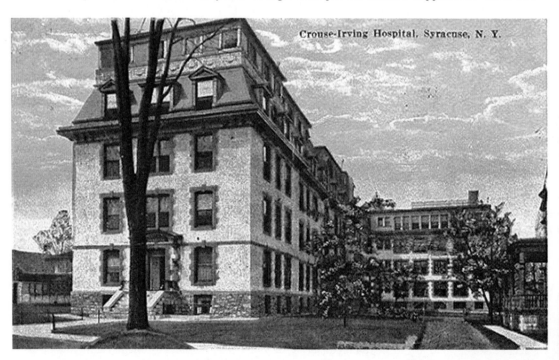

The Crouse-Irving Hospital in Syracuse, where Phil Hallen started working as an ambulance driver in 1952.

disability in the back of modified hearses and police wagons, the mayor's celebrity moved the issue off the anonymous headstones and into the headlines.

On November 4, 1966, the seventy-seven-year-old Lawrence was at the Shriner's Syria Mosque delivering a spirited address at a Democratic fundraiser when he was felled by a massive heart attack.[31] A quick acting nurse in the audience initiated CPR, keeping his body alive while a police emergency wagon careened to a halt outside the elaborate, faux–Moorish hall. What happened next was a dramatic example of the weaknesses in the emergency medical services that had been described only two months earlier in *Death and Disability*. The officers raced inside with their stretcher, heaved Lawrence onto the canvas, and bolted back to their rig while the nurse tried frantically to keep up, watching helplessly as he slipped into pulseless respiratory arrest. Reaching the police wagon she squeezed in back alongside her patient, only to find the inhalator/resuscitator was broken. There was barely enough room for her to move as she leaned over Lawrence and tried to resume CPR, but when the cruiser lurched forward and began its swaying, rocking race to the hospital, she was continually thrown off balance and was unable to continue her resuscitation efforts. For too many critical minutes, from the moment he was settled into the stretcher on the mosque's stage to the time he banged through the ER doors, Lawrence went without oxygen or circulation, and although he was swiftly resuscitated at the hospital the delay caused by the inadequate vehicle and poor equipment left his oxygen-starved brain permanently damaged. When he died two weeks later, without ever regaining consciousness, his death became a minor catalyst in the reform of his city's ambulance system.

Lawrence's death, and the publicity it received, worked on Hallen's mind. The backwardness of the city's ambulance services was an affront to the young reformer, but he was also

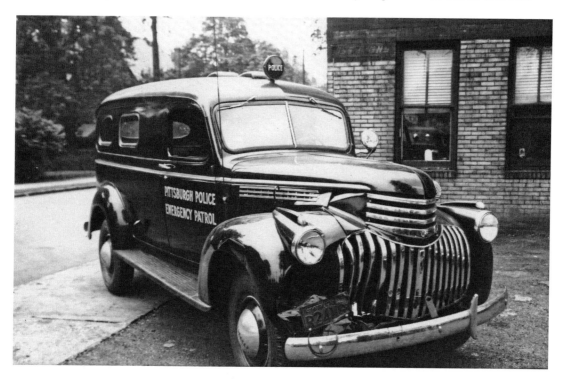

A Pittsburgh Police Department Emergency Patrol in 1947. Political pressure to maintain this rudimentary ambulance operation ultimately stymied efforts to create improved private services (Pittsburgh City Photographer, Archives Service Center, University of Pittsburgh).

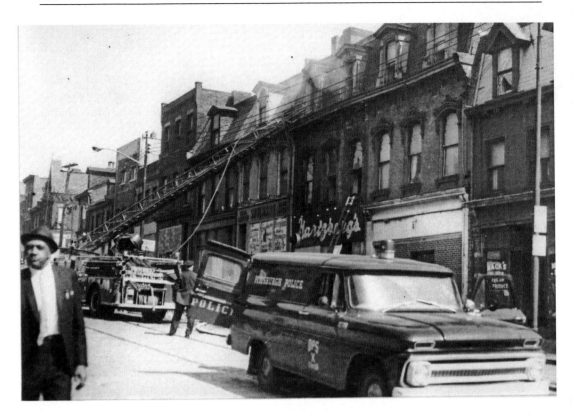

In this mid–1960s view of a business street in the Hill District, one of the two police emergency ambulances assigned to the area stands by at a fire (Carnegie Museum of Art, Pittsburgh; gift of the estate of Charles "Teenie" Harris).

troubled by the dismal condition of the inner city, where economic stagnation and restricted city services conspired to create a culture of futility. In his mind the two seemingly disparate issues swirled together until, in February 1967, influenced by the mayor's death and recent initiatives to bring new businesses to the African-American community, Hallen sat down at his typewriter and banged out "Preliminary Thoughts on the Development of a Private Ambulance Service in the Hill District," the memo that became the founding document for the world's first comprehensive civilian paramedic service.[32] At the time, the neighborhood known as The Hill was the city's most unprepossessing section, a poverty-ridden, mainly African-American enclave. In the 1920s and 1930s it had been an economically diverse neighborhood home to playwright August Wilson, ballplayers like Satchel Paige, and jazz clubs hosting luminaries like Lena Horne and Billie Holiday who flocked to the "The Harlem of the Midwest" when that sobriquet conjured comparisons to The Cotton Club and The Apollo. The war years saw an infusion of new residents during the great migration from the South, but then in the mid–1950s the heart of The Hill's commercial section was flattened to make room for a sporting arena and thousands more were displaced when entire neighborhoods were razed and grim public housing blocks took their place. Stripped of its once viable commercial center and rapidly losing its middle class residents, poverty, crime, and drug use shaped the street until, by the mid 1960s, a nearly self-contained universe of African-American civil life had imploded into a grotesque caricature of its own celebrated past. And as for medical services for the city's poorest citizens, if ambulance service in the rest of Pittsburgh was one step above homicide, in the Hill District it was a case for the Missing Persons Bureau. As a local white nurse noted:

> Let's face it—the poor areas of every city get the worst type of service in every way, and this includes ambulance service. First, there is no money in it. The people they are serving many times don't have enough money to buy groceries, much less pay for ambulance service. Also, there is the racial aspect. Most privately owned services have white drivers and white attendants. The poor areas are usually black, and on emergency calls you can run into some pretty tough situations—stabbings and shootings and the like. Many white attendants don't like these calls because of these factors.[33]

Since private ambulance services were largely unwilling to drive into the "dangerous" ghetto on calls they were unlikely to ever collect a fee for, by 1967 the two police ambulances assigned to the area received an average of seven emergency calls a day. While their response times were not unreasonable, the police crews only held certificates for ten hours of training—and since refresher courses were not required, some of those Red Cross certificates were almost old enough to have been signed by Clara Barton. In a city whose ambulance service was disgracefully out of date, Hallen knew that The Hill was singularly ill served.

Hallen envisioned his proposed ambulance service as providing both medical help and economic opportunity to a community with few examples of either. He saw ambulance work as the kind of exciting job that would appeal to men in particular, believing the service would target that "segment of the male population that does not ordinarily get touched by the typical work programs or social welfare programs in the slum areas," and that the medical training provided would ultimately put trainees in line for better jobs elsewhere, such as hospital work.[34] As he wrote in his first memo, he hoped the service would create "a new kind of business personality in the group," and he wanted the program to be owned and operated by local residents as an entrepreneurial exercise creating jobs for ambulance crews, managers, clerks—and given

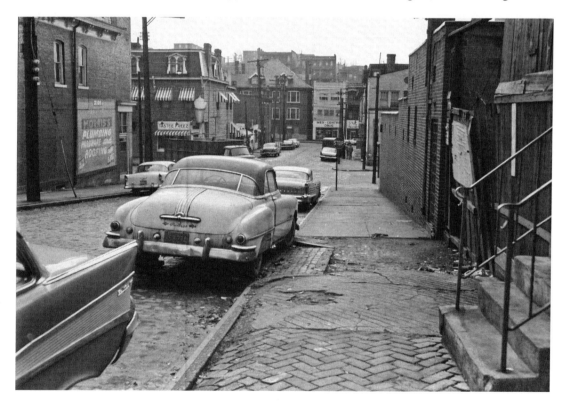

Pittsburgh's Hill District in the 1960s, shortly before arrival of the Freedom House Enterprises Ambulance Service (Pittsburgh City Photographer, Archives Service Center, University of Pittsburgh).

the likelihood the service would begin with second-hand ambulances, plenty of work for local mechanics, as well. Finally, he believed working on ambulances saving lives would give the crews dignity and pride, make them leaders in their community, and ultimately help eradicate racist beliefs that it was lack of ability keeping impoverished African-Americans segregated in economic sloughs.

Hallen took his idea to the University Hospital, obtaining an audience with the hospital president who, apparently seeing something in the idea, referred Hallen to Dr. Peter Safar, Chairman of Anesthesia and already a nationally known figure in the effort to introduce better resuscitation techniques into the emergency services. After several meetings, Safar, looking for a demonstration project for his ideas on out-of-hospital emergency care, agreed to sign on.[35] (Coincidentally, Gerald Esposito, the president of the Pennsylvania Ambulance Association, had recently contacted Dr. Safar about developing state-wide training and equipment standards for ambulance services, and he was quickly brought on board, lending his political and managerial expertise—to say nothing of his enthusiasm—to the nascent scheme.)[36] Given the proposed location in the Hill District, the logical community partner was the neighborhood's Freedom House Enterprise Corporation, founded by James McCoy, Jr., in January 1967 (only a month before Hallen committed his proposal to paper). McCoy wanted to use Freedom House

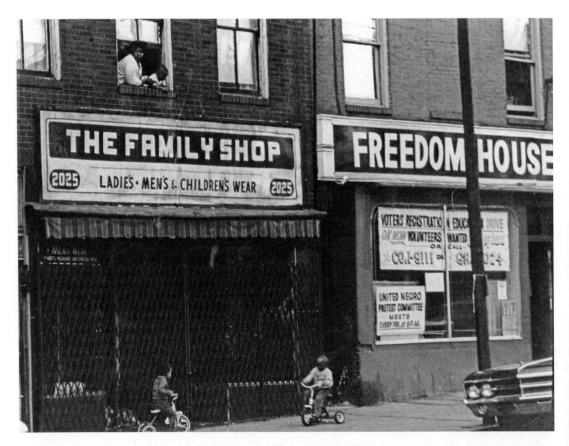

The original Freedom House headquarters in the late 1960s. A young group of community activists chafing at the restraints imposed by their more staid leadership acquired the property for meetings, christening their new home Freedom House because they were "free" to pursue bold plans without naysaying from elders (Library and Archives Division, Historical Society of Western Pennsylvania, Pittsburgh, PA).

to foster self-sustaining African-American businesses in Pittsburgh, and he quickly saw the tremendous potential in Hallen's plan and became an eager participant. Hallen's trips to the University hospital had also gotten his name into the social work department, where a part-time professor named Morton Coleman heard of, and approved, the idea—which was significant because when not teaching undergraduates, Coleman was an aide to Mayor Joseph Barr.

In the space of two months, then, Hallen's idea had attracted a quorum of motivated individuals who each saw in his scheme something they could use—for McCoy, the community activist, the ambulance service represented a novel minority business opportunity of the kind he had founded Freedom House Enterprises to support and develop; for Safar it was a chance to put into action his proposals for improved out-of-hospital resuscitation techniques; for Esposito it was a vehicle to test-run his ideas on new statewide ambulance standards; for Hallen and Coleman it was a chance to address racial disparity while creating a model for community and personal development; while for Mayor Barr it looked like a way to leverage an opportunity to improve services in a decrepit corner of his city. The need was acute, the enthusiasm genuine, and, three months after the idea first occurred to Hallen, the Freedom House Ambulance Service Committee held its inaugural meeting on April 15, 1967. In addition to the principals, the meeting was attended by representatives of the Mayor's Office, the County Medical Soci-

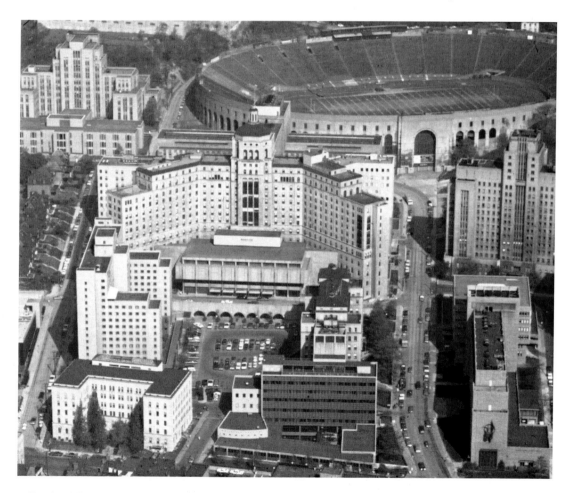

Presbyterian-University Hospital in 1968, when it first served as the operating base for the Freedom House Ambulance Service (University of Pittsburgh Archives, Archives Service Center).

ety, the Pittsburgh Police Bureau, and Presbyterian-University Hospital. (Perversely, with the sole exception of the university, each of these well-wishers would ultimately conspire to destroy the ambulance whose inception they so amiably witnessed: the mayor and the police bureau ultimately saw it, rightly, as a threat to the patrol jobs staffing the police ambulances, and the county starved the service of vital revenue by opposing its expansion outside the downtown core, lest it compete with suburban providers.) At the time ambulance attendant training was already being provided separately by the University's anesthesia department, the Allegheny County Medical Society, and the Pennsylvania State Health Department, but the assembled parties agreed their individual efforts were delivering too little to too few.

Of the three, the County Medical Society represented the largest reservoir of talent and likely political support, and so it was a blow when the head of the County Medical Association, Dr. David Katz, later announced that the association had no interest in aligning itself with a specialized service limited exclusively to the Hill District and would only support the service if it delivered services countywide and recruited employees from the entire metropolitan area and surrounding suburbs.[37] The difficulty with this idea was that the proposed ambulance service had been intended, from the beginning, not only to provide a new model of emergency care but also to develop the economic and social capital languishing in Pittsburgh's inner city. Since the program's community sponsor, Freedom House, had neither a mandate nor an interest in serving overwhelmingly white and relatively wealthy suburbs, the County Medical Society was reluctantly written out.

Although this withdrawal left Dr. Safar as the sole committee member with the expertise to oversee training, it was a task for which he was eminently qualified: after all, he had started developing his own theories on emergency responder training while working with the Baltimore Fire Department back in the 1950s. If this coincidence of need and expertise benefited Freedom House, it must also be said that Dr. Safar made sure that the terms of his cooperation were favorable to his own research efforts. In the end he exacted five promises from Freedom House before he would commit to the project: first, Presbyterian-University's emergency room was to be the preferred receiving site for ambulance calls, and University was the only hospital that would receive life-threatening injuries, including cardiac cases; second, all case data would become the exclusive property of Presbyterian-University hospital; third, he and the hospital would have access to follow-up records of transported patients regardless of destination; fourth, education of the crews was the exclusive prerogative of Presbyterian-University; and fifth, he would have a voice in ambulance design and the day-to-day operations of the service itself, as a sort of ex-officio program director.[38] For their part, the Freedom House Ambulance Service got access to Presby's facilities for training and the nearly undivided attention of Dr. Safar, one of the nation's leading experts on ambulance service, resuscitation, and emergency medicine, as well as being chairman of both the American Medical Association's Emergency Care Committee and the Emergency Committee of the American College of Surgeons. Still, any plan organized to tilt the majority of cases into Presby's ER, and which seemed carefully tailored to further Dr. Safar's personal research, risked alienating other hospitals, regardless of its underlying humanitarian mission. Anticipating this, the memorandum memorializing the Committee's meeting with Dr. Safar specified that Freedom House Enterprises, as the operator of the service, "must be prepared to both accept and defend this policy," and without this loyalty oath Dr. Safar would not participate.[39] Recognizing Dr. Safar's training as indispensable to the program, Freedom House Enterprises pragmatically, if somewhat reluctantly, acquiesced to Safar's terms at a committee meeting on June 17, 1967.[40] The FHE Ambulance Service was on its way.

After discarding a plan to stage the vehicles from an abandoned ambulance center on the grounds of the old Passavant Hospital, Freedom House decided to set up shop in the Presby-

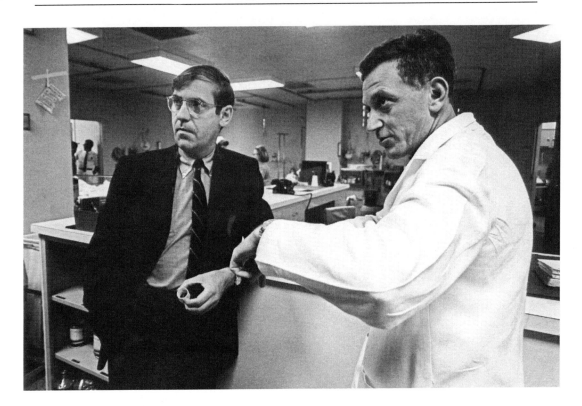

Phil Hallen and Dr. Peter Safar in the Presbyterian-University's ER. A decade earlier Safar introduced rescue breathing to ambulance crews by injecting willing Baltimore firefighters with curare in front of stunned professional audiences while trained laypeople, such as Boy Scouts, kept the paralyzed firemen alive with mouth-to-mouth resuscitation (Library and Archives Division, Historical Society of Western Pennsylvania, Pittsburgh, PA).

terian-University Hospital's Emergency Room. While an early grant proposal envisioned a fleet of ambulances, including a deluxe resuscitation ambulance with physician staffing (based on the 1966 Belfast "heart-mobile"), a wheel-chair ambulance for lucrative non-emergency transfers, and two traditional ambulance rigs, the more austere reality was that the service went into business with just two second-hand police wagons donated by the city (which also pitched in for gas, oil, and maintenance).[41] As the material side dwindled, enlistment ramped into high-gear while the summer of 1967 boiled off into the mists of autumn. Recruiting was done principally through the minority-targeted Opportunities Industrialization Center, but as October wound down and the first day of classes drew near there were so many vacancies that enthusiastic program personnel went into the neighborhoods to approach anybody who appeared to be African- American and unemployed—or who just didn't run away fast enough. Jerry Esposito, taking time away from operating his own ambulance service to assist with setting up the program, was quoted as saying "we went out onto Centre Avenue to finish our recruiting. We literally pulled them off the streets to meet our quota."[42] Whether they volunteered or were shanghaied, the pool of forty-three applicants was subjected to a gantlet of psychological tests, including personality inventories and in-depth interviews with a therapist, followed by serial interrogations by the project director, the project's medical advisor, hospital medical staff, the director of the university's inhalation program, and a representative of the university hospital personnel office.[43] When all was done, the twenty-five survivors entered training in November 1967—five months after program planning had started.[44]

According to the original plan, the "on-the-job training" would be preceded by three months of combined full-time work in the hospital, the lab, and the classroom. That three months ultimately turned into eight, however, due to a high rate of absenteeism, scheduling conflicts with instructors and staff, and the need for twelve of the trainees to only attend part-time while they completed adult education courses to earn a GED. (Since the program opened shop with only six weeks of funding, thanks to the Labor Department and a grant from the Kaufmann Foundation, the principals found themselves perpetually chasing additional funds to keep the project alive.)[45] As written, the clinical curriculum was almost absurdly challenging, and it is a testament to the abilities of the trainees, and the tenacity of their instructors, that so many made it through to the other side. The first thirty-five hours were devoted to completing the standard and advanced Red Cross first-aid courses (which together represented the peak of ambulance attendant training then officially available). Next came fifty hours of anatomy and physiology, taught by instructors from the nursing school. To keep the lessons engaging and as relevant as possible, the instructors used small animal dissection, manikins, x-ray films, and even raw tissue specimens from local slaughter houses to demonstrate their lessons.[46] The remainder of this preclinical course included seven hours of defensive driving, fourteen combined hours of medical ethics, professional deportment and hospital protocol, thirty hours of inhalation therapy, and over twenty hours of CPR training.

After Phase One, which itself was exponentially more training than any non-physician

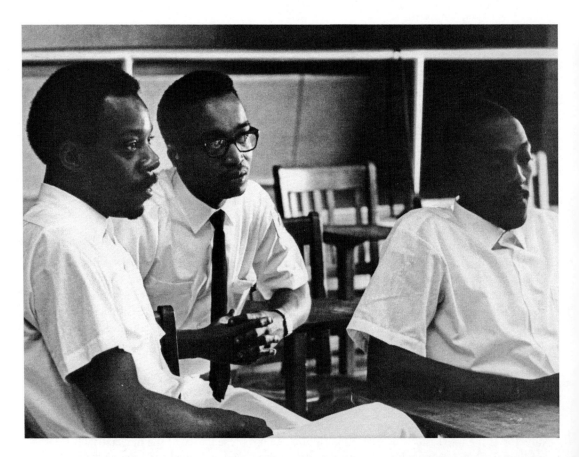

Freedom House recruits attending a lecture in 1967 (Library and Archives Division, Historical Society of Western Pennsylvania, Pittsburgh, PA).

civilian ambulance crew had ever obtained, came one hundred seventy two hours of Clinical Training, and this proved to be the most challenging portion of the program for the trainees as well as their instructors. The curriculum called for the following subjects:

1. Practical experience (six weeks)
    a. Operating room/anesthesiology
    b. Post-anesthesia recovery room (monitoring vital signs, venous infusions)
    c. Intensive care unit (monitoring vital signs, care of intubated patients)
    d. Morgue (gross anatomy review, forensic medicine)
    e. Emergency room (largely observation, some assistance with patient transfer and minor procedures)
    f. Delivery room (observation only)
    g. Inhalation therapy
    h. General medical wards (observation of nursing care and practicing patient transfer)
2. Lectures (one hour each)
    a. childbirth
    b. neonates and infants
    c. introduction to wounds
    d. skull and scalp wounds
    e. facial wounds
    f. chest wounds
    g. abdominal wounds
    h. genitourinary tract
    i. environmental emergencies
    j. internal medicine
    k. emotionally disturbed patients (hysteria, psychosis)
    l. legal issues (two hours)

Originally Dr. Safar had intended to make all of the trainees proficient in tracheal intubation—the challenging art of passing a rigid tube through the mouth, past the oropharynx, and then blindly into the tracheal airway—an activity that can be compared to threading a needle inside a dark room while wearing mittens. This potentially life-saving operation was related to Safar's own specialty of anesthesia, of course, but perhaps his insistence on mastery of the technique was related to his daughter's terrifying death from asphyxiation during an asthma attack when she was eleven years old—had an ambulance crew with the ability to perform this procedure been on hand they might have been able to save her life by prying apart the convulsing muscles and swollen tissues pinching her airway closed in those awful final moments. Whatever the motivation, his plan foundered on the innumerable barriers that seemed to plague this portion of the training. Safar had planned on letting the students become proficient by practicing on cadavers, but morgue staff at the hospital and local funeral homes balked, fearing the trainees would inflict disfiguring facial injuries requiring time-consuming restoration.[47] Deprived of cadavers, the only alternative was to practice on live patients during surgery, and, not surprisingly, Dr. Safar was the only anesthesiologist willing to let the trainees take a turn with his patients. (Patient consent was not required, it being possible at the time to simply assume those being treated at a teaching hospital had implicitly consented to being used for academic purposes, whether they were awake or not.) Despite his efforts, after two weeks of practice only one trainee was able to complete a successful intubation without coaching.[48] Similarly, efforts to teach the placing and administration of IV medication and fluids was simply too complicated for the time allowed, with only seven students completing this part of training. Of course, even if the training had been successful there was no legal basis for crews to undertake invasive procedures in the field, and doing so would likely have been construed as practicing medicine without a license.

Despite these technical setbacks the trainees moved onward through their clinical training, learning to estimate total blood loss by watching bottles of outdated blood being poured over white sheets, and studying how to deliver babies from films and lectures (the OB nursing staff proved particularly uncooperative when it came to permitting hands-on training). The third section of the clinical component involved forty hours working on an ambulance service, either a fire department rig in Baltimore (Dr. Safar's former hometown), a funeral home ambulance in Pittsburgh, or with the Citizens' Ambulance Service (a non-profit run by Jerry Esposito, the FHE's first project director) in Indiana, Pennsylvania. When the trainees came back from the field it was time to demonstrate that they were ready to perform independently on the street. The final exam consisted of each trainee being placed in front of a special training manikin and given a series of clinical findings: for each problem set they had to correctly diagnose the "patient's" condition, immediately initiate the indicated treatment, and demonstrate the correct transportation technique. No one graduated until they could complete the tasks 100 percent correctly, 100 percent of the time. The fastest and best did it in forty hours, while others took more than two weeks of full-time work before they could turn in the required perfect performances and graduate their clinical course. Finally, the initial round of training wrapped up with eight hours of Ambulance Service Administration Seminars, covering everything from public relations to the use of the two-way radio. It was the most comprehensive civilian ambulance training ever imagined: where other early advanced first aid training was often limited to heart-attack interventions, such as the groundbreaking work done in Miami in

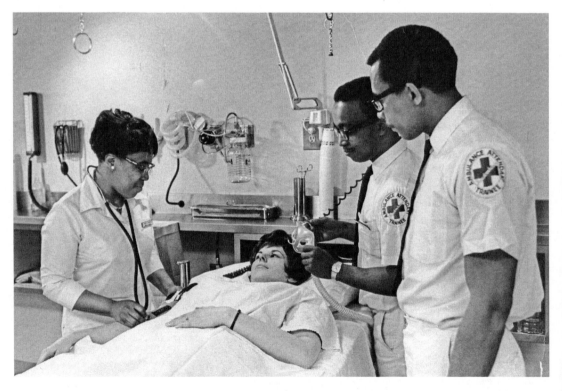

Freedom House trainees working in the emergency room at the Presbyterian-University Hospital, circa 1968 (Library and Archives Division, Historical Society of Western Pennsylvania, Pittsburgh, PA).

1966 with portable EKGs, the Pittsburgh crews were following a course of instruction that was recognizably the first draft of what is now routine paramedic/emergency medical technician training.

Since this arduous work was complicated by personality conflicts arising within a group often lacking rudimentary job skills, a strict disciplinary code was set up to ensure that the trainees, many of whom were skeptical of their mostly white instructors, comported themselves like professionals. Ultimately, to preserve a sufficient number of graduates, the rules were relaxed so that only the most outrageous violations resulted in dismissal.[49] Nor was all the conflict internal: wearing short lab coats the Freedom House trainees drew stares, sometimes hostile, in the largely white hospital when they reported for training in the emergency room, the anesthesia suite, and the operating theatre. More than once staff walked up to a trainee and, seeing the color of their skin and not the ambulance patch on their sleeve, asked "Are you with housekeeping? We need the floor mopped over here."[50]

Despite all the problems, of the twenty-five recruits who entered the program, twenty graduated from the first section and started nine months of on-the-job training under a $100,000 city contract to provide ambulance services to the downtown and Hill districts. The first call came on July 15, 1968, when the ambulance switchboard at Presbyterian's ER took a police call for a Freedom House Ambulance: a woman had gone into convulsions on a city bus, apparently slipping into unconsciousness. Jumping into their squadrol-style ambulance, the crew raced to the 3900 block of Forbes Avenue, swiftly loaded the seizure patient, and whisked her back to Presby's ER: with her complete recovery, the Freedom House Enterprises Ambulance

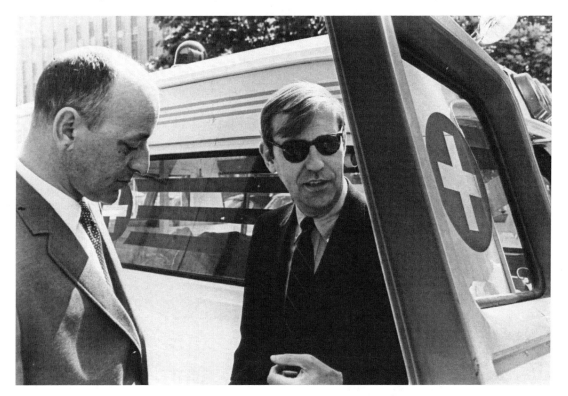

Gerald Esposito, director of the Pennsylvania Ambulance Association and an early supporter of the Freedom House Ambulance Service, and Phil Hallen in 1968, alongside one of the service's original ambulances: a former police "squadrol" repainted white (Library and Archives Division, Historical Society of Western Pennsylvania, Pittsburgh, PA).

Service was in business.[51] In its first year Freedom House made 5,868 runs, transporting 4,627 patients—an average of fifteen calls a day, with an enviable DOA record of 1.9 percent.[52] CPR was required in forty cases, and physicians accompanied the crews on just twenty-one runs, suggesting that, in common with their ancestors at Bellevue and their descendants today, the vast majority of ambulance calls were for non-life-threatening, non-urgent cases.[53] Which isn't to say that life as a Freedom House paramedic was mundane: in addition to the occasional heart attack or stroke, there were plenty of nights spent pulling overdose cases from filthy shooting galleries under the bleary gaze of stupefied junkies or rolling out to crime scenes. One evening the crew responded to a man who had been bludgeoned by a bottle-wielding jealous boyfriend—who returned to the scene to finish the job with a hatchet just as the paramedics were getting started.[54] Luckily, friends of the injured man made a timely appearance armed with pistols, and the assailant was persuaded to keep his distance as the ambulance crew loaded the victim. (Whether the crew came back a few minutes later for the sequel is unrecorded.)

For their part, the ambulance crews had discovered that sense of purpose and *esprit de corps* Phil Hallen had hoped for when he sat down and typed up his vision for an ambulance service eighteen months earlier. One of the men taking full advantage of the opportunity offered was twenty-four-year-old Arthur Davis, who had spent several years moving between jobs after dropping out of high school—"I have one of those funny minds," he explained, "I just didn't take to math and English. It was hard to catch on."[55] After washing dishes, die-casting, and working maintenance at a hospital, he signed up with the Freedom House project. A year later he was a paramedic, telling a reporter, "I've got an obsession about my job. I want to help people. It makes me feel good and proud that I can sometimes save a life. And for my mother, I'm somebody."[56] Another graduate, Dave Rayzer, expressed his pride at mastering a difficult art, saying, "I have professional status. I'm more or less a doctor's assistant, having been taught how to save lives and not to panic at the scene of an accident. I know how to control bleeding, calm people, assist a seizure patient."[57] In addition to the personal benefits accruing to the ambulance crewmembers, Hallen's goal of creating role models was also realized. David Thomas, born and brought up in one of the most impoverished areas of Pittsburgh, was twenty-one when he became a Freedom House Ambulance Services paramedic, and he marveled at the aura the job cast around him: "When I go into some of the poor, black neighborhoods, the kids gather around and talk to me. They are impressed to see a black man like myself in a responsible position. Their attitude is 'gosh, if he made it, maybe I can.'"[58]

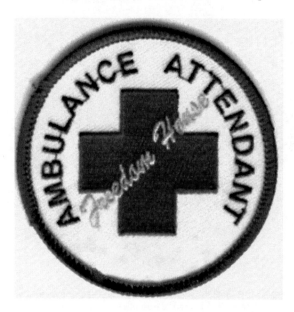

Freedom House Enterprises Ambulance Services badge.

Cuts and Bruised Egos

Despite a year's worth of success as both a medical system and a jobs program, the Freedom House Enterprises Ambulance Service was struggling financially in early 1969. Needing to bill around $50 a run to stay solvent, they couldn't collect this from their clients in the poorest neighborhoods in the city, and the state guaranteed them a mere $10 for patients receiving general assistance (they

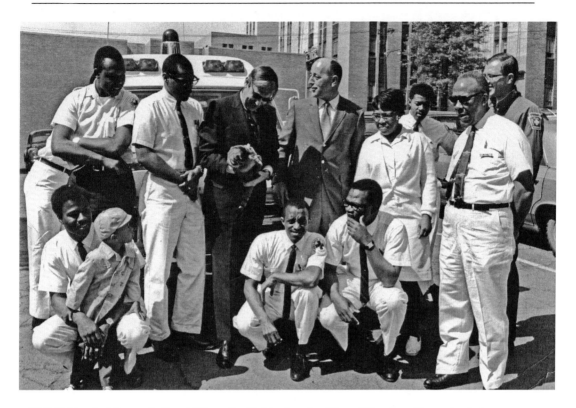

Phil Hallen (holding cat), Gerald Esposito (light colored suit), and Freedom House Ambulance crew members in the parking lot outside Presbyterian-University Hospital in 1968.

were also discouraged from fielding calls outside their assigned district where they might have picked up lucrative spot-cash jobs like transferring patients to and from clinic appointments—and where they would have been competing against the twenty-five white-owned ambulance services in the city at large).[59] With their paltry billing receipts not even the addition of the city contract could generate sufficient revenue to finance their operations, much less pay for equipment upgrades. Heroic fundraising efforts, led by Phil Hallen, pulled in sufficient money to bankroll a second class of nineteen trainees beginning in March 1969. A month later the service purchased two "mobile intensive care units": $13,000 orange and white Ford Econoline vans equipped with "everything a physician needs to support life in a life-threatening situation," according to co-designer Dr. Safar.[60] (At this point the program's legal counsel was skeptical that Pennsylvania's "good Samaritan" laws would apply to paramedics applying defibrillators or giving medications, so physicians continued to attend the most urgent cases along with the regular crews.) Up until now the program's biggest problem had been educating donors about what it was: now that its identity, its potential, and its ambitions were becoming clear, it faced its first real attack when the Pittsburgh's new mayor, Peter Flaherty, announced in 1969 that the municipal contract would be cut in half, to $50,000 a year, with an eye to terminating the payments altogether.

The mayor's Public Safety Director, James Cortese, explained that the city contract was only intended to push the program forward, with the intention that it would become a self-sustaining economic enterprise, a view embodying two distinct distortions.[61] First, it was impossible for the ambulance service to live off its receipts serving an impoverished inner-city neighborhood, but the city refused to grant them a wider franchise that would include neighborhoods whose residents could afford to be billed at a profitable rate. Second, by comparing the municipal contract to a set of economic training wheels, the administration suggested its only interest in the program was as an employment/anti-poverty scheme, failing to see it as a new model of providing municipal emergency services. This may have been an intentional misunderstanding, since the mayor had good reason not to encourage the FHE ambulance service: if he granted them a citywide contract, it would almost certainly mean the loss of one hundred twenty jobs on the police ambulances. That would not only mean the mayor would have one hundred twenty fewer supporters in his next election, it would also jeopardize the almost two thousand votes represented by the city's Fraternal Order of the Police, to say nothing of their voting-age dependents and the FOP's political allies.[62]

For his part, Dr. Safar was running his own medical counter-insurgency by pursuing grant money to broaden the ambulance service, but, as the money usually required matching funds from the city or the county, literally millions of dollars were taken off the table for want of a stake from local government. In defense, the city and county pointed out these grants came with sunset clauses, leaving the politicians with the responsibility to pick up the tab for enhanced services in perpetuity.[63] However, for ambulance activists like Dr. Safar, quality emergency service was an obligation of local government similar to police and fire protection, and arguing that it cost too much to do it right was the moral equivalent of saving money by laying off the fire department and encouraging citizens to form neighborhood bucket brigades. By January 1970, the program was looking at graduating its second class of trainees and wondering how it would pay their salaries with its diminished city contract, but a few months later Dr. Safar announced that he had received a $236,000 grant to develop a countywide emergency medical service based on the fledgling Freedom House Ambulance operation.[64]

Once again, the success of the program put it on a collision course with another well-established lobby opposed to its expansion, this time the one thousand members of volunteer fire and ambulance companies in the suburban communities of Allegheny County, to say nothing of the private funeral homes running profitable non-emergency transfer services. The two groups opposed Safar's standards for training and equipment as burdensome, expensive and, in the case of the private mortuaries, an unnecessary infringement on free enterprise.[65] Their adamant opposition found a staunch ally in County Commissioner Dr. William R. Hunt, a retired surgeon with strong ties to the volunteer and private ambulance services in the county dating back to his days in local emergency rooms: his nostalgic reminisces of their sincere but inarguably retrograde medical services appeared to cloud his medical judgment, as he fulminated that "it is important that the public realizes that there are differences of opinion by equally competent medical authorities as to the extent of sophisticated medical procedures that can be carried on in an ambulance weaving through busy city streets at fifty or sixty miles an hour."[66] Commissioner Hunt made this observation in 1973, when paramedic services were fully operational in major cities across the country, every professional medical association with an interest in trauma was endorsing advanced emergency medical technician training, and the federal government was busily drawing up ever more elaborate standards for ambulance design and crew training. The difference of opinion between "equally competent medical authorities" apparently referred to Dr. Hunt versus the rest of the AMA. (Of course, as a practical matter he was setting himself in opposition to Dr. Safar, and the hot-headed Hunt and the authoritarian Safar found plenty of opportunities to get in one another's way.) Other critics of the council argued that the ambulances were the city's responsibility—while Mayor Flaherty countered they were the hospital's responsibility (choosing to ignore the fact that the city paid one hundred and twenty policemen solely to provide ambulance services, and had been doing so for twenty years). The hospitals, for their part, pled poverty and asked for nothing more than to be left out of the debate entirely.

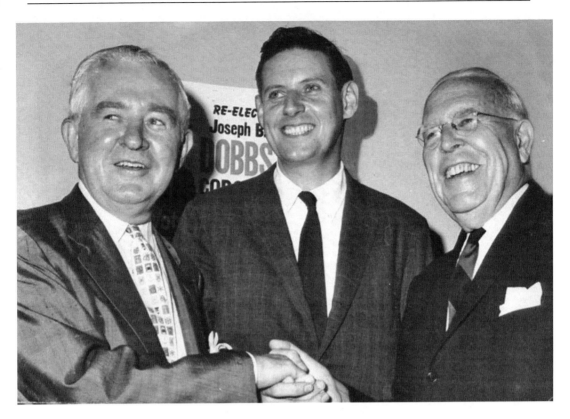

In 1965, Pittsburgh Mayor Joseph Barr posed (left) with Councilman Peter Flaherty (center) and former mayor and governor David Lawrence. A year later Lawrence was dead, with the poor ambulance care he received helping to inspire the creation of Freedom House Ambulance Service. While Barr supported Freedom House, he was succeeded in office by Flaherty in 1970, and the new administration was actively hostile to the group. (Jim Klingensmith. Copyright *Pittsburgh Post-Gazette*, 2008, all rights reserved. Reprinted with permission.)

By 1972, the regional reputation of the FHE ambulance service was so great that the downtown service was getting emergency calls from one end of Allegheny County to the other, even as it struggled to wring increased funding from the city and county commissioners. At this critical juncture the towering figure of Dr. Safar became a liability—his passion did not suffer fools, and his lack of diplomacy quickly turned opponents into enemies. In a later interview, Safar reflected, "My role ... was as a sparkplug and an expert. I served the role of hitting people on the head, so to speak, to bring the need of a modernized system to the attention of the community and government officials."[67] One of the heads he hit the most and the hardest belonged to Mayor Flaherty, who soon added a personal antipathy towards Dr. Safar to his initial distrust of the cost, and political liability, of turning over ambulance services to FHE at the expense of his police department. Even as this political wrangling kept the Freedom House ambulances off balance financially, professionally they continued to develop. By 1973, Freedom House, fueled by a series of grants, was running five orange and white vans with thirty-five paramedics on staff. The program had become fully integrated, with increasing numbers of women and white paramedics joining the crews since nearby Allegheny Community College had started offering a course for Emergency Medical Technicians (modeled on Safar's original work at Presbyterian-University Hospital).[68] With its new inclusive hiring practices and willingness to respond countywide, the FHE ambulance service was becoming a stand-

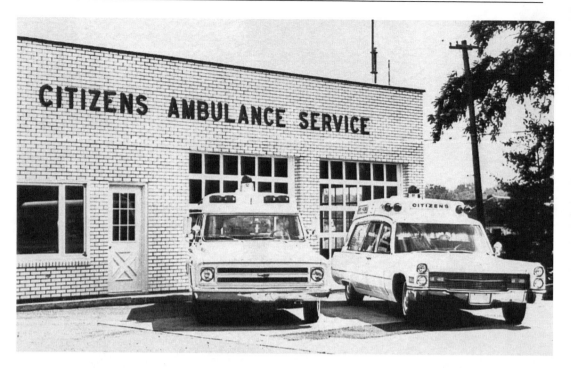

Citizens' Ambulance Service, operated by project director Gerald Esposito, was one of the field sites for the Freedom House trainees (courtesy Citizens' Ambulance Service, Indiana, Pennsylvania).

alone ambulance operation rather than a sometimes awkward blend of jobs program and inner-city medical service. Maturity brought no relief form its brittle finances, however, and Mitchell Brown, one of the earliest program graduates and by now Operating Manager, was aghast at the refusal to shift money from the inadequate police ambulance service, costing anywhere between $750,000 and $1.5 million a year, to the demonstrably superior FHE service. "The city really needs our services," he told a reporter. "It doesn't make sense for people to die or suffer unnecessary hardships because of untrained, poorly equipped private ambulance attendants, when we could be expanded and sponsored to serve the entire community with the best mobile medical units in the world."[69]

Finally, in April, 1973, a frustrated Dr. Safar sent a letter to Mayor Flaherty threatening to go public with the "hot political issue" of poor emergency care if the mayor didn't meet with him within seven days.[70] Calling police ambulance services "a crisis," Dr. Safar excoriated the level of care offered, complaining that if the mayor were a traffic case he'd be "picked up like a sack of potatoes, dumped on a canvas stretcher ... and rushed to the nearest hospital, perhaps choking to death on your own tongue, blood or vomit."[71] While the letter was signed by twenty-two community and medical figures, the colorful rhetoric was unmistakably Safar's. When three weeks passed without an audience, Safar distributed the letter to the local media, setting off a barrage of rebuttals by the city. Predictably, Police Superintendent Colville was livid at this assault on his own ambulance service: referring to the "sack of potatoes" remark, he asked a reporter, "Have you ever seen an orderly at Presby (Presbyterian-University Hospital) transfer a patient?"—a pointed reference to Safar's own hospital.[72] For his part, Mayor Flaherty gave numerous interviews in every available medium defending the police ambulances and castigating Dr. Safar as either an unwitting cat's paw of the mayor's political opposition or an egomaniac demanding personal control of the region's ambulance services. Daily

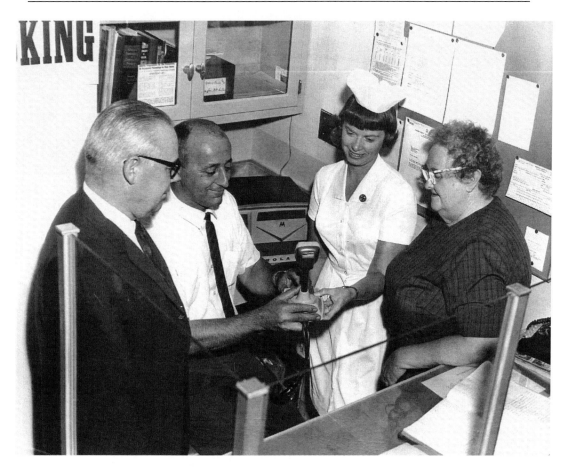

Gerald Esposito holding a microphone at the dispatch center for his Citizens' Ambulance Service. In addition to providing on-the-job training to Freedom House crewmembers, Esposito was the program's first project manager and a state advocate for improved ambulance services (courtesy Citizens' Ambulance Service, Indiana, Pennsylvania).

articles in the local press carried charge and counter charge, with Dr. Safar vehemently denying any motivation other than his decades' long crusade to improve emergency medical care. The service's perennial foe Commissioner Hunt also weighed in, echoing earlier remarks by the Police Superintendent that the hospitals had long ago abandoned their ambulance responsibilities and so were in no position to assume the moral high-ground: the ex-surgeon found it "regrettable that well-meaning proponents of better ambulance services in these communities have continuously promoted better ambulance service by defaming and insulting the very people who are providing what services we have now," especially since the current poor state of emergency services could be laid to "the short-sightedness of the very medical departments and medical community of which [these critics] are members."[73] In response, Dr. Safar noted that the police were trained little better than Boy Scouts, but the fault was not theirs—it belonged to the administration for not providing better.

As spring wore on, a series of articles by Dolores Frederick in the *Pittsburgh-Press* titled "The Great Ambulance Debate" covered the history of the various available services, the politics that had plagued reform since FHE first started five years before, and pointing out the millions of dollars in grants that had been lost due to the city and county's failure to commit to improved services. Her articles succeeded in bringing the debate out of city hall and into

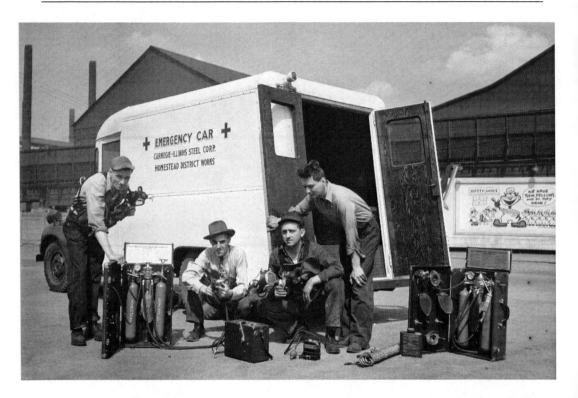

The Freedom House Ambulance was in the tradition of earlier local medical squads, such as this accident crew at Pittsburgh's Carnegie Steelworks. Freedom House, however, introduced an unprecedented level of professionalism and medical competence (William J. Gaughan Collection, Archives Services Center, University of Pittsburgh).

the living rooms of the people it actually affected, and under this barrage of press the public statements of the officials began to change: it became clear that the years of rancorous debate were drawing to a close, the blame and recriminations, the timidity about committing resources, all were giving way to a dawning realization that Pittsburgh, which only five years earlier had led the nation in emergency services, was now, inarguably, a joke with a deadly punch line. By the end of May it seemed Safar's gambit would pay off: Police Superintendent Colville agreed to look into certifying police ambulance crews as paramedics and upgrading their equipment, and by July even Commissioner Hunt reversed course and announced that the county would add ambulance dispatch to its emergency call system, opening the door to greater involvement.[75] Although change was coming, there would be no room for the FHE Ambulance Service since the city ultimately decided to reform the police ambulances, not replace them. After a year of negotiating and planning, a decision was announced in the spring of 1974 to provide enhanced training to the police ambulance squads and purchase new, van-type ambulances and specially equipped intensive care vehicles.[76] It was pointed out that the scheme saved a supposedly cash-strapped city no money since police officers were paid between $12,000 and $14,000 a year, while Freedom House paramedics averaged only $8,500: in addition, the police department would have to invest in an entire fleet of ambulances, estimated at eleven new vans plus five specialty rigs, while FHE was already operating five state-of-the art ambulances.[77]

At the time, Freedom House was still receiving $50,000 from the city for its services, but with no chance of renewal, and facing the last payment from a $200,000 federal grant on July 1, the service was in the untenable position of surviving on its nearly nonexistent billing capacity plus $95,000 pledged from various private sources.[78] The lights were dimming, but the men and women of Freedom House weren't about to shrug off their uniforms and shuffle meekly off to the unemployment office. They spoke up for their jobs with all the passion they had brought to saving lives and fighting an indifferent and hostile political system for the last six years. The eminently quotable Mitchell Brown, original crewman and current operating manager, had this to say about the prospect of policemen taking over emergency services: "How would you like to receive emergency medical attention from a policeman who has a stethoscope around his neck and a gun on his hip, the shoot and patch-up theory?"[79] (Mr. Brown's concerns reflected a distrustful attitude towards the largely white police force among African Americans in Pittsburgh. When the time came, however, officers on ambulance duty did not carry sidearms: their role was to provide medical care, not make arrests.)

The plan proceeded apace, however, and when logistical questions came up about staffing and equipping the new police service, the antipathy between Mayor Flaherty and Dr. Safar made its final appearance. Despite Safar being one of the world's leading experts in ambulance design, resuscitation, and emergency service operation, the mayor refused to seek his help in planning the new police service, instead asking the staff of a new for-profit hospital, Central Pavilion, to provide technical and medical advisory services: he even offered them an exclusive contract for overseeing the service, a proposal vetoed by the city council.[80] Ultimately, after answering more than 40,000 calls in seven years of operation, the end for the Freedom House Enterprises Ambulance Service came on October 15, 1975. A week later Mitchell Brown gave an impromptu eulogy in a *Pittsburgh-Press* interview: "We were the first. We developed a little known area—emergency ambulance care by trained technicians—into a successful model which has been copied by other municipalities across the country.... People always try to say crazy things about us, that we ran crap games in the vehicles or even that we sold dope in them, but the charges were unfounded. We were good, and the people—all the people—came to recognize that fact."[81]

Afterwards

Facing pressure from the medical community and a vocal segment of the general public, the city begrudgingly extended an offer to the Freedom House crews to apply for spots on the municipal police rigs, as civilian employees—assuming they were willing to complete a course in Advanced First Aid. The insult, like asking an astronaut to take a kite-flying class, was the final indignity for some of the crewmembers. Of the thirty Freedom House paramedics on service at the end, five refused to apply for the new jobs. Of the twenty-five crossing the street to work on the police ambulances services, the entrenched racism in the city government and dissatisfaction with working conditions and standards wore them down, and within a year, half of the former Freedom House crewmembers had quit.[82] (One who didn't was John Moon, a graduate of Safar's Presbyterian training course, who persevered to become the assistant commissioner for emergency services.) Some of the men found work elsewhere, like Mitchell Brown, the once caustic-tongued operations manager, who left Pittsburgh in the mid–1970s to run Cleveland's EMS services, ultimately rising to the rank of director of public safety. Others simply dropped back into their old lives, vanishing into anonymity, their only legacy the thousands of lives they had saved, their only memorials those men and women they passed on the street who, but for their dedication, would have lived only in memory.

In addition to launching the medical and public service careers of many ex-crewmembers, the Freedom House project made numerous contributions to the development of the modern EMS system. To raise funds, the Freedom House Ambulance crews had barnstormed the coun-

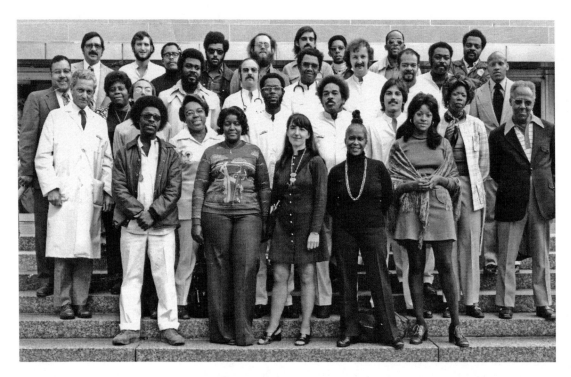

Freedom House crew members in the early 1970s, with Nancy Caroline in the front row, center (Library and Archives Division, Historical Society of Western Pennsylvania, Pittsburgh, PA).

try, visiting charitable foundations in Kansas City and New York and attending a health fair in New Haven, always earning unstinting praise from professional audiences and educating them on the potential of similar training programs elsewhere.[83] Accordingly, one of the most important outcomes of the program was its role in demonstrating the need for the nascent specialty of emergency medicine. It had been years since physicians had ridden ambulances as part of their training, and the minority who understood the importance of creating paraprofessionals for ambulance work were generally unclear about how they could effectively contribute to the training. Dr. Safar actively recruited physician colleagues to go out with his teams, to the benefit of both the crews and the doctors pried loose from what one physician described as the "relatively calm and secure enclave" inside the hospital.[84] The most notable of these participants was Dr. Nancy Caroline, a 1971 graduate of Case Western Reserve Medical School, who made eleven hundred runs with the Freedom House ambulances starting in 1974. As she later remarked, "my job presumably was to teach these troops the sophisticated techniques of advanced life support, but I had a great deal to learn from them, too. The first time I climbed into a sewer to do a resuscitation, I realized there were a lot of things they never told me in medical school."[85] Later, Dr. Caroline used her experiences with Freedom House to rewrite the national emergency medical technician curriculum under a contract from the U.S. Department of Transportation: she eventually emigrated to Israel and helped create a modern, national ambulance service under the auspices of the Magen David. She was only 58 when she succumbed to multiple myeloma in 2002, leaving a legacy of brilliant innovation in emergency medicine.[86]

Judged by history, the Freedom House Ambulance Service accomplished much in its brief span. From its first flush of enthusiastic support to its prolonged struggle with a political and social structure that, in the words of Phil Hallen, "didn't want to see unemployed black people at the top of the medical system," the service operated with a dignity and professionalism that should have guaranteed its longevity.[87] While at the start some physicians resented taking reports in the ER from an African-American with a high school diploma and a white coat, by the end of its run the service, the first in America to meet all of the ambulance standards of both the American Society of Anesthesiology and the National Research Council of the National Academy of Sciences, had won the respect of medical professionals and citizens alike. Even the police department, their political rivals from earliest days, came around, and by the early 1970s the family of an officer needing emergency medical attention was most likely to request a Freedom House ambulance: as Mitchell Brown said at the death of the service, "We were good, and the people—all the people—came to recognize that fact." In the end, the property of Freedom House passed away, but the example it set simply moved onto a national stage. Sadly, coming from an unfashionable and unphotogenic city, the service never received the attention lavished on later paramedic squads in larger media markets like Seattle, Los Angeles, and Miami, and its story disappeared even as its influence gathered strength.

Finally, in a remarkable post-script, in 2008 a Freedom House Enterprises Ambulance Service documentary by paramedic and independent film producer Gene Starzenski had its world premiere in Pittsburgh, bringing renewed attention to the service (before moving to Los Angeles, Starzenski had worked as both an ambulance attendant and a hospital orderly in Pittsburgh, and had seen the Freedom House crews in action). Among the guests of honor at the lavish debut was Phil Hallen, and, inspired by the enthusiastic reception, the indefatigable creator of the original Freedom House service turned his attention to creating a brand new emergency medical technician training program for Pittsburgh's inner-city youth—creating the possibility of an improbable Hollywood ending to the story that started with his typewritten proposal in 1967, a tale proving to be as enduring as any in the history of the ambulance.

While Pittsburgh's Freedom House Enterprises Ambulance Service was certainly the first to offer the level of training expected of modern emergency medical technicians and paramedics, they were not the first to apply techniques, like running intravenous medications or using defibrillators, that were formerly restricted to physicians but which are now the *sine qua non* of the emergency medical responder. Unfortunately, Pennsylvania laws permitting paramedical interventions lagged, and in the interim other ambulance services slipped under the velvet rope separating first aid from invasive medicine. Leading the way were two disparate groups: municipal firefighters in Miami, Florida, and the ambulance volunteers of Haywood County, North Carolina. Whether working in remote mountain hollows or a glittering tropical city, each team pioneered techniques that are now considered core competencies in paramedic and emergency medical technician training and, like Freedom House, they played an influential part in creating the modern paramedic movement.

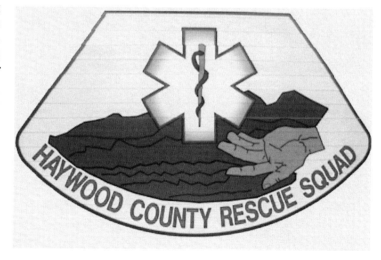

Haywood County EMS badge (courtesy Haywood County Rescue Squad).

Ridgetop Rescues

The mountains of western North Carolina impose a geographic isolation on its scattered towns and hamlets, and this, along with the rigors of upland rural life, has for generations produced men and women who are resourceful as individuals and self-sufficient as communities. It is hardly surprising, then, that when the national medical establishment was looking to redress deficient emergency medical care in the mid–1960s, Appalachian Haywood County reached further, faster, by recognizing the particular needs of its remote population and not quibbling over legal authority or statutory authorizations.

Haywood County's original rescue squad was, like so many others, created in response to a terrible loss. It was the summer of 1958 and a hard thunderstorm had passed over, bloating a creek emptying into Lake Junaluska, a little northeast of Waynesville. A young girl was walking across a sewer pipe bridging the creek when she lost her footing, fell in, and was swiftly swept away and drowned.[88] When word reached town of her death, one of the first to hear the news was a handsome, rail-thin sheriff's deputy with strawberry blond hair named Gene Howell. An Army vet whose parade-rest posture cast a long shadow from his spare, 6'4" frame, the news of the child's death angered him: none of the adults who were there when she was pulled from the water knew first aid, and it was an unanswerable question whether she might have been successfully resuscitated if they had. Howell's wife Charlene remembers her husband had always been a "go-getter," and now he put himself to work going from storefront to storefront in his little town, drumming up interest in a volunteer rescue squad, talking to his friends and his co-workers, determined to build a living memorial to a girl who had gone down into the deep for want of skilled aid. He was a persuasive man, and soon others were carrying the banner forward, and on July 29, 1958, the first meeting of the Haywood County Volunteer Rescue Squad took place.[89]

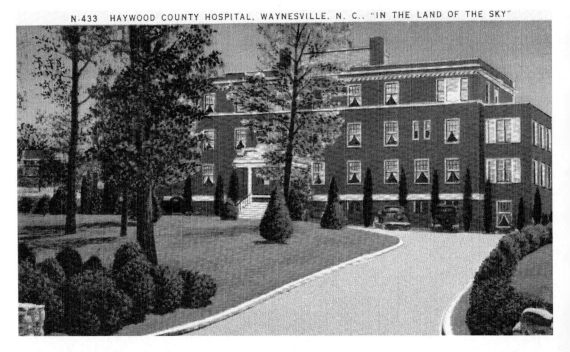

Haywood Hospital, shortly before Dr. Feichter arrived. In 1968 the facility became one of the training grounds for a groundbreaking paramedic service.

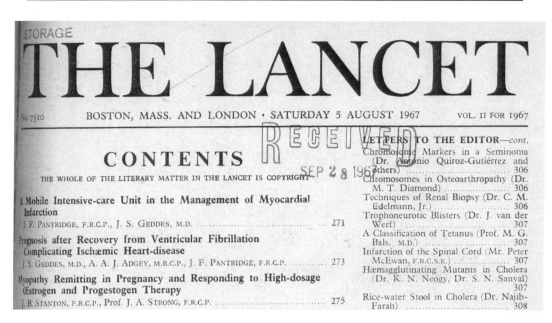

The *Lancet* article that inspired Ralph Feichter to create the world's first volunteer paramedic squad in Haywood County, North Carolina. (Reprinted from J.F. Pantridge and J.S. Geddes, "A Mobile Intensive-care Unit in the Management of Myocardial Infarction," *The Lancet* 2, no. 7510 (1967): 271–74. Copyright 1967, with permission from Elsevier. Copyright Elsevier Properties S.A., all rights reserved.)

At the time there were perhaps six thousand souls in Waynesville, out of a county population of close to forty thousand, and the only ambulance services were provided by local funeral homes.[90] Marty Stamey, born on the Rescue Squad's first anniversary and later its Waynesville captain for seven years, recalls that the mortuaries would "throw someone screamin' in the back, and if they died they'd just take 'em to the funeral home instead of the hospital."[91] Determined to do better, the little squad scraped up enough funds to buy an old panel truck as their first rescue rig, which they soon replaced with station-wagons that they converted into ambulances by putting in their own cabinet work, stationing one ambulance in Canton and the other in Waynesville.[92] Deputy Howell's wife Charlene was an early member of the Ladies' Auxiliary, raising funds for equipment with square dances ("mountain folk love to dance," she recalled in an interview, "so that's always a good way to raise money"), and whenever a car show or a gathering of any size came to town the Auxiliary sold plates of corn-bread and soup-beans, hot-dogs and hush-puppies, from an old panel truck converted into a rolling kitchen, the proceeds financing equipment and defraying the squad's expenses.[93] Training was the standard Red Cross First Aid course, which after the first year was augmented by occasional lectures from some of the local physicians.[94] One of these was an internist named Ralph Feichter, a thin, bespectacled gentleman with combed-back hair and long legs that carried him swiftly down the hospital corridors with his lab coat blown wide open behind him.[95] Quiet, unfailingly kind, and devoted to his little community, Dr. Feichter's combination of intelligence, stamina, and respect for the Rescue Squad's volunteers formed the foundation for one of the most audacious experiments in ambulance history.

In 1965 Dr. E.B. Goodwin, a family practitioner, came to Haywood County and volunteered to provide training for the rescue squad alongside Feichter. Some years later Goodwin remembered how in 1967 Dr. Feichter read an article in *The Lancet* about a Belfast Hospital operating a mobile cardiac intensive care unit that delivered physicians and nursing staff to a

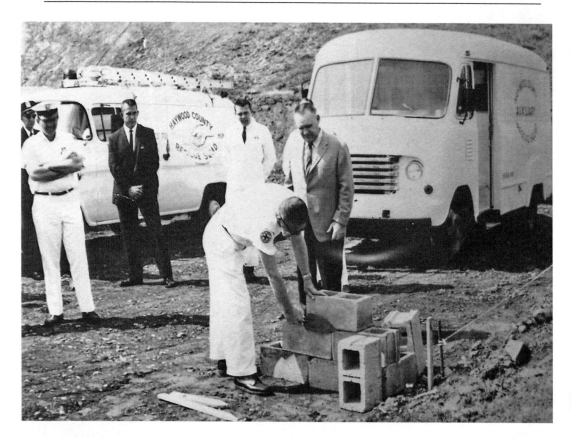

The Haywood Rescue Squad's first "crash truck" was the 1959 GMC seen on the left. The auxiliary van to the right was often used as a concession vehicle at conventions and fairs, raising funds by selling dinners of soup beans, corn bread, and hot dogs (courtesy the Haywood County Rescue Squad).

patient's home in order to stabilize them before transporting them to the hospital: the service was dramatically reducing the lag time between onset of symptoms and treatment, and appeared to be substantially reducing the number of deaths due to heart attack.[96] Deciding he needed to see this for himself, Feichter simply bought himself a ticket to Ireland, called in some unused vacation days, and left. When Feichter returned he announced that Haywood County was going to be home to the first mobile cardiac intensive care service in the United States, and the Haywood County Rescue Squad ambulances were going to be the centerpiece.

Needing proper equipment, he successfully applied for a state grant to purchase portable defibrillators for the two squads then operating in Canton and Waynesville, telling the state that *"the concept was that Dr. Goodwin and I would carry radios and we would try to get to the scene of the coronary [first] and come back with the ambulance."*[97] In short order the futility of this scheme became obvious, since the physicians' own work-load made it impossible for them to be on 24-hour standby, and swinging by the ER to pick up an RN would create staffing shortfalls and add yet more delay. If it had been audacious to plan America's first mobile cardiac intensive care ambulance with the meager resources of a hospital whose critical care unit amounted to a single bed with a heart monitor, Feichter's back up plan was even more astounding: he would go ahead and train laymen to provide cardiac resuscitation and stabilization out of the back of an ambulance, with or without medical supervision. While this course was clearly dictated by the limited medical resources of the county, it took a rare physician to undertake it—Dr. Feichter was energetic and capable enough to organize this unprecedented operation, but he also had sufficient faith in the members of his rescue squads to master what had always been considered the exclusive province of the physician.[98] When asked later whether they had been worried about the absence of any legal authority for their bold scheme, his colleague Dr. Goodwin just laughed: they were more concerned about people dying on the long drive in from a sequestered hollow or up and over a distant ridge.[99]

It took over a year for Feichter and his colleagues to gather their equipment and put together, or, more accurately *invent*, a curriculum. By April 1969, they were ready to begin training, and for three months squad members eagerly attended classes on placing cardiac leads, reading heart rhythms, administering IV medications, and the use of the defibrillator.[100] The crewmen learned to start IVs and "cut down" to a vein if they couldn't reach it with their needles, practicing on patients in the hospital's intensive care unit and on cadavers in Winston-Salem.[101] Leading the teaching was Dr. Feichter, of course, assisted by Dr. Goodwin and, representing surgery, Dr. F.G. Wenzel. The squad's Hewlett-Packard heart monitor was reportedly the size of a footstool and, with a battery life measured in minutes, it had to be plugged into the nearest wall socket after it had been lugged inside the home.[102] The ambulances were also equipped with telemetry units so physicians at the hospital could read the heart rhythms and radio instructions back to the crews in the field and, as Dr. Feichter put it, "as soon as we had the telemetry, we considered the ambulance to be an extension of the hospital."[103] Practically

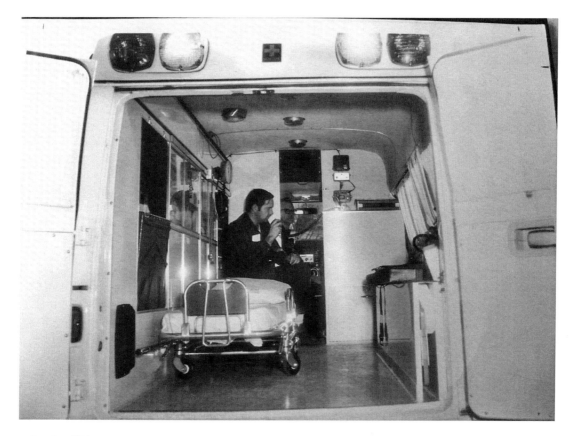

By the 1970s the Haywood County Rescue Squad was operating with well-equipped ambulances like this one, purchased with funds raised from the community (courtesy the Haywood County Rescue Squad).

speaking, however, these telemetry units were being dragged across a county whose topography could rise and fall two thousand vertical feet in the space of a few miles, and more often than not the ambulance crews found themselves in the radio-shadow of one peak or another, working the case alone, without medical supervision of any kind. In such instances they faithfully adhered to a set of standard protocols that instructed them how to proceed when confronted by a variety of abnormal heart rhythms: carried in each rig, these standing orders were dutifully signed by each member of the County Medical Society.[104]

When they started services the crews had twelve drugs they could use in the field, but their interventions were not limited to cardiac cases. One veteran of the original service recalls that in the spring of 1969 they were taught how to provide fluid resuscitation in cases of severe blood loss, as with a major head wound, and how right away they were reviving diabetic patients by giving insulin shots to the hyperglycemic and starting an IV with glucose and water "if they were cold and clammy, [because] we knew they'd had too much insulin then."[105] Unlike the standing written orders for cardiac cases, there were no signed protocols for other emergent conditions, and if a crew was unable to reach the hospital by radio there was nothing to fall back on but their own judgment, relying on the lessons taught them by Drs. Feichter, Wenzel, and Goodwin. In so doing, the Haywood County Rescue Squad entered history in 1969 as the first civilian, lay ambulance crews to employ invasive medical techniques, including intravenous access, to non-cardiac cases in the field.

Response to the new service was so favorable that a second course of training was offered in the autumn of their inaugural year.[106] By the mid–1970s the rest of the country was catching up to the Haywood rescue squad, and the members were eager to improve their capabilities with better equipment. Accordingly, sometime around 1976, their founder, Gene Howell, went to the county's biggest employers, A.C. Delco and the Champion Paper Mill, and got them to institute a voluntary payroll deduction to finance an equipment upgrade.[107] (For many years these same plants paid employees their hourly wages when they left work on an emergency call.) The success of the Haywood County experiment eventually influenced state policy, as North Carolina went on to adopt many of Haywood's techniques and training when setting up state EMT certification standards. Not surprisingly, many Haywood County veterans went on to shape the new field of paramedic medicine: Gene Howell, who had started it all back in 1958, was one of the state's first certified paramedics and was the North Carolina Emergency Medical Services Coordinator from the early 1970s until his retirement in 1991; Marty Stamey, who shared a birthday with the Haywood Rescue Squad and who learned intubations as a fifteen-year-old orderly working with Dr. Feichter, went on to serve seven years as captain of the Rescue Squad, and in 1986 he was one of North Carolina's original flight paramedics, flying out of Asheville until 1992, when he left to become Haywood County's EMS Director.

Much has changed since the Haywood County Rescue Squad debuted the world's first fully operational civilian intensive care ambulance service, breaking ground for the full-fledged paramedic services that swiftly followed them. In 1981 they took in their first female crew member, an ER nurse named Frances Cagle who was nominated by her fellow crew-members to a captaincy shortly after she started. Today, the squad operates five ambulances along with two heavy-duty crash trucks and three support vehicles that are used primarily for tractor-trailer accidents along Interstate 40. Fitting for an outfit that was created in response to a drowning death, the squad maintains a swift-water rescue crew—one of whose members is a 77-year-old veteran of the original squad, now with fifty-one years in service.[108] The Volunteer Rescue Squad's fifty or so members respond to over one hundred emergency calls a month, as well as many "convalescent" trips between home and hospital, or to transfer a frail patient to a clinic appointment. It isn't easy running a volunteer rescue squad with a mandate as large as Haywood County's, and as Captain Walter Brookes observes "we get by on what we can make,

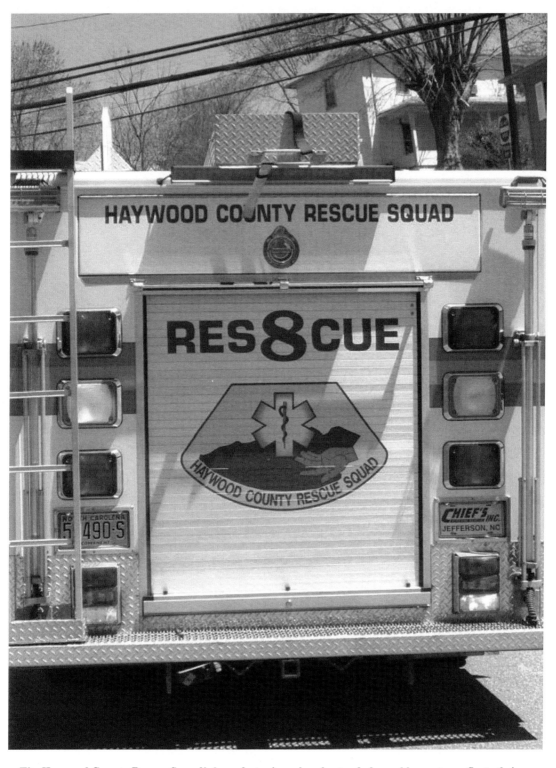

The Haywood County Rescue Squad's logo, featuring a hand extended over blue water, reflects their roots in water rescue, as the inspiration for their founding was the death of a young girl swept away near Lake Junaluska in 1958 (courtesy the Haywood County Rescue Squad).

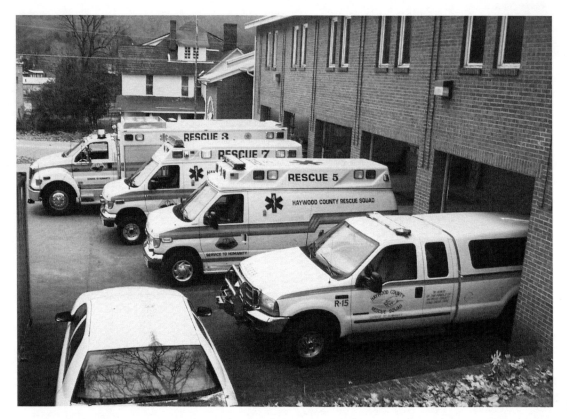

Haywood's Rescue Squad has kept pace with the times, continually upgrading their ambulance and rescue equipment to the modern state of the art (courtesy the Haywood County Rescue Squad).

take, or steal, but it's our mountain heritage: people are just used to helping one another." After almost sixty years of continued service, the Haywood County Rescue Squad still carries out its original mission, and their pride comes not just from being the first volunteer ambulance company in the world to carry out invasive resuscitation techniques on non-cardiac cases in the field, but from the excellence with which they have served their community and the moral courage of founders who believed that any person with the motivation to help their neighbor could, with guidance and training, master the critical care skills once deemed the prerogative of the physician.

Surfside

A slightly earlier innovation appeared in Miami, where, starting in 1966, the city fire department rescue squad debuted radio EKG telemetry: unlike the unobserved reaches of Haywood County, the big city crews lacked sufficient anonymity to simply ignore restrictive laws, but, on the other hand, their media-friendly location gave them considerable influence nationally. Things really started in 1964, not long after Dr. Eugene Nagel was hired as an assistant professor of anesthesiology at the University of Miami. A scuba-enthusiast, Nagel made the acquaintance of some off-duty rescue divers from the municipal fire-department and started spending the occasional evening with the crews of Rescue-1, giving informal tutorials in closed-chest massage and elements of advanced first aid.[109]

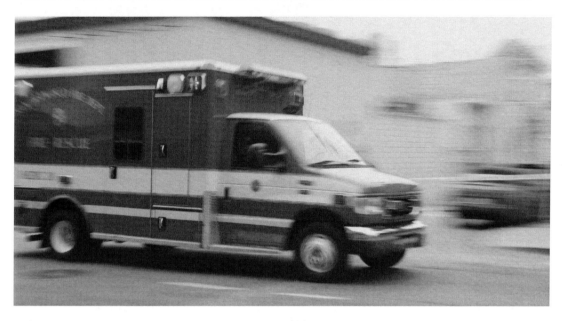

Contemporary Fire-Rescue ambulances are descended from a 1966 experimental program in Miami, when the city fire department first equipped its rescue squads with portable telemetry units (photograph by Aaron Kohr).

Two years later, in 1966, a future colleague, Dr. Jim Hirschmann, was experimenting with providing cardiology consultations from a hospital ship off the coast of West Africa by reviewing radioed EKG signals. When he returned to Miami his experimental work reached Dr. Nagel (who had been an electrical engineer before going to medical school), and in 1966 the two men got to work outfitting the men of Rescue-1 with a portable EKG telemetry unit. Working with various manufacturers they cobbled together a fifty-four pound kit wedged into an aluminum suitcase, which was portable, alright—if you were a husky fireman.[110] When the leads were placed on a victim's chest the unit radioed its signal to the city's Communication Division, which relayed the telemetry by telephone wires to Jackson Memorial Hospital.[111] Receiving sets in the surgical recovery room and the offices of the Anesthesiology Department allowed physicians to read the EKG and give instructions to the ambulance personnel by radio while the hospital prepared itself for the arriving case (the crews had no authority to give meds, intubate, or defibrillate the patient). The tech wizards behind this innovation even entertained the idea of a completely automated system, with a computer processing the incoming signal and, based on the EKG's pattern, selecting a pre-recorded audiotape of physician instructions for broadcast to the crew in the field.[112] Encouraged by the initial success, Nagle went straight to the fire chief and asked permission to train the crews to use a defibrillator. The response was emphatic, but not particularly encouraging. As Nagle later recalled in an interview with Mickey Eisenberg:

> I told the fire chief I wanted to train the guys in defibrillation.... A big, tall, 6'3" Irishman by the name of Lawrence Kenney he had been quite tolerant of me up till now. He took his finger and he punched me in the chest and drove me back about three feet with his one finger. "This is a fire department, not a hospital; these are firemen, not doctors. I don't want you to forget that." Every time he would say something he would punch me again in the chest with his finger, which hurt a lot. I think I probably got the idea.[113]

(This resistance often appeared when fire departments began devoting scarce resources to this new mission: a veteran of the Haywood County Rescue Society remembers going out to

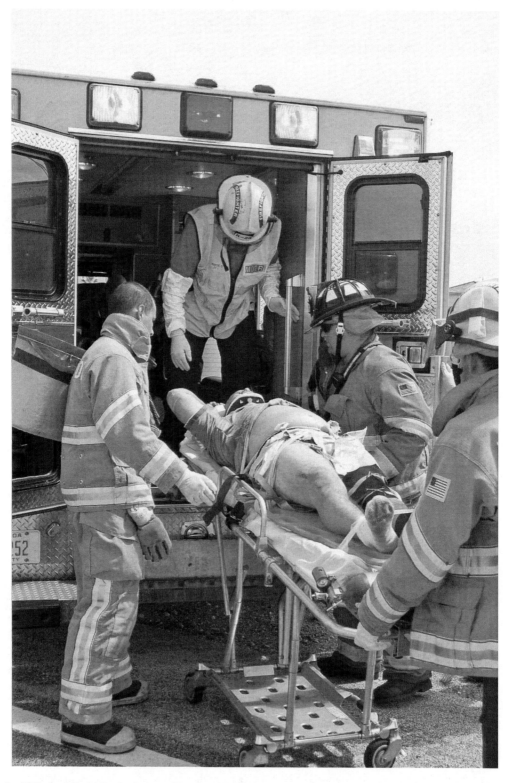

In 1973 the Miami-Dade County Fire Department developed its own paramedic squad, modeled on the city of Miami's innovative program. Today both agencies provide world-class medical service in the community where modern fire-rescue operations began. (Courtesy the Miami-Dade Fire Rescue Department)

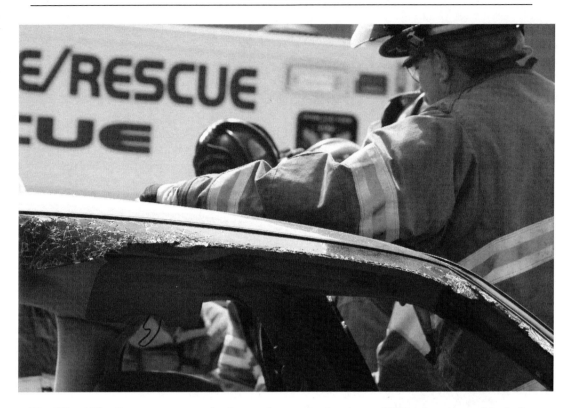

The Miami Fire Department was the first such organization to use EKG telemetry and train its personnel to modern paramedic standards. Today, the majority of all calls to fire departments are for medical emergencies, testifying to the success of Eugene Nagel's original idea (photograph by J. Bryson).

Los Angeles County shortly after L.A. began providing paramedic services and hearing a chief complain about having some of his crews tied down on a medical call when a big alarm came in: "The chief told me 'I can explain a patient dying of a heart-attack better than I can explain a house burning down or a business burning down,'" he recalled later.)[114] After a year with no catastrophes the Miami program decided to make its experiment known, giving a ground-breaking presentation on radio-telemetry at a regional medical conference in 1967.[115] To get the message to an audience wider than medical conventioneers sitting in a conference room in Miami, the resourceful promoters grabbed some headlines, and proved the reliability of their instruments, by broadcasting the heart rhythms of Miami's "Miss Fire Prevention, 1967" all the way to Culver City, California.[116] By 1968 the crews were tired of simply being disc-jockeys on WEKG, broadcasting to their audience of one, so in November Dr. Nagel started a formal course in advanced emergency medical care. The Rescue-1 squads were given twenty-two hours of classroom instruction and fifty-four hours of hospital and laboratory training, covering anatomy, physiology, cardiology, gross pathology, patient assessment, endotracheal intubation, and radio communications, among other relevant topics.[117] The training was similar to the program the Freedom House Enterprises crews had completed a few months earlier, in June 1968, although Miami's didactic component was about one-half as long as the Pittsburgh curriculum. By the end of 1968 the squads were equipped with defibrillators, but the county drew the line at invasive procedures, even under radio direction from a physician. Tired of jousting with the timid politicians, Nagel decided to show the commissioners what he was talking about. He scheduled a meeting and, abruptly,

I lay down on the commissioners' huge teak conference table and said, "Let's imagine that I've collapsed in your chamber." Then I brought in the paramedic unit. They looked at my EKG, said, "Start an IV," and radioed the hospital for approval. As soon as the hospital answered back with the okay, they stuck a needle in my arm and started the drip, right there on the table. The commissioners finally consented, but we were dragging our chiefs, the department, and the city every step of the way. For each improvement, we had to convince them that procedures like defibrillation and intravenous fluid therapy were reasonable, safe, and logical.[118]

The demonstration paid off, and by June 1969 Miami's revamped Rescue-1 had the legal authority to put their training in cardiac resuscitation to use, including defibrillation and IV cardioactive meds and fluid boluses (coincidentally, this was the same month that Haywood County debuted its own paramedic-style services, although in Haywood they weren't restricted to cardiac interventions). As the press began playing up their activities the program began to pull in overwhelming support from politicians, physicians, and members of the general pub-

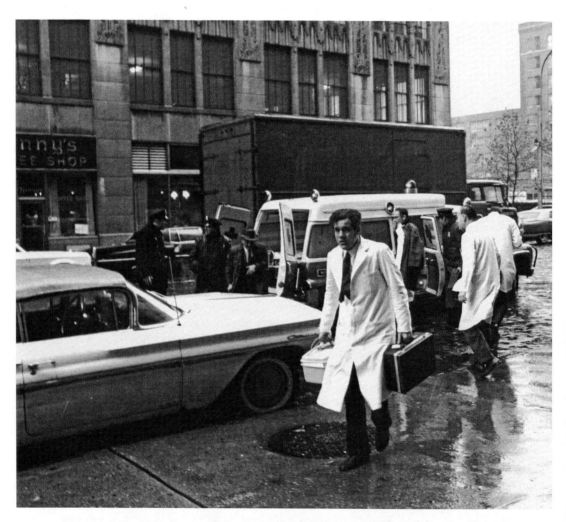

After visiting the Royal Belfast Hospital mobile cardiac care unit, Dr. William Grace organized a similar team at Manhattan's St. Vincent's in 1968. Bucking the paramedic trend, it relied on physicians, RNs, and EKG technicians. Since "time is heart muscle," staffers had four minutes and thirty seconds to get to the ambulance after a call came in, with latecomers left behind (Library of Congress, Prints & Photographs Division, Look Magazine Photograph Collection, Job 68-3971).

lic, all of whom now saw the program as an unqualified success.[119] The year 1969 ended with Miami buying a stock recreational van, raising the roof to standing room height, tricking out the interior with custom cabinetry bursting with medical equipment, and finally modernizing its ambulance fleet to keep pace with the advances it was making in the field of emergency medicine.[120]

While Pittsburgh's FHE ambulance service was the first to employ a training model corresponding to our current understanding of a paramedic, it was Miami in 1966 that introduced radio EKG telemetry and the volunteers of Haywood County, North Carolina, who, in the spring of 1969, introduced full-spectrum invasive interventions on ambulance calls without direct physician supervision, giving IV infusions and applying defibrillation years before the wisdom of their innovations was sanctioned by the solons in Wilmington. Ultimately, by combining imagination with hard work and disdain for the status quo, each of these services dared to reimagine what the ambulance could be and put their dreams on the street, to the everlasting benefit of those they served.

Heart Mobiles

Virtually simultaneously with the breakout services in Haywood County and Miami, other jurisdictions began developing their own mobile cardiac care units, although these originally hewed close to the Belfast model by relying on physician staffing. The first American hospital to appropriate Pantridge's model was St. Vincent's in Manhattan, which brought out a physi-

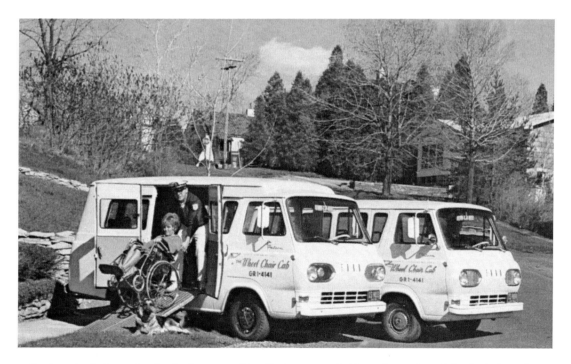

Eastern Ambulance Service in Syracuse, New York, operated this early version of the "cabulance" to transfer clients to medical appointments or on other errands. While the 1960s rate structure seems shockingly low—only six dollars one way and a dollar for each flight of stairs after the first—their service was not reimbursable, limiting their charge to what an average person could afford out of pocket (courtesy Eastern Ambulance Service).

cian crewed mobile cardiac care unit in 1968. More influential was the Columbus, Ohio, "Heartmobile" in 1969, staffed by EMTs with a staggering 2,000 hours of training and resident physicians.[121] Operated by the fire department, this mobile intensive care unit frequently found itself idling outside the hospital lobby while the overworked resident on-call struggled to break free from the wards and race downstairs to meet them. After a year of these frustrating delays the paramedics officially ditched the doctors and started operating solo, with radio contact to the ER as required: by 1971 the successful program was operating with a full staff of no fewer than twenty-two EMTs and was beginning to handle general medical cases as well as cardiac emergencies.

Similarly, in December 1969 Dr. Michael Criley, head of cardiology at Harbor General Hospital in Torrance, California, looked at Pantridge in Belfast and the pioneering work in Miami and wondered if something similar couldn't be brought to the seven million potential patients living in Los Angeles county. While he wondered, Walter Graf—head of the local chapter of the American Heart Association and the personal physician of the Chairman of the County Board of Supervisors—put his political connections to good use and persuaded his influential patient, Kenneth Hahn, to appropriate funds for L.A.'s first "heart mobile."[122] Unfortunately the new mobile unit was totaled while crossing an intersection in Inglewood, putting the American Heart Association out of the paramedic business. Criley picked up where Graf

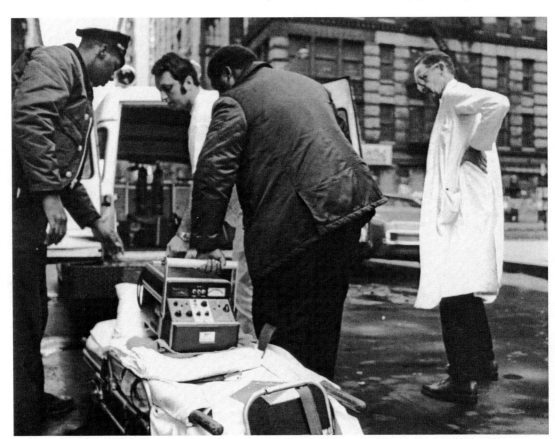

The founder of the first physician-based mobile cardiac care unit in the United States, Dr. William Grace (in glasses), responds to a possible heart attack, assisted by Dr. John Chadbourn (in white coat). (Library of Congress, Prints & Photographs Division, *Look* Magazine Photograph Collection, Job 68-3971.)

had left off, and ultimately persuaded Hahn to fund a second experiment. This time the project was given to the fire department—which initially wanted nothing to do with the job, feeling ambulances just got in the way of fighting fires. Nonetheless, the fire chief ultimately acquiesced to the scheme, realizing there was no profit alienating the most powerful political figure in the county. For his pains he was given a second-hand Forest Service station wagon with a defibrillator in the back and the optimistic logo "Rescue Heart Unit" stenciled onto the quarter panels.[123]

At first the medics who staffed the unit required a nurse to ride along and supervise their use of the equipment and the administration of any drugs, a restriction that was lifted in 1970 after Governor Reagan signed the Paramedic Act, officially making paramedics "physician

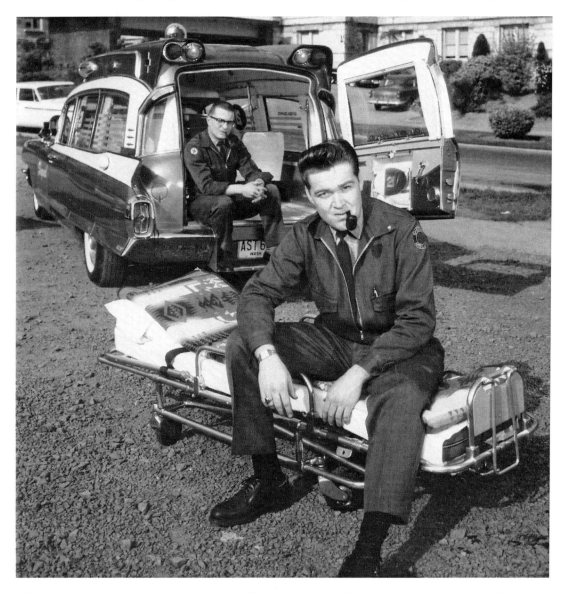

Shephard Ambulance crewmembers Eddie Haddock and Jim Farmer outside Seattle's Providence Hospital in 1963 (Bob Peterson, Seattle Times Collection, Seattle Museum of History and Industry).

extenders" who could perform advanced medical procedures in the field under the radio or telephone supervision of a physician or nurse.[124] A few years later the service achieved national fame when it became the subject of the popular television series *Emergency!*

At the same that Los Angeles county and Columbus were launching their services, the Seattle fire department was en route to making its own contribution to the paramedic cause. Seattle, clinging to a series of steep hillsides overlooking tidal mud-flats, was long a town where civic life was dominated by local business interests, and in its formative years was not considered particularly progressive in its politics. Not surprisingly, the city's original ambulance service had been limited to a single police wagon and a carry-all used by the Department of Health to supply its smallpox hospital, although between 1899 and 1925 the city operated a separate emergency ambulance staffed by a physician from the municipal hospital downtown.[125] For general purposes the citizens relied on local funeral homes and a few private ambulance companies, and in 1925 the city mothballed its ambulance and paid a politically connected firm $1,000 a year to operate two emergency ambulances during the day, moving one of the rigs to the Public Safety Building at night for "hurry cases" occurring after dark, and promising that an intern from the city hospital would be made available as needed for the night runs.[126]

During the 1930s the city fire department built up a small fleet of "aid cars," which in keeping with the time were intended mostly for the use of firefighters, but which would respond to any urgent civilian call: while this technically represented competition with the Shephard Ambulance Company's emergency ambulance contract, they were being paid by the year, not the call, so they had little financial incentive to raise a kick, nor is there any evidence that the fire department was fielding large numbers of calls. By 1947 the annual contract with Shephard was gone, and the city reimbursed any local firms that were left with unpaid charges after an emergency call: in the early 1950s this arrangement evolved into an informal agreement between the city and two private ambulance companies, Shephard and Rainbow, to handle all emergency cases, with the city treasurer regularly reimbursing them for unpaid fees incurred on emergency calls. (Consistent with Seattle's relaxed approach to handing out money to friendly contractors, no one got around to actually getting this on a legal footing until an ordinance was finally passed in 1967—a decision precipitated by a brawl between ambulance crews over a patient, resulting in a formal division of the town between Shephard and Rainbow, a statutory rate structure, and installation of sealed taximeters in all ambulances to make sure they didn't overcharge on mileage.)[127] By now the fire department was operating eight GMC carry-alls as "aid cars"—plus one station wagon assigned to firehouse with an unusually low ceiling in its garage, and, in order not to upset the financial arrangement between Seattle and the private companies, the fire department ambulances were discouraged from actually transporting civilians to the hospital unless their condition was so dire that delay might lead to death or serious injury: instead, the crews were expected to call one of the private firms and provide essential first aid to the patient until the Shepherd or Rainbow ambulance arrived to deliver them to the nearest infirmary, at the prevailing rate.[128]

In 1967 Dr. Leonard Cobb, chief of cardiology at Harborview (the county hospital whose art deco silhouette overlooks Puget Sound from the heights of Capitol Hill), read Pantridge's article about the Belfast "heart mobile" and, like his colleagues in Los Angeles, Columbus, and Haywood County, decided that this was a business he wanted to get into.[129] By this time fully one third of the Seattle Fire Department's calls were medical, and while most of these calls wound up being referred to the private fleet, a fair number were cardiac emergencies requiring the fire department aid cars to execute immediate transportation, a situation that made Chief Gordon Vickery quite amenable to Cobb's proposal to upgrade the fire department ambulances into heart-friendly emergency vehicles. The grant applications started going out in 1967, and when the first check finally arrived in 1968 they purchased their new vehicle: a

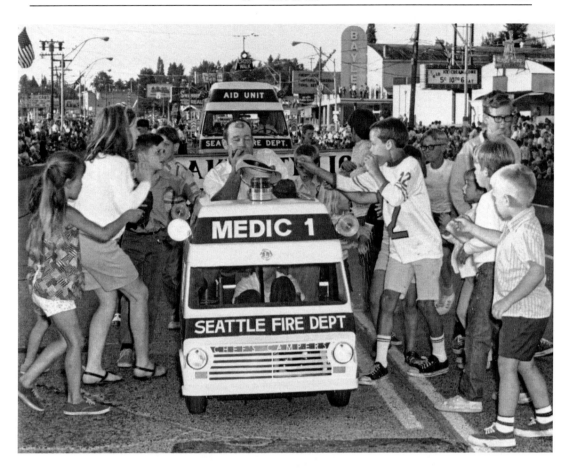

The Seattle Fire Department quickly followed Miami's lead, launching Medic 1 in 1970 with a renovated Winnebago nicknamed "Moby Pig." A year later financial shortfalls threatened the service until the fire department raised thousands in donations with a public campaign, including this appearance in a local parade (courtesy the Seattle Museum of History and Industry).

round sided mobile home (complete with kitchenette) that the firemen nicknamed "Moby Pig."[130] Obviously some remodeling was in order, and with the help of the local firemen they converted the caravan into a cardiac care unit, with a central stretcher area surrounded by a full suite of monitors, defibrillator units, IV materials, and everything else that could be required.

In October 1969 preparations were complete and the fire department hired fifteen paramedic trainees for what was now called "Medic One." After the crew had been trained in EKG reading, defibrillation, emergency cardioactive medications, and how to start and run an IV, Medic One was ready to go live in March 1970. One of its hallmarks was the concept of tiered response—a fire unit would respond to the first call for aid and only summoned Medic One if the situation warranted their intervention, in the meantime providing sufficient care to stabilize the patient at the scene (alternatively they would still call Shephard or Rainbow if the case was non-critical). For the first nine months of its operation the unit answered calls with a Harborview physician on board in addition to the medics, but as had happened in Columbus the extra staffing effort was soon considered to be unnecessary, and by early 1971 "Moby Pig" was responding with an all paramedic crew and physician back-up available by radio.[131] Unlike in Los Angeles, where the fire department had been a reluctant participant, the SFD had been an enthusiastic partner from the beginning, reflecting their forty years of experience operating their own ambulance fleet: it proved a prudent investment, as Chief Vickery declared Medic One to be the best public relations program his department had ever undertaken.[132]

A different model took hold in Portland, Oregon, one that eschewed physician staffing from the outset and was destined to become the prevailing standard of advanced ambulance care in the decades to come. The "Rose City" had, since at least the early 1940s, been the scene of a few notable ambulance innovations—not only had its fire department pioneered the all encompassing "disaster car" concept with its legendary Jay W. Stevens Disaster Unit, but local emergency mainstay Buck Ambulance had made a name for its progressive policies by adding oxygen to its entire fleet during the Second World War. By the late 1960s Leonard Rose was a cardiologist at the Good Samaritan Hospital in town, and like many of his colleagues he had read about Belfast in *The Lancet* and been intrigued by its possibilities. In early 1969 Rose started a training course for the employees of Buck Ambulance, using the facilities of Good Samaritan as his own improvised "cardiac college." His students were already trained above the norm for ambulance crews of the day, thanks to Buck's forward thinking management, and Rose taught them the elements of cardiophysiology, EKG reading, and how to use a portable defibrillator.[133] The ambulance crews proved apt pupils, and the program was a success, helping to demonstrate to an ever larger audience the possibility of training private ambulance crews to a high standard of emergency care—and showing the way forward for more such training.

Whatever their format, unless built on the backs of volunteers, these programs were not cheap, but a closer look at one such program suggests not only the expenses involved, but also

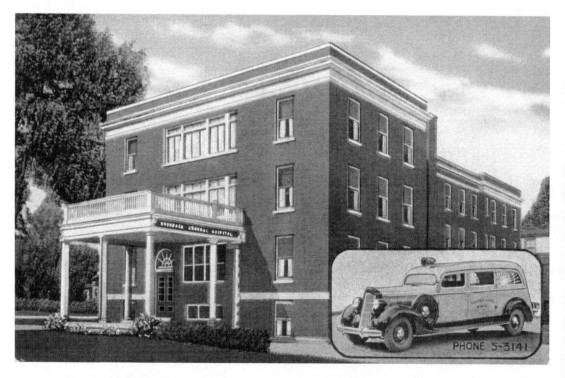

In the late 1930s the Onandaga Hospital in upstate New York proudly included its resident ambulance on this postcard. Such services were good advertising for the institution and also brought in extra business. Hoping to capture similar values, a few hospitals in the early 1970s re-launched their own ambulances during the new vogue for paramedic service.

the potential financial benefits that encouraged their development. Turning to Manhattan, the New York Hospital had proposed the city's first ambulance service in 1869, only to see the operation go to Bellevue after losing the lease on their principal property. One hundred years later, in 1973, the New York was ready to make local history again by introducing the city's first full-scale paramedic program, with a capital investment of $230,000, inclusive of five ambulances, equipment, and training costs (representing over $1 million in 2008 dollars).[134] At a time when a basic ambulance call was billed at $40, the New York Hospital charged $150 for paramedic services to cover the higher salaries and equipment expenses, but with a collection rate of only 50 percent the paramedic ambulances inevitably lost money. Still, Dr. Melville Platt, associate director of the hospital's professional services, was adamant that the program would continue, saying "Even if it continues to be a losing operation, we would never consider eliminating the paramedic program. It is a necessary community service."[135] In addition to its status as a necessary community service, the paramedic operation had an unexpected financial benefit that helped offset its weak billing profile: because patients arrived in a more stable condition, Platt reported that the hospital saw its absolute ER expenses decrease, even as billable visits increased from 3,107 in March 1972 to 3,765 a year later. (This likely represented a noticeable increase in overall profitability, and not just for the emergency room, since the article noted that between 10 percent and 15 percent of a hospital's total billing was derived from admissions through its ER, suggesting that even a "losing" ambulance service could generate profit for the infirmary.)

Ultimately the majority of hospitals found operation of their own paramedic services an unwelcome administrative burden, and as soon as equivalent community providers entered the market most were happy to divest themselves of the operation (hospitals, once the majority provider of ambulance service in the largest cities, were down to 6 percent by 1989, for example).[136] In whatever form, however, the trend towards more advanced pre-hospital care was clearly in place, and while the earliest programs had been patterned on the limited interventions of the Belfast "heart mobile," within a year or two the majority of services had evolved into full medical providers.

Training Standards

With so many successful advanced training programs in operation by the end of the 1960s, from Pittsburgh to Miami, and from the Appalachians to the Cascades, in 1970 the DHEW and DOT jointly commissioned guidelines for an Advanced Training Program for Emergency Medical Technicians/Ambulance, to be created by the National Academy of Sciences' Subcommittee on Ambulance Services. Once again, the chairman for the project was the ubiquitous Dr. Farrington, and their report, "Advanced Training for Emergency Medical Technicians/Ambulance" released in September 1970, represented the first attempt to provide a national curriculum. As seen, the country was awash in a variety of advanced training programs and reaching a consensus on what a paramedic ought to be looked like a long slog: as Nancy Caroline put it, "Ask any ten people for a definition of a paramedic and you're likely to get eleven answers—even if you ask ten paramedics themselves."[137] As a practical matter, a paramedic was anyone who had completed a course claiming to confer that credential—and as Caroline pointed out that could mean a few days of clinical skills work tacked onto the end of the Dunlop Course resulting in "glorified EMT-A's trained only to initiate intravenous lines," or it might mean "highly trained firemen doing transthoracic cardiac pacing and cricothyreotomy in the field" after undergoing nine months of intensive training.[138]

By October 1972 the Springfield Hospital Medical Center in Massachusetts had taken Farrington's 1970 guidelines and, under a DOT contract, roughed them into a pilot course that was sent to one hundred fifty agencies for road-testing. Two years later the recommendations from forty services were collated and forwarded to Nancy Caroline at the University of Pittsburgh, along with a contract to refashion the original coursework into a modular program that could train students to various intermediate levels of proficiency, culminating some 500 to 800 hours later with certification as a Paramedic (or, more specifically, EMT-P, to distinguish them from the EMT-A, who had completed the 81 hour Dunlop course).

In September 1975 Caroline turned in a fifteen module course that could be offered in its entirety or as an *ala carte* training system based on the local needs. (A year later additional changes to the trauma, pediatric, and psychiatric emergency sections were made by the University of Kansas, and it was only in 1976 that the final course was approved by the federal Interagency Committee on EMS and released into the wild.) Ultimately, Caroline's course (which by now was the province of the Department of Transportation's Highway Safety Division, HEW having largely ceded pre-hospital care to the roads department) had the following fifteen components, representing for the first time a consensus view of what a paramedic should be capable of (and, not surprisingly, it reflected what Caroline's colleagues at the Freedom House Enterprises Ambulance Service had been training to do since 1967):

1: role of the paramedic
2: human systems and patient assessment
3: shock and fluid therapy (initiation of peripheral IV lines)
4: pharmacology, including calculation of dosages
5: respiratory system (use of external airways; methods of delivering supplemental oxygen; suctioning the nose/mouth/trachea; removal of foreign bodies)
6: cardiovascular system (running an EKG, identifying dysrhythmias, CPR, defibrillation, and administration of cardioactive drugs)
7: central nervous system (immobilizing spinal injury, transfer of spinal injury patients; management of seizures and the comatose)
8: soft tissue injuries: including amputations; lacerations; control of bleeding with direct pressure, tourniquets, and use of anti-shock trousers.
9: musculoskeletal system: sprains, contusions, and fractures, including splints.
10: medical emergencies, including status asthmaticus, burns, and electrocution.
11: obstetric/gynecologic emergencies
12: pediatrics and neonatal transportation
13: emergency care of the emotionally disturbed
14: rescue techniques, including vehicle stabilization, access, disentanglement, and extrication
15: telemetry and communications

With customary modesty Caroline made light of her work preparing the course work, writing:

> What's so special about the USDOT curriculum—aside from the fact that it comprises nearly 2000 pages and takes two people to lift it? Nothing, really. Any curriculum and any teaching strategy which brings the student to the desired skill and knowledge objectives will do. The USDOT course merely defines those objectives in precise terms and offers one possible strategy for reaching them.[139]

Of course, by "merely" defining the critical objectives in comprehensible terms and delivering a coherent system for teaching them, Caroline put down the marks that future paramedics would have to hit when they stepped onto the national stage. She knew that not every community could afford, or would even necessarily need, crews possessing the full complement of skills she had enumerated, but she also understood that before the paramedic could claim to be a profession it had to have a recognizable standard: it was her contribution to make sure that standard met the bar set by her friends and co-workers at Freedom House, and to ensure that whatever happened to the historic ambulance service in Pittsburgh, its principles would survive intact. She benefited from trailblazing done by Deke Farrington in his lectures to the Chicago fire department in 1963 and his almost single-handed creation of the EMT-A course, the contributions of surgeon's groups and government officials who tried to prioritize the skills required, and the assistance of all who tried out the first drafts and contributed suggestions. In the end, however, it was Nancy Caroline who took the responsibility of fashioning these raw materials into a workable program for the education of the American paramedic.

While the debate over what constituted optimal training appeared to be winding down (and the optimists plotted global licensing requirements, universal reciprocity, and a single national curriculum for emergency medical technician training), the struggle over the ambulance and its equipment continued. Clearly, the nature of the training would have an effect, since the more training required, the more the ambulance itself would have to morph in order to provide the space and the equipment for the crew to perform their interventions: after all, just eight years earlier the concept of a civilian paramedic had been unknown and the most elaborate recommendation for ambulance equipment that the American College of Surgeons could conceive of would have fit comfortably into the back of a station wagon. Now that the scope of pre-hospital care was being reimagined, it was time to redraft the platform on which these services would be delivered. At this point in the late 1960s, the growing influence of Swab's modular

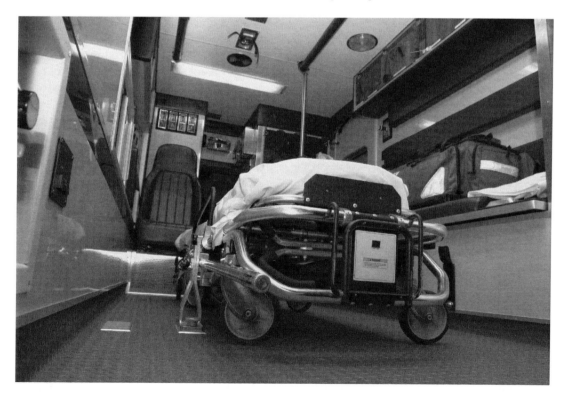

A modern ambulance interior reflects the reforms of the 1960s and 1970s, when space requirements, equipment standards, and improved training transformed the ambulance (photograph by Nancy Louie).

ambulance aside, the majority of ambulances were still "professional cars" patterned after hearses, albeit with raised rooflines. Once again the initial voice for federal leadership sounded in the pages of *Accidental Death and Disability,* which noted in 1966 that "the bodies and fixed equipment of ambulances and rescue vehicles are produced by the conversion of passenger-type vehicles or are fabricated to fit assembly line chassis, and are usually expensive in outward appearance, but impractical for resuscitative care."[140] A follow-up in 1967 concluded, glumly, "anyone wishing to do so can purchase any type of vehicle he wishes, call it an ambulance, and charge for transporting the sick and injured, regardless of the appropriateness or quality of the service."[141]

Vehicle Standards

While the majority of medical attention was being devoted to the question of how ambulance crews should be trained, this criticism of their working space was not lost on the Department of Transportation, which was marshaling its energy to assume a new federal role in regulating automotive safety under authority of the Automobile Safety Act of 1966, the companion to the Highway Safety Act. In the intersection of these two campaigns, for safer motor vehicles and better trained ambulance crews, and in the context of the scathing reports that had come from the Academy of Sciences, in 1968 the DOT asked the National Academy of Engineering (a subdivision of the National Academy of Sciences) to prepare a report concerning recommendations for ambulance design.

The committee members represented the entire range of disciplines associated with ambulance design and operation — there were engineers from General Motors and Chrysler, physicians like Peter Safar and J.D. Farrington, industry representation from the Ambulance Association of America and the Oregon State Ambulance Association, specialists in air conditioning, heating, and other niche fields, as well as academics, government administrators, and state and federal experts in injury control or the operation of emergency medical services. As members of various subcommittees and in plenary sessions they met several times over nine months, and held an open forum at an ambulance exhibition in Columbus, Ohio, in January, 1969, where they not only had the opportunity to inspect recent designs but took questions from an audience of over one hundred highly invested exhibitors and attendees.[142] Given the variety of backgrounds represented, the diversity of viewpoints, and the discrepancy between those with practical experience in ambulance construction and operation and those whose interests were aspirational, it is not surprising that the chairman later noted, drily, "as the Committee activities progressed, very free and frank dialogues developed."[143]

From this free and frank dialogue the committee was able to identify a little more than one hundred elements that it felt were critical to a vehicle's ability to function as an acceptable ambulance, and it was these elements which formed the bedrock of its design recommendations, covering size and space requirements, mechanical performance, electrical systems, vehicle identification, communications equipment, climate control, supplies, and safety requirements. In addition to these, the committee identified four other elements that were critical to proper function but for which no recommendation could be made without further testing. These

Opposite: A turn-of-the-century ambulance interior contrasts with its modern-day equivalent: The simple rig with its cot, cramped patient compartment, and rudimentary supplies has evolved into a rolling emergency room equipped for the stabilization and treatment of the most serious medical emergencies (Library of Congress, *Chicago Daily News* **negatives collection, DN-0004686 [1907]; Pamela Moore [2005]).**

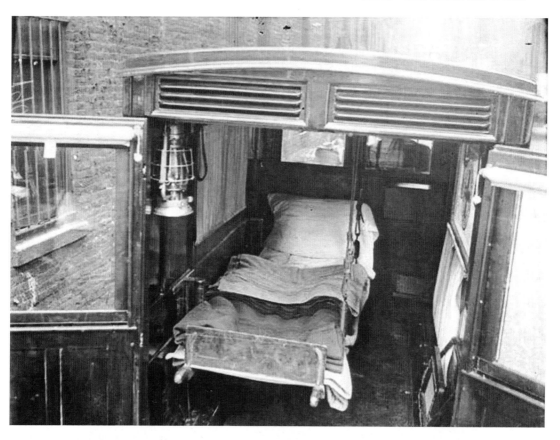

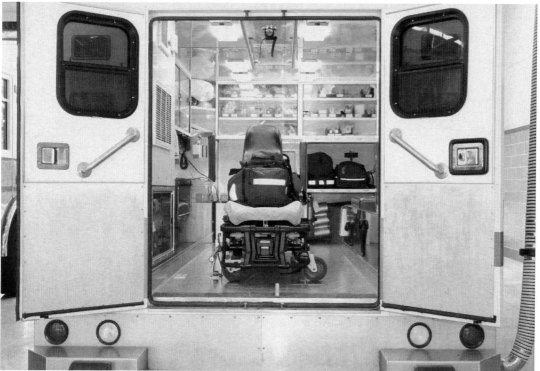

deferred features were the color and intensity of the warning lights, noise and vibration tolerances, the smoothness of the ride over various conditions, and the optimum braking requirements.[144] On an individual level, the committee tried to preserve some flexibility in the design standards to allow for innovation and experiment, and generally followed a rule of matching its most inflexible instructions to the most critically important components.

Broadly speaking, the resulting report, turned over in June 1969, provided for vehicles sufficient to transport two litter patients and two crewmembers inside the cabin, with enough headroom for an EMT to hang an IV bottle and lean over a stretcher and administer CPR. Addressing a deficiency found in the majority ambulances of the time, two-way radios were required, as well as walkie-talkies, an intercom, and a public address system. The committee also provided equipment guidelines and recommended national standards for identification, including blue and white beacon lights and "Omaha orange" crosses on a white background for the roof, rear, sides, and front of the vehicle, with the word "ambulance" placed below each insignia and written in reverse on the hood for the benefit of those looking into their rear-view mirrors. In all, it was a comprehensive document and laid the foundation for the first federal standards for ambulance vehicles, although contrary to the author's expectations these criteria were never legislated at the national level, their precepts being limited to vehicles purchased by federal agencies or those receiving federal funds. Still, this report's completion fell one week after the one hundredth anniversary of the Bellevue service, and was a fitting monument to usher out the first century of the modern American ambulance and point the way forward to the most dramatic decade in ambulance history.

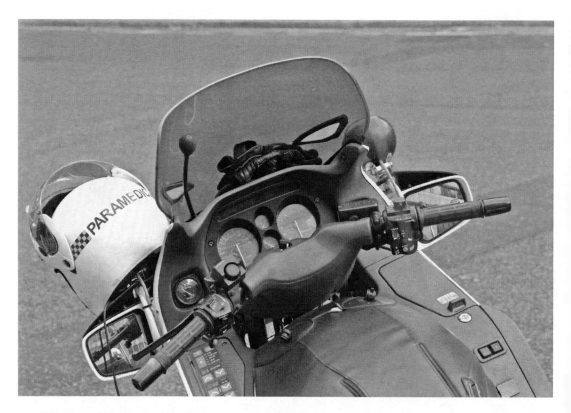

The idea of the Derbyshire "flying squad" lives on through National Health Service paramedics staged on motorcycles, allowing them to reach patients ahead of the ambulance and initiate medical care while awaiting transportation and more intensive interventions.

Flying Squads

While authorities in the United States attempted to improve ambulance service by mandating bigger, more elaborate rigs staffed by well-trained non-physicians, those in Great Britain attempted a different model. Starting around 1955, the Derbyshire Royal Infirmary began deploying "flying squads," dashing outfits consisting of surgeons, with or without nursing and anesthesia, responding rapidly to accident scenes on summons from a first responder (either a traditional ambulance attendant or the police). Reportedly inspired by German "mobile operating theatres" dealing with catastrophic high-speed accidents on the *autobahnen*, the Derbyshire flying squad was widely imitated and persisted into the early 1970s, when it was supplanted by paramedic services resembling those popularized in the United States.

Rather than responding in their own ambulances, the early British flying squads were transported by the local police, all equipment being broken down into boxes capable of being carried by one person and the entire assembly fitting into the "boot" of one or two cars. Upon receiving a call for the flying squad, the police commonly dispatched two patrols to the hospital while simultaneously sending riders ahead to clear traffic from crossroads as the squad approached. As a supplement to the regular ambulances the services were used sparingly: for example, the Derbyshire Squad responded to an average of nineteen calls per year, varying from accidents in mines and industrial plants to roadway smashups.[145] While largely supplanted by conventional emergency medical technicians and ambulance services by the mid–1970s, this was far from being a failed scheme, as some aspects of this plan have been incorporated into modern American ambulance operations. Specifically, the expense of putting Advanced Life Support staff on every ambulance is prohibitive: just as British surgeons were called to back up basic ambulance crews in the most serious cases, so some ambulance providers now station single ALS crew members around a municipality "on call." These solo "flying squads" carry their gear in personal vehicles and are available to race to a scene when their particular abilities are urgently needed, recreating the dramatic appearance of their British predecessors.

• 14 •

An Incomplete Revolution: 1970 to 2000

"The health industry is fully in favor of progress—but change is out of the question."
—Gerald Looney, 1973. *Journal of Emergency Services* 6:6—"Getting What We Pay For."

After swift progress in pre-hospital emergency care in the late 1960s, with multiple cities introducing advanced ambulance services and an escalation of federal investment in emergency services, 1970 opened with another auspicious omen: the University of Cincinnati (where America's original hospital-based general ambulance service began in 1865) announced the country's first Emergency Medicine residency. Since the late 18th century the emergency room and the casualty ward had been intimately associated with ambulance services, and in America particularly the frequently scattershot staffing of emergency rooms with rotating doctors from various specialties perpetuated the myopic view that emergency care—in the hospital or out of it—required only the most rudimentary training or skill, as its purpose was flying the patient to the hospital where whatever ophthalmologist, pediatrician, or sleep-deprived trainee who happened to be on-call could temporize any egregious injuries while a specialist was rousted from bed to come in and take charge of the case.

Slowly surgeons, and later cardiologists, had realized that the better the initial care the more sanguine they could be about the outcome, and since the 1950s they had lent increasingly vocal support for improved ambulance services. Now the new credential of "Emergency Medical Physician" promised an entirely fresh stream of allies with a vested, professional interest in the improvement of pre-hospital care—and, despite the recent changes, the ambulance services sorely needed champions. The scattered innovation and increased federal attention in the mid to late 1960s had resulted in isolated services achieving unprecedented levels of care, but in the national aggregate the emergency medical services continued to be uneven. As Merlin DuVal, the Assistant Secretary for Health, Department of Health, Education, and Welfare explained in 1973:

> There are communities where the transportation system is extremely good; others where the quality of ambulance training is very high. Some where communications are first rate; others where emergency rooms are very good. The trick is to get them all together.[1]

Even at the most literal level, ambulances were seldom really ambulances—in 1974 fully 64 percent of American's emergency vehicles were actually station wagons (25 percent), panel trucks (10 percent), or hearses, "carry-alls," and vans (totaling 29 percent).[2] While communities like Portland, Miami, Pittsburgh, and Haywood County, North Carolina, had pioneered exemplary emergency medical care services, they remained the notable exceptions in what remained a largely under-resourced field.

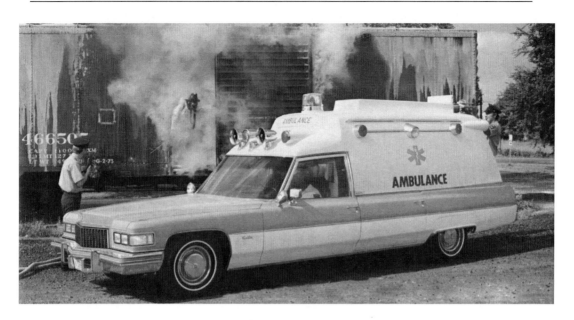

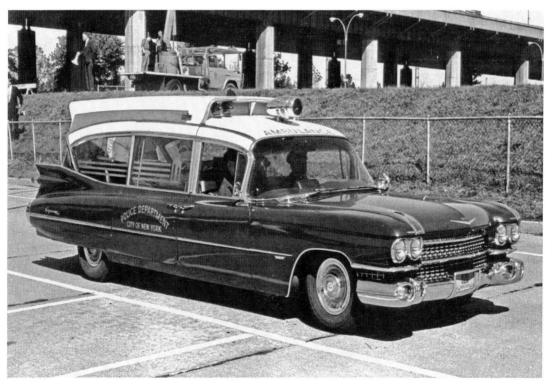

Top: This brochure cover for the 1975 Criterion ambulance captures the excitement of emergency medical service, as well as showcasing the dramatic lines of the late-model "professional car" ambulance (courtesy Miller-Meteor/Accubuilt). *Bottom:* In the early 1970s the New York Emergency Services Unit used this ambulance for police officers and their families, funding its acquisition and operation with money raised from the ranks. Due to uneven regulation, private ambulance services were inconsistent, making a reliable and quality service like this one much in demand. (Copyright 2001, New York City Police Department, all rights reserved. Used with permission.)

Not only was the physical equipment of many services clearly deficient, a 1973 exposé written for *The New York Times* by David Andelman revealed how the goal of universal access to quality emergency care was impeded by a lack of uniform standards and training, lax enforcement of what standards did exist, and the shoddy way in which emergency services were coordinated between the "crazy-quilt pattern" of volunteer, municipal, and commercial ambulances in operation.[3] For example, Suffolk County, on the western end of Long Island, had ten commercial ambulance companies, twenty-eight volunteer corps, and fifty-six volunteer fire departments offering aid car services—an average of one ambulance company for each square mile of dry land, and each with its own telephone number. (At the same time a report by the Robert Johnson Foundation noted that while Kansas City residents could sleep better knowing they were surrounded by forty-five different ambulance services, wading through seventy-eight different emergency telephone numbers to reach them was a nightmare.)[4]

Keeping track of all these companies was, apparently, too much for the local authorities. Staying on Long Island for the moment, the article noted that New York had a litany of regulations on ambulance service (covering everything from minimum head-room and type of oxygen cylinders to the number and size of gauze bandages carried), but even in relatively affluent Suffolk County forty-seven percent of ambulances were not up to code, and one third of ambulance crewmembers either had no first aid training at all, or had only completed the Red Cross basic eight-hour course—far below the forty-hour Advanced First Aid Certification required. Still, the Empire State outstripped Connecticut, which by 1973 had yet to pass a single state standard for ambulances or their crews. Not all was disastrous, however, as the article concluded that New York City, Baltimore, and Jacksonville had assembled first-rate emergency response systems, with high standards, consistent enforcement, and inter-agency cooperation: had the *New York Times* remembered the United States was bordered by the Pacific as well as the Atlantic, they might have added Los Angeles, Seattle, San Francisco, and Portland to their list of high achievers.

"Sadism Rides the Ambulance"

This contrast between the woebegone and the wondrous, the untrained attendant riding in a converted hearse in Connecticut and the Los Angeles paramedic transmitting EKG signals to a cardiologist at the county hospital, fueled the reform movement gathering force in Washington, D.C., and, to a lesser extent, in state capitals and city council chambers. By the end of the 1960s the improvement in technology, the growth of strict legislation (on paper, at any rate), and public and political attention to the scope of the need had all combined to raise the bar for reformers and conscientious operators alike. At the same time, the sheer number of communities adopting a laissez faire attitude towards the emergency services meant that, by 1970, the chasm between the best services in the United States and the worst gaped as wide as it ever would in the history of the ambulance. In time, individual communities would face these comparisons and many would react; in time Congress would consider the enormity of the inequalities and attempt to intercede, but in the interval countless thousands would be abandoned to the worst emergency medical care that greed could create and poverty endure.

A well-documented case study in how the best ambulance service of the era could coexist with the worst comes from Chicago, whose diverse experiences with aid cars provided a tiny simulacrum of the nation as a whole. By 1968 Chicago's fire department was operating the country's first municipal medevac service for trauma cases, ambulance crew members held Red Cross Advanced First Aid certificates and received regular training from the local chapter of the American College of Surgeons, and the department had been singled out in a government report as one of the eighteen leading ambulance fleets in the country.[5] As was typical of the day, Chicago was also home to a host of private ambulance companies, and the contrast between the municipal service and some of these entrepreneurs would, when realized, shock a city not known for being squeamish. It was hardly a surprise that private firms, subsisting on the out of pocket payments of their customers and needing to turn a profit, could never match the investment put out by a city drawing taxes from the fourth largest metropolitan area in the country, but what few understood was how utterly decayed the bottom rungs of the quality ladder had become. In the blighted neighborhoods and slum sections of Chicago the shoddy ambulance operator went about their work with impunity, confident that the poor were either too ignorant to know how badly they were being treated, or were too disaffected to make a noise that anyone uptown would ever hear. For decades they were right. Year after year they extorted money from desperate families, demanding cash up front before transporting a man literally turning blue on the living room floor or a girl hemorrhaging from a miscarriage; year after year they paid their employees less and less, invested less and less in equipment or services, and no doubt grew amazed that there was never any retribution, divine or earthly, for their increasingly brazen depredations.

By 1970, however, the Civil Rights movement had exposed the conscience of the nation to the burdens imposed on minority groups due to outrageous inequalities in public services and discriminatory business practices: as a result, reforms were pursued across a spectrum of government and private enterprises, from new citizen commissions monitoring police operations to increased oversight of lending practices at neighborhood banks. It could hardly be a coincidence that at this critical moment, when patience for substandard service was at its lowest ebb, that the most reputable of Chicago's private ambulance firms began worrying that the lowest representatives of their profession might commit some newsworthy outrage producing the kind of publicity that leads to increased regulation or even government take-over of a suddenly recognized "public utility." Accordingly they conferred with one another and sent a discrete deputation of whistleblowers to the Better Government Association with word that their down-market rivals were engaging in wholesale fraud, extortion, patient abuse, and negligent practices—and that as good corporate citizens they wanted to be as far away as possible from the bull's-eye when the inevitable reforms were levied. From the Better Government offices the complaint found its way to the newsroom of *The Chicago Tribune,* and a couple of young reporters, William Jones and William Recktenwald, wound up spending two months working undercover at a series of low-rent (but astonishingly profitable) ambulance firms in Chicago, assisted by George Bliss, a special investigator for the Better Government Association.

The first the city knew of the incipient scandal was a full page teaser ad appearing in the paper's June 6, 1970, edition, a murky photo of a blurry ambulance on a dark street, promising readers a startling weeklong expose to read over their coffee and cereal. As promised, the story officially broke in the June 7th sunrise edition, its lead sentence setting the tone for the deeply personal reporting to follow: "They are the misery merchants and they prowl the streets of our city 24 hours a day as profiteers of human suffering." The rest of the article quickly laid out the specifications of the indictment—ambulance crews paying off policemen and firefighters in exchange for calls to collect welfare patients, fraudulent claims, stealing from hospital emergency rooms, and "sadistic treatment" at the hands of men whose most charitable defense was gross negligence compounded by incompetence, and whose heaviest charge would be perversity, racism, and greed. The investigation's targets were the bottom feeders of the city's broad array of private entrepreneurs, all operating in the poorest, and predominantly African-American, sections of the metropolis and each of which was supposedly supervised and regulated by the Board of Health and the Motor Vehicle Bureau.

Per these regulations an ambulance attendant was required to pay a $5 annual fee to the

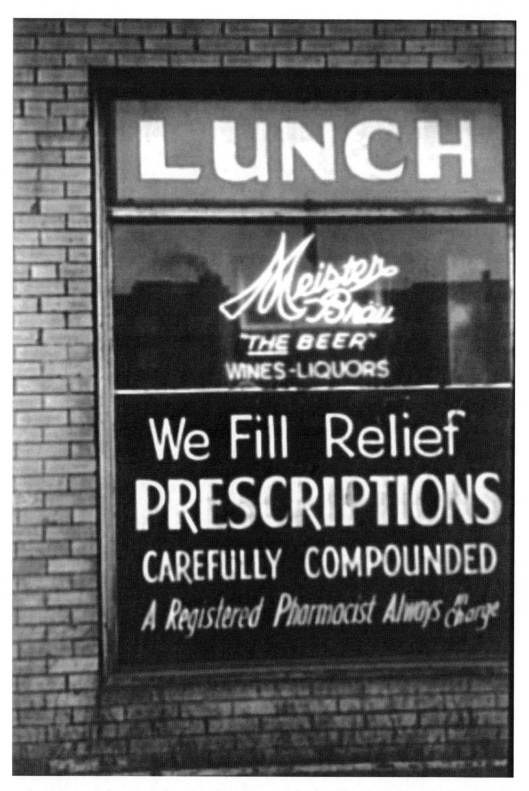

This combination lunch counter, bar, and pharmacy was emblematic of the often dubious health care found in Chicago's poorest, segregated neighborhoods in the late 1960s and early 1970s—which included its local ambulance services (Edwin Rosskam, Library of Congress, Prints and Photographs Division, USF33 005193-M3).

Vehicle Bureau, show proof of a negative test for tuberculosis, get clearance from the police department, and pass the forty-hour Red Cross Advanced First Aid course. As a practical matter, assuming they paid the five dollar fee and had the rest of the paperwork in hand, applicants were given their "hard card" (the laminated license declaring them a certified ambulance attendant) as soon as they registered for the First Aid course—not after completing it. Of course, by giving the card up front with no mechanism to verify that anyone had sat through a single first aid lecture, much less passed, the city effectively waived the training requirement.[6]

Not that it mattered. The investigators soon realized that few of these shadowy ambulance operators ever asked to see anyone's "hard card," and indeed in one case Jones was hired over the phone without even the pretense of vetting. Once on staff, one shop was very much like the other: a grueling world of "24 hour shift stacked on 24 hour shift," as Jones described it in the first installment, pay that was as low as eighty-seven cents an hour, vermin infested garages, and the cheapest equipment that could be bought—or the best that could be stolen from an emergency room. (Most of the sheets, pillow cases, and towels in the backs of these ambulances were stenciled with the names of the city's major hospitals. When one reporter asked the obvious question of whether all the bedding in an ambulance had really been swiped from the hospital whose name was emblazoned on the linens, the driver said yes, and then reached under his seat and flourished a stethoscope saying "Where do you think I got this?")[7] At one firm petty theft was a job requirement, with a weekly contest to see which crewmember had stolen the most supplies from local emergency rooms—and rewarding this Artful Dodger with a handsome $25 bonus.[8]

Since the 911 phone system was still a distant dream, private firms got jobs by advertising in the yellow pages and waiting for the phone to ring—or by working out special arrangements with hotel clerks, factory bosses, police officers, and firefighters that made sure their company was notified whenever a likely looking injury, heart attack, or other medical emergency turned up. The going rate was $10, which was slipped to the cop on the beat, the lead fireman at the scene, or the helpful hotel clerk—in turn, the ambulance companies charged between $36 and $40 for a straight case, plus extra for oxygen and night calls. Competition was tough, and firms worked hard to build up a network of "friendlies" in various districts: one Southside manager for Scully-Walton was beside himself when they got a call from a cop in a precinct formerly sewn up by a rival, saying "This is a milestone for us. The 7th (police) district has been completely tied up with Mid-America. Maybe we can start to get more of their business."[9] Brokering these calls was especially lucrative for the bent harness bull, as the police patrols were most likely to arrive first at a scene—but once they chanced upon a victim on the street, they could be quite casual about collecting their fee, since once the patient was stowed in the back of a police van they were money in the bank. In one instance an older man with a seizure disorder fell and broke his hip, and a police patrol responded to the scene. They shoved him in the back of their low roofed wagon, but when a few other matters turned up requiring their attention almost two hours passed with the delirious man rolling around in back before they got around to calling their pet ambulance firm for the transfer. Jones was undercover that shift, and watched the other crewman pass along a sawbuck before they dragged their patient out of the squadrol and heaved him into their ambulance for the long delayed trip to the ER: to avoid creating trouble for their police friends, the attendant lied on the admission slip and said they had picked up the patient at a neighbor's house.[10]

(Other sources were cultivated as well to ensure a steady stream of patients, and supervisors spent a great deal of time trying to nail down exclusives: Jones reported being at one shift-change when a hard-charging supervisor announced the latest "contracts," telling the men "Listen up, you guys, if any of you get a call from [a north side hotel] it's a $10 drop to the room clerk," and adding that from now on they would be getting all the ambulance calls from

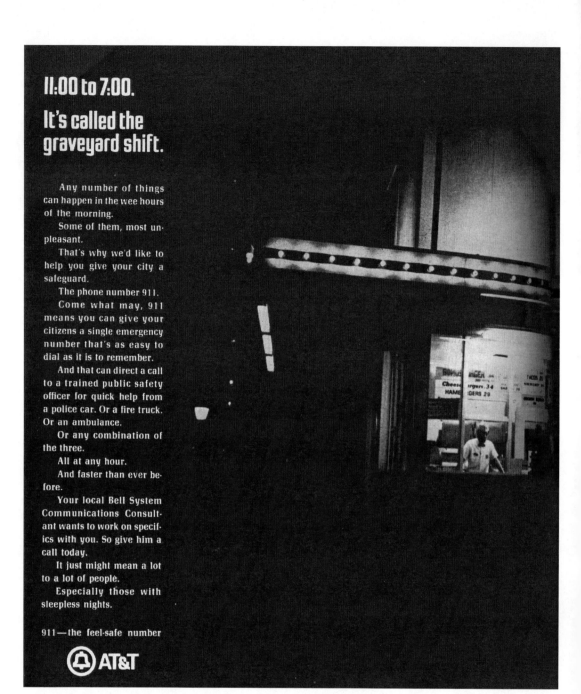

The creation of a central emergency telephone number eliminated the shady advertising practices and illegal kickback schemes that governed which ambulance company got the call in Chicago. This advertisement appeared in 1970, the same year the city's ambulance scandal made headlines in the *Tribune* (copyright AT&T, all rights reserved).

a certain factory in the north end, but they were not to pay off on the spot because "I take care of that myself."[11])

For those at the mercy of these services (representing perhaps twenty percent of the private market in Chicago, according to estimates of the more reputable firms) there was little recourse.[12] If a person provided a welfare card, thus ensuring state payment, they were guaranteed a ride into the hospital—although since the firms charged $1 a mile, it might not be the closest one.

If you couldn't produce a welfare card, the shady firms all enforced a strict cash in advance policy, no matter how serious the case. In the most notorious instance in the weeklong series, the investigators set up a sting operation to document just how far the firms would go to enforce this "no bread, no bed" policy. Renting rooms in a rundown boarding house, they phoned a local service and requested an ambulance to transport a heart attack case. When the crew arrived they saw Bliss, the BGA investigator, lying on the floor, moaning and gasping for breath, with a distraught Jones standing over him.[13] Setting the stretcher down, the attendants demanded $40 in cash before taking Bliss to the hospital. Jones, pretending to look frantically through his pockets, could only come up with $2, which he put down on the kitchen table while begging them to take his friend, babbling on about how Bliss had a job and would be sure to pay the bill.

The crew, obviously skeptical, asked to use the phone and called their boss: he reminded them that this was a cash call, and if there was no money up front they should walk out. Hanging up the phone they hoisted Bliss off the floor and dropped him into a chair at the kitchen table, where with admirable verisimilitude he pitched forward, his head falling on his arms, a ghastly rattle sounding in his throat. Without saying a word one of the attendants casually reached past him, scooped up the $2 from the table and, picking up his end of the empty stretcher, the two men stalked out into the street. (Meantime, Recktenwald and a photographer had been hiding in an adjacent room, photographing the little drama through the slats of a venetian blind.) As another ambulance attendant later explained to Jones, if someone can't pay "they can go in a blue star ambulance. That's the police. If they're bad enough the police will take them. And if they don't move them while they are sick, they do remove stiffs."[14]

And what did the patient, or the state, get for their $40? If the previous customer had bled or vomited, the next one in the cab got a clean sheet, otherwise they used the same linen as the last patient (or the last eight, as the case might be). Treatment en route was apt to go by the boards. In one instance Jones was in back with a woman with an apparent heart attack: she was struggling for breath, so his partner slapped a mask on her face and turned on the oxygen—for a few seconds. He promptly turned it off again, but left the mask over the woman's nose and mouth so she could enjoy the benefit of the placebo effect on the ride in, and he could bill the state an extra $10 for "providing" oxygen during transport.[15] That whiff of air was probably more than Jones himself could have done, since in jobs with more than half a dozen firms not once were any of the investigators given formal training in how to operate the oxygen tanks before going on duty. In fact, none of their co-workers were in any position to teach them anything at all about first aid. While employed by Mid-America Ambulance, Jones was paired with an ex-cabbie who had been in the ambulance business for seven months. Between calls they sat on old automobile seats in a converted service station, Jones usually dozing while his partner read comic books. One day, having run out of pictures to look at, Jones' coworker got bored enough to give an impromptu demonstration of the rig's emergency equipment. He got off to a bad start by accidentally blowing up a regulator bag trying to demonstrate how the oxygen tank worked, then picked his way through the rest of their supplies, winding up his "lesson" by holding up an inflatable splint and telling Jones, apologetically, "I don't know what it is, myself."[16] Readers were left to conclude that, in the worst services, the ambulance was nothing more than a $40 cab ride.

What kept these carrion feeders fat was a billable system pouring one million dollars a year into Cook County for ambulance services provided to the indigent and those on Medicare. Since these ambulance companies were stealing supplies from hospital emergency rooms, paying their expendable workforce under a dollar an hour, saving money by dispensing with training, and avoiding the problem of uncollected fees by charging cash up front, there was a comfortable margin to be had. To make that margin even more attractive, there was always the prospect of padding the billing sheets submitted to the state for welfare cases. Here, many of the crooked ambulance firms found a friend in the managing director of "Welfare Billing Service," a cheerful entrepreneur who had spent five years as the Illinois State Director of Welfare Payments before quitting his job in 1968 after realizing the real money was in the private sector. Trading on his public service experience, he sent circulars to Chicago area ambulance services, physician offices, and clinics, proclaiming "You and I know welfare business is good business. Increase your income from welfare and Medicare. Be represented [in the Chicago aid office] by someone who knows ALL the ins and outs of welfare." [17] He encouraged his ambulance clients to submit partially blank forms, so he could complete them in ways that would maximize their return—say, by routinely adding a $2 night surcharge without checking to see if the patient had actually been transferred after dark or not, or automatically charging the state's maximum reimbursement rate for a service even if the company's cash rate was actually lower—billing the state $10 for oxygen when the company's posted rate for paying customers was only $6, or charging $40 for transportation when a company only billed $36.[18] (The practice of differential charging is still very much a part of medicine—hospitals will routinely bill an uninsured patient much more than they charge insured patients for the identical service: the justification is that insurance companies negotiate such steep discounts that the hospitals have to charge the uninsured much more money to make up their losses.)

When asked about these practices, the civil servant turned corporate titan was chattier than his lawyer would have ultimately liked. He helpfully told a reporter "When you're talking about a dollar, you're not talking about much money, my friend. I just took it upon myself to raise [the bills.] It looks bad, I agree, but there's nothing wrong here."[19] He then proceeded to explain how he was actually doing the state a favor, because while his bills were bogus, they cost *less* than the expense of rejecting accurate bills filled out incorrectly by the sub-cretin clients. As he put it, "it may seem like I increase the cost of welfare, but this is just not true. You see, since I know how to fill out the forms correctly, it actually saves the state money because the computers don't reject them and create a lot of extra bookkeeping." State auditors proved an unforgiving audience, alas, and in the ensuing investigations he and his ambulance company clients were wriggling in the same net. In fact, within 72 hours of the first article hitting the street the Board of Health launched a series of raids, and by the end of the week three of the worst businesses were suspended from taking welfare cases pending review of their license status.[20]

While inarguably extreme, there is nothing to suggest that Chicago was unique. It had an excellent city system, a number of reputable and creditable private services, and had ambulance statutes on the books: what it did not have was a reliable enforcement mechanism or an effective monitoring system. In one sense the strict free market libertarian could argue that the system worked—the good providers, fearing loss of business, exposed the bad, but the free market had taken years to police itself, and even then it had taken state action to finally put an end to the existing abuses. In the meantime countless individuals suffered unnecessary harm and death, and absent meaningful regulatory oversight critical components of this vital public service would continue to be at the whim of the most predatory providers.

The Revolution Will Be Televised

> *It's just like that TV show* Emergency!
> —Comment by the wife of a stroke patient as the paramedics carried her husband out of their New York City apartment in 1973.[21]

Chicago's experience demonstrated the possibility for superior service and wholly inadequate ambulance operations to co-exist in the same city. In large part this was due to ignorance—the average person's knowledge of ambulance service was entirely experiential, and since the denizens of America's poorest neighborhoods had exactly zero access to foundation reports and government white-papers extolling the virtues of paramedic services in Miami and Seattle, popular outrage was hard to muster absent the occasional muckraking report by investigative journalists. Absent a universal health care system the first step in achieving nationwide change in the ambulance services was simply exposing each community to the existence of alternatives, and in that three network era of visual oligarchy, when it was still possible for a popular program to be seen by a majority of Americans at the same time, producer Jack Webb (of *Dragnet* fame) brought a vision of advanced emergency medicine to the nation through its televised proxy, the Los Angeles paramedic team of Gage and DeSoto on the series *Emergency!*

The original idea for the show came from Los Angeles producer and writer Robert Cinader, who had developed the popular television police procedural *Adam-12* and had gotten the idea while working on *Dragnet 1967* with Jack Webb. When the studio decided to expand the franchise by developing a show about a rescue squad they tapped Cinader to develop the pilot. Looking for a place to start his research he called Dick Friend, the Public Information Officer

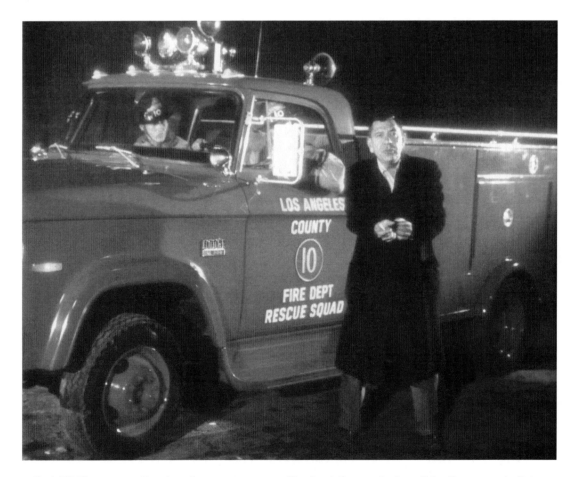

Jack Webb next to a Los Angeles county paramedic rig at the conclusion of the *Emergency!* pilot (in the actual series this truck was replaced by the fictional Rescue 51). This vehicle was not configured for patient transport, so crew members rode along in a county or private ambulance when additional medical care was necessary en route to the hospital (the Estate of Jack Webb).

for the Los Angeles County Fire Department in May 1971, and after explaining that he was working on a television script about rescue work for NBC, Cinader was referred to James Page, a captain in South Los Angeles who had been assigned to implement county-wide paramedic services.[22] By 6 o'clock that very night Cinader was sitting at the kitchen table in Fire Station 7 listening to Page pitch the department's paramedic squads as the ideal focus of the new series.

He was apparently quite persuasive, because Cinader decided to base his new show right in Page's firehouse, and promptly made himself a regular fixture there as he soaked up all the verisimilitude he could absorb. Years later Page remembered how Cinader would sit behind him in the Battalion Chief's red sedan, burning his way through handfuls of "foul smelling" cigarillos en route to whatever misadventure had summoned the rescue squad.[23] A committed "background" man, Cinader soon developed a more than professional interest in the paramedic services, and he spent hours sitting around the kitchen table playing poker with the crew, grumbling whenever he lost and was sentenced to go "into the tank" and wash the company's dishes.[24] His effort paid off, and the development script he turned in was enthusiastically received and picked up by Jack Webb's Mark VII Entertainment for production and distribution over NBC. (Cinader was not only an executive producer for the show, but his experiences and research made him such an expert in the field that he was appointed to the Los Angeles Emergency Medical Services Commission, serving until his death in 1982.)[25]

An evolution of the advanced fire department rescue ambulances of the 1930s, the rescue unit featured on the show was a paramedic truck assigned to a city fire station. As portrayed by Randolph Mantooth and Kevin Tighe, the paramedics of Squad 51 responded to a satisfyingly eclectic variety of medical emergencies, always wearing their billed steel firefighter helmets. In keeping with California law at the time, the paramedics could only perform medical procedures under the supervision of a physician: this was accomplished by keeping in radio contact with the unflappable Dr. Brackett (Robert Fuller) back at Rampart Hospital, ably assisted by steely calm Nurse Dixie McCall (played by Julie London, Jack Webb's ex-wife).

With its indelible images of well organized, well trained, and thoroughly equipped paramedics handling every imaginable emergency, the show became enormously popular, and it is no exaggeration to say that it, more than any other force, introduced the bulk of America to the merits of paramedic services. As it happened, its vision of medically trained firemen zipping down city streets and placid suburban neighborhoods saving lives was more fantasy than reality for most Americans when it premiered in 1972, when a government spokesman noted that fewer than five percent of emergency responders were qualified to perform the advanced life saving techniques on display Saturday nights at 8:00 on NBC (surviving counter programming that ranged from the formidable *All in the Family* to the forgettable *Holmes and Yo-Yo* and *Bridget Loves Bernie*).[26] By the time *Emergency!* went off the air on September 3, 1977, it is estimated that fully half of all Americans were within ten minutes of a fully equipped paramedic unit. Just like on TV.

However, not everyone who tuned in Saturday night was won over, with the owners of private ambulance firms frequently complaining that the program was an uncritical portrayal of government-run ambulance services that might brainwash Americans into voting for universal health care and other outrages. Disgruntled ambulance entrepreneurs complained to the producers and argued their case in letters to the editor of EMS journals protesting, in the words of one disgusted businessman, that profit-making services delivered the same—or better—care than the "socialized medicine" portrayed on *Emergency!* and the world would be a better place if tax dollars stopped funding ambulance service as if it were a public utility like the police department and the fire bureau.[27]

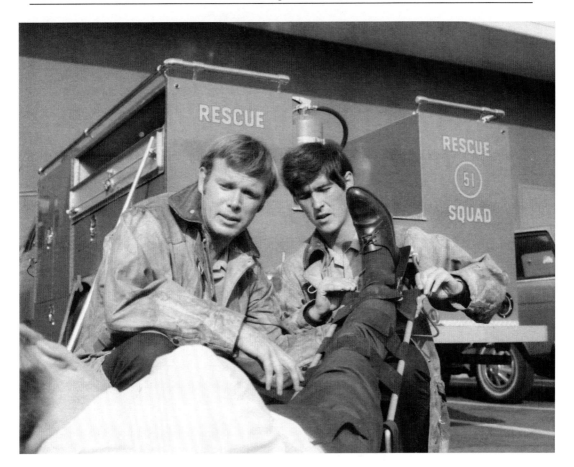

Kevin Tighe and Randolph Mantooth achieved national fame playing paramedics Roy DeSoto and Johnny Gage on *Emergency!* Visible in the background is Squad 51, which like all the early California paramedic trucks was not yet equipped for patient transport (the Estate of Jack Webb).

Leaving aside the question of who was in a better position to cure the ills of the American medical system, the necessity for *someone* to improve the state of pre-hospital care was becoming clearer, as a 1971 study found that each 30 minutes of delay in the definitive treatment of the seriously injured raised the mortality rate by 300 percent.[28] This particular review looked in detail at the early paramedic service in Jacksonville, Florida, where after three years of operation the fatality rate among the accidentally injured fall 28 percent (from 1.55 percent to 1.11 percent), while the rate in surrounding rural counties rose from 4.21 percent to 4.3 percent. Faced with this combination of steadily advancing research on the benefit of improved emergency medical service and increased public awareness of the issue, in 1972 President Nixon directed the Department of Health, Education, and Welfare to identify optimal ways to organize the nation's emergency medical services. He announced the mandate in his State of the Union address that year, promising more federal dollars would be spent to research "new systems of emergency health care that could save thousands of lives annually."[29] Reflecting a more conservative view of federal benefits, Nixon ultimately proposed, and delivered, five federally funded demonstration projects whose outcome would be made available to the states to interpret and apply as they saw fit: it was not his intention to dictate outcomes, only to support basic research that could inform decision making by private enterprise and local government.

Change and Crisis

While America's fractured state of emergency medical services awaited the outcome of this field work, the ambulance fleet itself was undergoing a sea-change. Between 1965 and 1972 mortuary ambulances declined from 50 percent of the market to 11 percent, according to a 1973 Rand Report.[30] At the same time, 20 percent of America's ambulance services were provided by volunteer groups, and fully 34 percent were delivered by local government agencies—overwhelmingly police and fire departments, augmented by municipal hospitals and a comparatively smaller number of boards of health.[31] For the first time in history, the plurality of ambulance services, some 35 percent, were now provided by private specialty firms, drawn into the field by the expansion of government reimbursement programs like Medicare and Medicaid and filling the gaps left by the many hospital and police ambulance services that were leaving the field as their funding priorities shifted. While the nation's ambulance services, and by extension the entire emergency medical field, remained decentralized, uncoordinated, erratic, and suboptimal in terms of training, equipment, and distribution of service, the authors noted that the chaotic scene on the ground was unlikely to be called to order by the cacophony emanating from Washington: the Congressional hearings, enabling legislation, and financial appropriations of the late 1960s had left in their wake almost a dozen agencies, divisions, and commissions with jurisdiction over parts of the emergency medical system but without any effective means to collaborate. For example, between 1966 and 1973 the Department of Transportation had spent $48 million on various aspects of emergency care while at the same time HEW had divided $78 million between ten different programs of its own: by not coordinating their projects, the two agencies had wound up duplicating effort, replicating failed programs that the other had previously discarded, and set aside virtually nothing to sponsor the sharing of their results to avoid future inefficiency.[32]

At the same time, by early 1973 there were enough exemplary ambulance services getting national publicity to arouse the ire of local communities who perceived themselves as receiving sub-standard care—and with less than 5 percent of the country's ambulances meeting the available standards for equipment and staffing, the substandard communities represented the largest share of the electorate.[33] It was therefore telling that, in the depths of the Cold War, the *Journal of Trauma* attempted to create a "Sputnik" moment by crediting the U.S.S.R. with operating, on a national level, a more sophisticated ambulance service than the United States. A 1973 editorial pointed out that a universal emergency phone number (03) had long been established across the Soviet Union while the United States was in the infancy of its own 911 system, and that since the early 1920s special emergency ambulance squads had been routine in the Soviet Union's largest cities.[34] Anyone dialing the medical emergency number was triaged by a dispatcher and, if deemed necessary, a *skoraya* squad could be sent from the hospital, helmed by a physician and rounded out with nurses and feldshers—the latter being the approximate equivalent of an EMT. Each ambulance was fitted out for the intervention required, including mobile cardiac intensive care units, neurology squads for stroke, and even special pediatric ambulances with all-female crews.

In comparison, the editorial cited research that every year as many as 25,000 Americans were permanently disabled due to improper handling by inadequately trained ambulance crews and rescue squad members, and repeated the well worn fact that half of all heart attack victims died before reaching the hospital—while delivering the startling assertion that of 29,000 heart attack cases picked up alive by Moscow's ambulance squads, only three had died en route to the hospital. (Of course, since the Soviets claimed to have invented helicopters, penicillin, moveable type, Vitamin C, and television, Kremlin censors weren't likely to blush over fluffing up a press release to a Western medical journal with a bit of hyperbole. Still, propaganda aside,

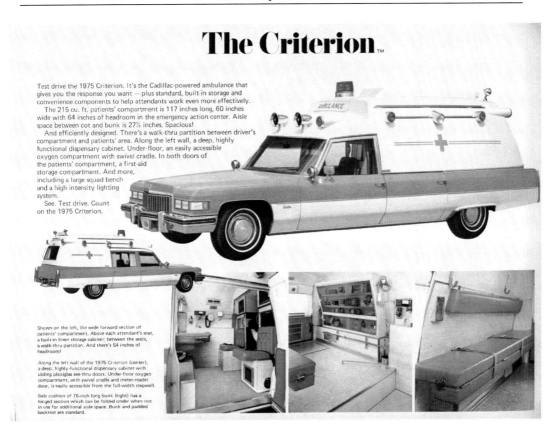

This 1975 Criterion ambulance schematic represents the near apogee of the "professional car" style ambulance, with its elevated roofline, dispensary cabinet, linen cupboard, and "action wall" for telemetry equipment. By 1978 manufacture of this configuration had yielded to the squad and van-style ambulances familiar today (courtesy Miller-Meteor/Accubuilt).

it was tough to argue that heart attack victims were better off when an ambulance crew was ignorant of CPR, or that the absence of supplemental oxygen on underequipped mortuary ambulances was saving lives.) The editorial went on to note that the United States already possessed the "technical capability, the raw manpower, and the money to address the problem effectively," but seemed to lack any sense that this was a crisis, rather than the unfortunate but acceptable byproduct of decentralized, market-driven health care services, a sorry state of affairs that would, some day, sort itself out when someone figured out a way to make enough money at it.[35]

Such un–American pessimism aside, in Congress a few Senators had adopted the cause and were mustering the last vestiges of the Great Society to deliver a big solution to a big problem. As David Boyd, soon to be the director of the EMS Division in the Department of Health, Education, and Welfare, put it:

> [the] current consensus is that only a comprehensive EMS program, logically planned and staged, will develop and mature so that all patients in need will receive the most appropriate care in the pre-hospital, hospital, inter-hospital, critical care, and rehabilitation phases. An EMS system must then develop a sound sequence of comprehensive program activities on a regional basis if the needs of all potentially emergent patients are to be properly anticipated and receive adequate response.[36]

With a little assistance from America's favorite paramedic duo, this bold experiment was about to get under way.

The Emergency Medical Services Act of 1973

In a bid to create that logically planned and staged comprehensive emergency medical services program (and to put the Soviets back in second place), Congress passed the Emergency Medical Services Systems Act of 1973, an ambitious attempt to drag emergency medicine forward, by force if necessary. President Nixon, skeptical of "big government" and wanting to wait and see what became of the five test programs funded in 1971, vetoed the bill as premature and overreaching. Congress, in a demonstration of how popular the reform idea had become, easily mustered the two-thirds majority needed to override the veto and the bill became law in the fall of 1973. The program's principal sponsor was Senator Cranston of California, and shortly after the Senate passed the bill the first time, he had written to Jack Webb to thank him for the role *Emergency!* had played in creating popular support for the legislation:

> We unanimously passed a bill that, among other things, would promote the training of paramedics to staff ambulances and emergency rooms in hospitals across the country. I introduced the provisions in the bill dealing with paramedics and emergency medical services in hopes that our nation will make greater use of the thousands of experienced, able young men who have returned from Vietnam with the medical skills America needs so desperately. They are to get top priority in the training pro-

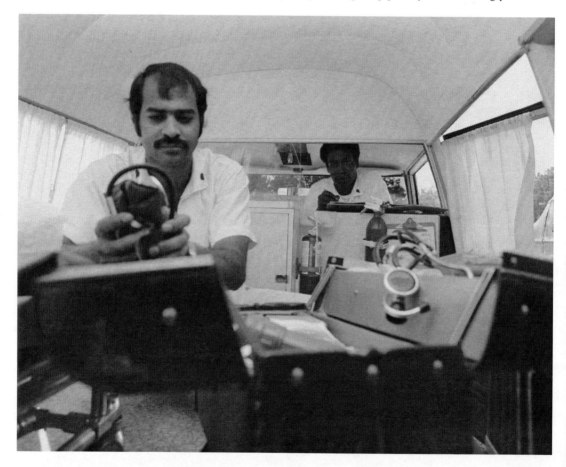

Interior view of a hearse-style ambulance used at Fort Bragg, North Carolina, in 1976. Spc. Ramradthan Rambally takes inventory in the back, while Spc. Jerry Grant checks the electrical equipment. A year later the last of these "professional car" ambulances would be made and the industry would convert to van and modular styles (Dick Johnson, DefenseLINK/DOD).

grams. Jack, your *Emergency!* series fired the public imagination and was the harbinger for a medical idea whose time, I believe, has come. In the midst of a severe shortage of doctors, nurses and trained emergency personnel, 175,000 die each year because they do not get adequate medical care in an emergency. Another 25,000 are left permanently disabled because of inept handling by untrained ambulance attendants. *Emergency!* has dramatized the potential of the paramedic. I hope the House of Representatives and the President will now follow the lead of 100 Senators—and Jack Webb![37]

The EMS Systems Act, as its name implied, was designed to consolidate the underfunded and under-resourced components of local emergency medicine (from ambulances, emergency rooms, specialty hospitals, and rehabilitation centers) into regional EMS systems where economies of scale and pooled resources could be employed to provide the kind of service that Jack Webb (and Congress) wanted America to have. While the transition would be funded by HEW grants for specific programs, the intention was that each regional system would become self-sufficient—and indeed, the very language of the statute defined a regional system as a grouping of sufficient size to be economically self-sustaining. Operation of the regional system would be vested in public or non-profit agencies coordinating services and communicating with the federal agencies providing support.[38]

To assuage fears that the bill would create a socialized medical bureaucracy under federal control, the number of grants each regional system could receive was limited: one award for planning, two for establishment of services, and a maximum of two grants for system expansion. After decades of watching local services wax and wane in their quality, Congress tried to ensure that minimal uniform standards would be created and maintained by requiring that regional systems pre-qualify for grant money by agreeing to meet fifteen criteria, including having system-wide communications, open access to emergency care, public education in first aid and EMS services, and developing a disaster plan.

In an effort to mediate between the frequently feuding DHEW and DOT, both of whom had interceded in ambulance and pre-hospital care operations, the Act drew a line in the park-

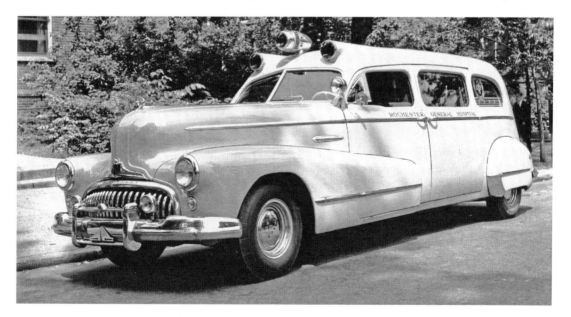

This stunning example of a 1940s Buick sedan-style ambulance operated by Rochester General Hospital in upstate New York was beautiful to the eye, but it could never have accommodated the equipment and work space demanded by modern emergency medical service workers (courtesy ViaHealth Archives Consortium, Rochester, N.Y.).

ing lot, mandating that DHEW funds were not to be spent on pre-hospital services unless DOT funds were insufficient to correct deficiencies identified by a state EMS agency. Overall, after years of individuals and individual communities taking the lead on discrete problems such as what equipment to carry in ambulances or how to coordinate dispatch in their city, the direction of reform had shifted to a "systems" approach, and the talk would predominantly be about regionalization for the next several years. As the director for EMS in the Massachusetts Department of Public Health commented at the time, "on a national basis, a couple of years ago people seemed to talk [only] ambulances: people are now talking medical direction and systems and health care organization."[39] The directors of emergency medical services in New York City apparently had great faith in the ability of the new law to create a lasting improvement in emergency health care, optimistically writing a few years later that "just as we regard equipment, vehicles, chrome and red lights as outmoded issues in 1977, so in 1987 we may regard organization, regionalization and evaluation as 'old hat.'"[40]

Unfortunately, if anyone in the long history of the ambulance has ever been wrong about more things in fewer words they had the good fortune not to be talking to a reporter at the time. In reality, thirty years later the topics of organization, evaluation, and allotment of resources are as far from solution as they were in 1972. First, the 1973 act's plan to create rational self-perpetuating regional EMS systems delivering optimum care foundered on the harsh economic realities of a nation reeling through an OPEC fueled recession. Government resources declined as incomes fell, and worried ratepayers had little inclination to fund a potentially expensive new civic utility. The three hundred EMS regions that had been identified across the United States found it impossible to become wholly self-sustaining, and extensions were repeatedly sought on their operational grants—even as many failed to meet all of the required objectives in the original bill. A 1977 GAO report admitted that, overall, services had improved, but pointed out that "self-sustaining regional systems, which retain area-wide control of resources and facilities, has not been completed, as intended by the 1973 legislation."[41] (In fact, of the EMS regions identified only twelve were self-sustaining by 1977, while two-hundred thirty-eight others remained dependent on federal aid.)[42] In 1976 the act was amended, in part to require grant applications to provide evidence of local government's willingness to provide economic support for the program after the federal money was withdrawn. Programs were also required to show that their regional plan included participation by public, private, and volunteer organizations currently providing EMS services, and it was hoped that these additions would "establish a firm basis for continued operation of the EMS system after eligibility for federal support had ended," in the words of Senator Cranston, the original sponsor of the 1973 EMS Systems Act.[43]

Unfortunately, the amendments had little impact. Three years later, in 1979, the GAO drafted an update for Senators Cranston and Kennedy, who had spent the better part of a decade attempting to rationalize and improve emergency medical care. The report's gloomy conclusion was that "EMS regional management organizations are not adequately planning for their financial self-sufficiency, nor are they obtaining firm financial commitments from local governments to continue regional systems at the conclusion of federal funding, although plans for financial self-sufficiency and local government endorsement of these plans are required by the 1976 amendments."[44] The problem was that no one at the federal level wanted to pull the trigger on programs, even when they were failing to meet the mandates of their grant, and so funding was going out to programs that had no viable plan to sustain themselves and creating instant "welfare states" out of the supposedly autonomous EMS districts: in an analysis of thirty-four programs receiving expansion and improvement grants, the GAO found that only six had developed the required post-subsidy financial plan, and not one had obtained the ostensibly mandatory community endorsements that were supposed to ensure the program's post-grant survival.

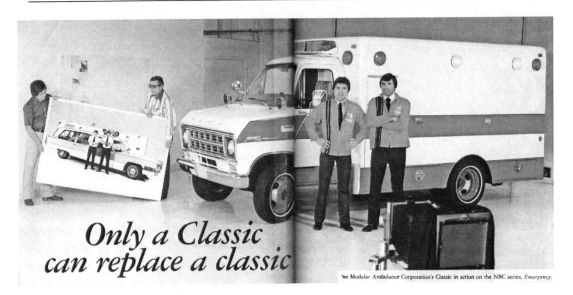

The transition between the old professional car ambulances and the modern silhouette is dramatically captured in this 1976 advertisement for the Modular Ambulance Company.

As the GAO noted, it would be impossible to tell whether the 1976 mandates would work until HEW actually enforced them.

In the Garage

While the macro-debate about how to organize the entire system of emergency medical services was being waged in Washington, the ambulance itself was receiving much needed scrutiny. The 1966 Vehicle Safety Act had paved the way for federal standards for ambulances, but the shift of focus to macro-systems and the push and pull between the Department of Transportation and HEW had led to a slower than expected roll-out of defining standards. The most comprehensive standards, as we have seen, were assembled by the Committee on Ambulance Design Criteria under the aegis of the Department of Transportation's Highway Safety Program, and after the initial 1969 draft had been revised in 1971 and 1973 the proposals were sufficiently vetted and comprehensive to serve as a broadly acceptable industry standard. Despite the plenary nature of the committee and its laudable motives, the idea of firm requirements for ambulance design alarmed some who felt the underlying principal was self-defeating. Dr. Fred Vogt, a committee chairman with the University Association for Emergency Medical Services, voiced the misgivings of many when he wrote "the debate to resolve issues involving standards will be influenced by personal preferences, lack of knowledge of the full scope of the problem area, desire to get something written and over with, and certainly pecuniary interest on the part of certain manufacturers" and implied that once set, standards could actually stifle further reform and development as the combination of inertia and vested interest impeded changes.[45]

Nonetheless, the continued use of hearse-style ambulances whose interior confines were ill-suited to provision of CPR, hanging intravenous fluids, or administration of invasive life saving procedures, to say nothing of the high percentage of station wagons and panel trucks functioning as jerry-rigged aid cars, was sufficiently prevalent that the federal General Services Administration felt it was time to set a procurement standard to ensure that the government, at least, was spending its money on ambulances that were worthy of the name.

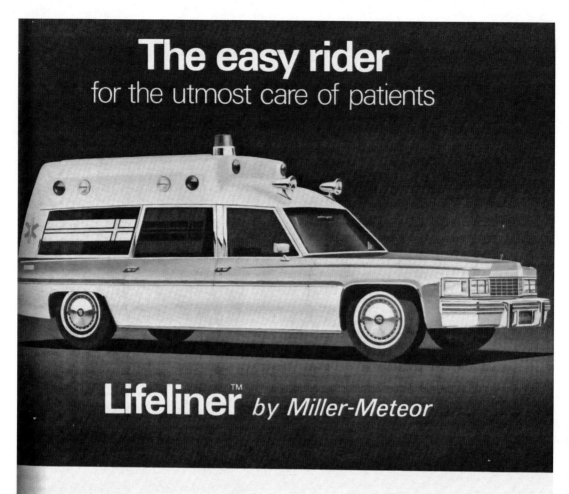

The easy rider
for the utmost care of patients

Lifeliner™ by Miller-Meteor

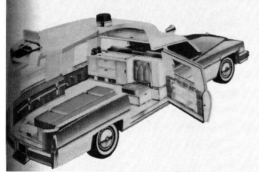

The Lifeliner ambulance—powered by the Cadillac chassis specially engineered for heavy-duty service—has the matchless riding comfort, quiet operation and dependable performance required by professionals who observe the highest standards in care of the sick and injured. Soft, stable ride provides protection from travel-induced aggravation of injuries and assures comfortable, restful transfer of patients over long distances.

Aerodynamic lines. Handsome, steel-reinforced fiberglass roof has vertical areas for flush mounting of warning and loading lights. The loading lights have special lenses that direct illumination downward.

Partition between driver's and patients' areas has sliding window, overhead linen compartment and electrical console. Oxygen is piped from compartment for "M" tank beneath floor. Spacious dispensary cabinet puts emergency supplies at attendants' fingertips, and there are numerous additional storage areas. Highly efficient air conditioning and heating system. *Everything* is designed for maximum convenience and comfort.

Ask your Miller-Meteor Ambulance Distributor for a Lifeliner demonstration now, or contact—

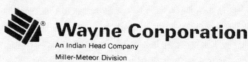 **Wayne Corporation**
An Indian Head Company
Miller-Meteor Division
125 Clark Avenue
Piqua, Ohio 45356   Telephone (513) 773-3824

Unable to compete with the modular and van ambulances in terms of space and out of compliance with the new federal standards, manufacturers of professional car ambulances fought a rear-guard action by stressing their vehicles' smooth, comfortable ride and attractive appearance, as in this 1977 ad for Miller-Meteor (courtesy Miller-Meteor/Accubuilt).

Accordingly, in 1974 the GAU used its rule making powers to transmute the Committee's revised ambulance standards into the new "federal specification" KKK-A-1822, setting minimum requirements for any ambulance purchased with federal dollars. While the 1822 rules were limited solely to ambulances paid for with Treasury funds, any manufacturer who ever dreamed of selling an ambulance to the federal government—or to any program receiving federal dollars to purchase equipment—had no choice but to reconfigure their assembly line. Speeding the conversion process were a number of states who promptly adopted the federal standards by incorporation, making it necessary for any ambulance purchased with local government dollars to likewise meet the new requirements from Washington and further curtailing the market for off-spec vehicles. By 1977 the last of the professional car/hearse style ambulances were rolling off the assembly lines, and the era of the Cadillac limousine ambulance was officially laid to rest. Implementation was largely by attrition, particularly with smaller firms and volunteer squads where equipment budgets were modest, and as late as 1978 fully one third of America's ambulances were older models falling below the new industry standard, although the transition become exponentially swifter with each passing year.[46]

When originally released in 1974 the new ambulance guidelines represented a quantum leap in ambulance engineering standards, consisting of precise specifications for literally every inch of interior and exterior space, versus previous recommendations which had been limited to how many inches of head room, how many cubic feet of storage space, and what was the minimum amount of equipment to pack in. By comparison, the 1822 specs had something to say about every design element from headlight to bumper, as well as including numerous "functional" tests that had never been formally regulated before: for example, ambulances now had to pass the "school-bus test" and support their own weight when flipped onto the roof, to avoid pancaking on top of a luckless patient—and crew. Certified ambulances had to provide at least sixty inches of headroom, two inches of flame retardant insulation in the walls, and not less than thirty cubic feet of storage space. Building materials, configuration, and performance all had to meet precisely defined tolerances, providing a measure of predictability—and performance—that had previously been the province of only a handful of high-end machines.

Physically, the KKK-A-1822 ambulance specifications provided for three designs: Type I was a transferable modular ambulance on truck chassis, Type II a customized van, and the Type III was a replaceable modular unit on a van chassis, rather than the truck chassis of the Type I. While the straight-ahead van ambulance was the cheapest off the showroom floor, the two modular configurations were considered the more economical over the long term, since the most vulnerable part of an ambulance was its transmission. It was estimated at the time that even the most deluxe hearse-style conversion ambulance only had a four year span before the transmission gave out: realistically, the time and expense of trying to rebuild the transmission was such that it was more cost effective to just replace the old ambulance, transmission and all, at a cost of anywhere from $17,000 to $20,000. On the other hand, a top of the line modular ambulance cost about the same as one of the luxury Cadillac professional cars, but when a modular chassis gave up the ghost the bodywork, still virtually new, could simply be swapped onto a new chassis and bolted down, at enormous savings over rebuilding the worn parts or replacing the vehicle entirely.[47]

The new designs quickly won converts, and the fears of naysayers that rigid standards would smother future innovation under *le mort main,* the "dead hand" of old ideas, proved to be more apparent than real, as the specifications have been repeatedly revised to keep them current with the lessons of experience and are regularly reviewed by manufacturers, providers, and medical experts. This process of constant adjustment quickly highlighted the enormous complexities confronting ambulance designers now that their product was to be measured by the yardstick of the possible, not confined to the shapes of what had gone before. Where once improvements to ambulance equipment had focused on making sure there were splints and clean sheets in back, by the middle 1970s the issues confronting a regulator were exponentially more complicated. Just on the issue of communications the issues to be decided included telemetry standards; assigning radio frequencies (after deciding on VHF versus UHF); telephone services, including acoustic couplers and demodulators; developing the vehicle battery and alternator standards required to power ambulance communication equipment, and how to make systems interoperative between various hospitals and multiple providing agencies without interfering/bleeding over to neighboring users. All of these issues required local, state and federal FCC involvement, to say nothing of manufacturing standards and training issues. Clearly, things had come a long way even since the mid–1960s, when reformers had been content to advocate for more bandages and a working resuscitator.

As the 1970s drew to a close it was clear that the decade had been a profoundly challenging one for the ambulance and the emergency services in general. An attempt had been made to systematically reform the nation's entire emergency medical delivery system, an effort built around regional organizations overseen by government or non-profit agencies and held to detailed mandates designed to deliver superior care. The experiment had foundered, however, on the inability of local communities to find the political will and financial commitment to sustain them. After the fact many looked back on the plan and felt it was too hierarchical, and that a scheme that built from the community up would have had a better chance of permanence, even if it would have meant that individual programs would likely have been below the optimal standard envisioned by the boldest reformers.[48]

In the background of these system-wide changes, the ambulance itself had undergone a tremendous evolution, driven in part by a desire to make it a suitable environment for the new generation of advanced emergency medical technicians. To keep pace with this strong interest for training beyond that offered by the Department of Transportation's 81 hour BLS course, the number of paramedic training programs expanded rapidly, even as attempts to create a nationally recognized curriculum and standard credentials stalled. As it was, by 1977 eight thousand paramedics had graduated from America's two hundred-plus training programs, after having completed coursework that might have been as short as one hundred hours or as long as twelve hundred (at the same time, approximately 260,000 people were employed as basic life support emergency medical technicians or drivers).[49] While the issue of training became one of diversification, the adoption of the A-1822 ambulance standards boded fair to standardize the national ambulance market for the foreseeable future.

Across the 49th Parallel

Signal as these developments were, they did not represent the universe of ambulance design and operation, of course. While impossible to examine ambulance developments across the globe, it is interesting to see how another jurisdiction handled the question of emergency medical reform at the same time—in this case British Columbia, where a service environment nearly identical to that prevailing in the United States evolved in a wholly different direction. For background, it is often a surprise to many in the U.S. that while Canadian provinces have been adopting various forms of public funding for selected health services since the late 1940s, the country, unlike England and most European states, has never had a national health service. Instead, it created a modified form of universal insurance which has always excluded significant service lines, such as dentistry, mental health, and emergency medical services—while individual provinces have extended coverage to these areas, British Columbia is the only province that has ever created a single-provider ambulance service.

Prior to its assumption of ambulance service in 1973, pre-hospital medical care in British Columbia was delivered by the same mix of private, volunteer, and municipal services found in the United States—and likewise the quality of the services varied enormously. There was stiff competition between services in the few large markets, such as Vancouver, while in the much more numerous rural areas service was frequently sparse and underdeveloped, and poor working conditions contributed to a high turn-over rate and discouraged professionalism (for example, in the late 1960s the Vancouver crews at Metropolitan Ambulance were paid $90 for an 86½ hour week of 24 hours on and 24 hours off, with one double shift tacked on each month: their rivals at Associated Ambulance worked 114 hours a week at about the same scale.)[50] In all, most B.C. ambulance jobs appeared designed to attract motivated, committed individuals and then ruthlessly grind their best intentions down into a smooth veneer of exhaustion.

In 1973 a commission convened by the Minister of Health published "Health Security for British Columbians," a report critical of the fragmented and uneven quality of ambulance services offered in British Columbia and recommending that the province take responsibility for pre-hospital care and "the fractionated ambulance services ... be amalgamated under one jurisdiction." (Of course, this was the same year that Congress passed the EMS Act, a diluted approach to the same goal—creating regional, integrated pre-hospital services, albeit within the framework of wholly private services.) In response to the commission's report an Emergency Health Services Commission was created, and under its authority the British Columbia Ambulance Service was launched on July 4, 1973. While a provincial entity, ambulance services are not technically covered by the provincial health plan: nonetheless its operation is subsidized by the province and its rates are, by American standards, shockingly low—for example, in 2007 it charged a flat rate of $80, regardless of the intensity of care required or the distance

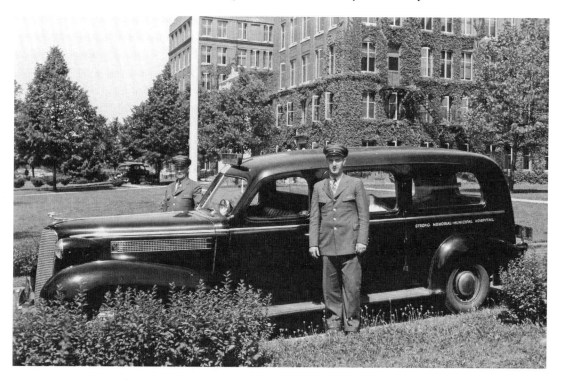

A glance back: A sedan-style Cadillac ambulance operated jointly by Strong Memorial Hospital and the Rochester Municipal Hospital in 1940, a few years after physicians were taken off the service (courtesy of the Edward G. Miner Library, University of Rochester Medical Center, New York).

traveled. In scale it is one of the largest ambulance providers in North America, serving almost 4.5 million people with five hundred ground ambulances and 3,200 emergency medical technicians, as well as an advanced medevac service. One advantage of its unified operation is the ability to perform detailed outcomes research, which has made it unusually successful in its quality improvement initiatives, such as an evaluation and training project in 2007 that led to a twenty percent increase in successful cardiac resuscitations.[51] Similar efforts have lagged in the United States, by comparison, where enormous variations in survival rates for out of hospital cardiac arrest continue to be observed between communities but whose etiology and precise definition has been elusive in the absence of standardized records and shared information.

Ultimately, during the 1970s ambulance services on both sides of the border were taxed with how to finance themselves, how to improve the care provided, and, ultimately, how to fit themselves into the increasingly complex and fractious interface between the art of medicine, the politics of administration, and the battlefield of business. As always, the story of the ambulance in America was a particularly complex one, with its various parts moving forward at a different pace, even as the sphere of regulations governing its operation was being refined into a narrower compass: where once the country had thousands of different ambulance services, some outstanding, the majority poor, now the differences were less geographical and more reflective of strong progress in some areas of national standardization (vehicle configuration and equipment) and relative confusion in others (training of crews, dispatch, and communications). By 1980 the emergency medical services had experienced nearly fifteen years of intensive growth, change, and challenge. What came next was the inevitable counter-reformation, as the spotlight that had burned from the Capitol steps was at last dimmed, and what candle power remained was focused on other, newer problems in the universe of emergency medical care.

The 1980s: Retrenchment

The election of Ronald Reagan in 1980 symbolized the ascendancy of a superficially more "decentralized" approach to government and tolled a terminal change in the grand scheme to systematize the emergency medical system. In 1981 Congress passed the Omnibus Budget Reconciliation Act which, among many other provisions, dismantled the grant programs of the 1973 EMS Systems Act, abandoning regional EMS funding and its broader goal of uniform EMS standards, training, and equivalent services as they might be planned by a central agency. Instead, funds earmarked for emergency medical services under the 1973 Act and administered by DOT and the successors to HEW (itself dismantled in 1979) were bundled into Preventive Health Block Grants—along with other federal dollars once designated for rodent control, fluoridation of water supplies, and other public health initiatives. After a brief period of mandated support for EMS, each state would decide how much of the block grant went to ambulances and how much to stronger teeth, fewer rats, and any other health issue it faced. On the one hand, this meant states were free to create local solutions for local problems: on the other hand, the federal government was busy making sure the block grants were getting smaller and smaller and that states were required to finance larger shares of programs such as Medicaid, putting pressure on states to cut back on costs wherever possible. Naturally, governors and state legislatures varied in their overall competence and their particular interest in pre-hospital services, and so some EMS programs went to pieces and others got stronger, depending on who was minding the store and how good they were at their jobs.[52] Partly in recognition of the failed federal effort to stimulate creation of self-sustaining regional EMS districts providing optimal care, and certainly recognizing the impact that the incipient withdrawal of funds would have, in 1980 representatives from all fifty states organized into the National Association of State EMS Directors in an effort to lobby for federal funds, to provide coordinated and rational direction to future policy initiatives, and to learn from one another's successes and mistakes.

In 1984 the GAO report "States Use Added Flexibility Offered by the Preventive Health and Health Services Block Grants" summarized how decentralization had affected the quality of services at the state level. In its accounting the GAO provided detail on emergency medical services, pointing out that "most states have assigned EMS a low priority and have reduced funding to this area," but noting that a few states had actually used the block grants to shift more resources to EMS and expanded their geographic reach and scope of service. As an aggregate, however, federal dollars allocated to EMS declined by 19 percent between 1981 and 1983, with two states, Florida and Kentucky, withholding all federal funds from their emergency medical providers, declaring such services a wholly local responsibility.

Two years later the GAO was back, with a new report dedicated exclusively to EMS and the states. In a small sample of six states the authors found that funding for the emergency medical services had reversed its slide in the early 1980s and was on the uptick. This return to funding was not, however, accompanied by notable improvement in quality. Specifically, less than 50 percent of the country had access to 911 services almost twenty years after its roll-out in Alabama, advanced life support ambulances continued to be a rarity in rural areas, and many communities had failed to develop any protocols to identify which ambulance patients should not be taken to the closest hospital, but instead should be driven to a possibly more distant specialty center (such as a regional burn unit or Level 1 trauma center) in order to begin definitive treatment immediately.[53] Stymieing progress was the continued lack of cooperation among emergency medical service providers and inadequate funding at the state and local levels. As one frustrated EMS provider noted, if your stove catches fire "twelve men and $200,000 worth of equipment show up right away," but communities continually balked at paying more taxes to provide a service that could save their life if they had a heart attack or were involved in a serious motor vehicle accident, despite the fact that many more of them would experience these critical health events than would ever wake up to find their house on fire or have a gas main explode under their front lawn.[54]

While funding issues continued to bedevil ambulance services, a more systemic problem

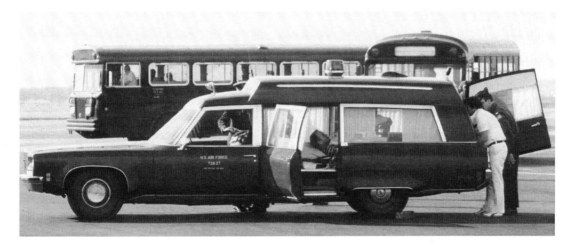

Replacing older styles of ambulance was often done by attrition. Here, an early seventies hearse-style Oldsmobile ambulance is used at a U.S. airbase in 1981 to transfer Major General Ogenbrood to a hospital after he had been wounded during the assassination of Anwar Sadat in Cairo (Don Sutherland. DefenseLINK/DOD).

was creating new logistical challenges for their operations, as America's safety net of trauma hospitals began to unravel. By the mid–1980s hospitals had begun to drop out of the trauma care system, as their capacities were overwhelmed and they faced less and less reimbursement for increasing amounts of ever more expensive trauma care (largely because those most likely to be victims of traumatic injury were the same young males who were least likely to be insured). In Congressional hearings it was reported that across the country trauma centers were withdrawing from the regional systems once considered the cornerstone of modern EMS care: in Los Angeles, eleven out of twenty-three centers had de-listed as trauma centers due to heavy financial losses; Dade County, Florida, started the decade with eight trauma centers—by 1990 seven had quit, leaving Jackson County Memorial as the only trauma center for a county of almost two million people; Hermann Hospital in Houston had withdrawn after losing $7 million in 1989; MedSTAR Trauma Center in Washington withdrew after $8.9 million in losses providing care to major trauma and burn cases in 1989.[55] (Contrast this with the experience of the New York Hospital in the early 1970s, where their cardiac ambulance brought in coronary cases, which were much likely to strike older patients, and thus insured under Medicare, as well as having the collateral effect of improving visibility of their ER for routine cases, which could be selectively admitted for higher utilization of their bed space.)

For ambulance crews this dramatic loss of available facilities meant driving further to deliver patients, resulting in more expense, longer turn-around times, fewer vehicles available for emergencies, and crews strained by providing heroic measures for sustained periods. Recognizing the crisis, Congress passed the Trauma Care Systems Planning and Development Act of 1990 (Public Law 101–590), aiming to improve coordination and communications within the regional trauma systems. Even more importantly, it allowed states to apply for waivers to use a portion of the Act's funds to reimburse hospitals for uncompensated costs of trauma care, which was the only way to ensure that after establishing your improved communication plan you would have someone around to pick up the phone on the receiving end. (The act was allowed to expire in 1995, and the search for adequate trauma coordination and reimbursement continues to frustrate local emergency medical providers.)

The 1990s: Holding It Together

Of course, not all the action was occurring on Capitol Hill or in claustrophobic hearing rooms for state and federal oversight agencies. While surgical groups had long been advocating ambulance reforms, after the federal government stepped in with the Automotive Safety Act of 1966 and the EMS Act of 1973, private firms and industrial groups began to take a more aggressive interest in the national standards debate. An influential example was the creation of the Commission on Accreditation of Ambulance Services (CAAS) in 1990, which had its antecedents in an earlier ad hoc group assembled in 1982 by the American Ambulance Association to promote the kinds of high quality industry standards that might shape (or even be substituted for) federal or state regulations. In 1990 this group met with representatives from the Emergency Nurses Association, the International Association of Fire Chiefs, the National Association of Emergency Medical Technicians, the National Association of EMS Physicians, and the National Association of State EMS Directors to promulgate formal accreditation standards, which were first applied in 1993: as of 2007, over 100 agencies in the United States and Canada had become accredited, including several of the largest regional providers, such as Rural/Metro in New York and Florida. As the corporate ambulance world became more proactive politically, the era of small, locally operated independent ambulance providers was making way for nationally operated chains. The harbinger for this shift was the listing of American

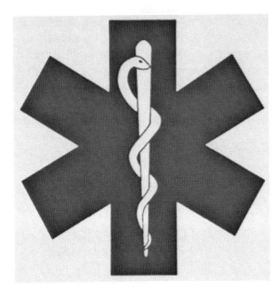
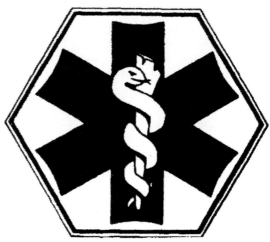

In 1963 the American Medical Association created the smaller image as a "universal medical identification symbol" to notify physicians that the wearer had a significant medical condition. In 1977 the federal government adapted the symbol, tinted it blue, and made it the official "Star of Life" logo that designates ambulances meeting its KKK-A-1822 design standards.

Medical Response on the New York Stock Exchange, which raised cash for an initial round of acquisitions and expansions that set it on track to become the largest ambulance provider in the United States with two hundred fifty operations in thirty-seven states and the District of Columbia.[56]

With the federal government pulling out support from above, local services giving ground to national chains, states struggling to regulate ambulance services and ensure adequate operations, and an unfolding crisis for trauma hospitals that was having a collateral effect on EMS operations, in 1996 the National Highway Traffic Safety Administration published *EMS Agenda for the Future*, an ambitious plan laying out fourteen goals considered essential to create an optimal emergency medical services system. At the time, the back of the envelope estimate for America's pre-hospital medical care system was $6.75 billion a year, or approximately $27 per capita.[57] Among the fourteen expressed goals of the document were expanding research in order to identify what was working and what was not; to improve coordination between providers at all levels of care; to devise consistent and adequate financial support for EMS; to deepen public awareness of the critical nature of EMS; and to standardize and improve training and management of pre-hospital emergency providers. To those with a sufficiently long memory, these goals were suspiciously similar to the ones enumerated in *Death and Disability* in 1966 and recapitulated in the 1973 EMS Act and its amendments in 1976.

Not only were the goals the same, the barriers to their implementation remained unchanged as well: a fragmented, diversified medical system lacking an entity capable of directing operations, much less providing the financial wherewithal to pay for the services increasingly in demand. At the federal level, by 2001 four agencies were involved in supporting and promoting EMS improvements: the National Highway and Traffic Safety Administration, the Health Resources and Services Administration, the Centers for Disease Control and Prevention, and the U.S. Fire Administration. Without authority to impose standards or enforce requirements on how EMS systems should operate, the agencies could only provide technical support, guidance, and some funding to the thousands of local services. For example, in 2000 NHTSA provided $4.9 million for a variety of EMS improvements and HRSA provided $4.2 million to facilitate development of EMS systems in rural areas: given that total spending on ambulance and pre-hospital emergency services was then in excess of $7 billion per year, the scale of these investments can be put into perspective. While the federal government also maintained significant indirect influence on ambulance operation with its Medicare reimbursement rates and the 1822 standards on ambulance design and manufacture, the overarching supervisory role it had once assayed in the 1973 EMS Act had been put aside. Once more the ambulance was a local issue, the domain of states, of counties, of cities and rural townships, and if its problems belonged to all, improvement was left to whomever cared enough to consider it.

Contributing to the general malaise, in terms of popular visibility the emergency medical services were deep in a lull. *Emergency!* had gone off the air in 1977 (although it returned with new TV movies until 1979), and the EMT all but vanished from the pop culture landscape, going the way of all those DeSoto and Gage lunchboxes. Not that the franchise wasn't cannibalized by networks hoping to jack up their Nielsens—after it went off the air a few thematically related programs broke on the scene, although mostly quickly perished.

Mother, Juggs & Speed (1978) was a broad comedy built around a private ambulance company in Los Angeles whose pilot episode ran as a summer special, before sinking out of sight. It was based on a reasonably successful 1976 film, *Mother, Jugs & Speed*, starring Raquel Welch, Bill Cosby and Harvey Keitel, a feature that took a beating by critics who found its blend of dark drama and slapstick less an urban variant of *M*A*S*H* than a forced and unfunny farce that whipsawed itself by overplaying the extremes. In a scathing review the *Los Angeles Times* predicted it would "bore even the ozone crowd with a backseat to turn to," a now cryptic reference to the famously undiscriminating drive-in movie audience.[58] The critic misread the public appetite for Raquel Welch in a t-shirt and Larry Hagman as a necrophiliac ambulance attendant, however, and the film turned a profit before being reanimated as a forgotten TV series.

The original film continues to have a devoted following among EMS workers, and those old enough to have seen it on the big screen are often able to quote the more memorable lines, such as the ambulance company owner telling his dispirited crew that while the economy is going sour, "Thanks to muggings, malnutrition and disease, we still have a chance to make a buck!" It would be twenty years before a major studio released another film centered on ambulance service, when Martin Scorsese's *Bringing Out the Dead* came out in 1999. Despite a strong cast, including Nicolas Cage and John Goodman, and moderate praise from the critics, it suffered brutally at the box office—taking in barely one half of its estimated $32 million production costs on domestic ticket sales, and after a month on the street barely pulling in $100 per screen even on weekends.[59]

240-Robert (1979; after a fifteen month hiatus, three more episodes were screened in 1981) was the closest take on *Emergency!* This drama centered on three members of the Los Angeles search and rescue unit, but weak ratings doomed it to a half a season in 1979, with three additional programs released with a largely new cast in early 1981. It is remarkable that the show didn't succeed, with such inspiring episodes as one where an earthquake strikes southern California, leaving the male leads trapped in a slowly flooding underwater cave with a gorgeous model, her equally attractive female photographer—and a voracious moray eel ("Earthquake," 11/19/79).[60] If only every episode had been able to match this combination of *Jaws,* Irwin Allen, and *Charlie's Angels,* the program might still be on the air.

Rescue 911 (1989–1996), unlike its sibling, *Cops,* used re-enactments and interviews instead of *cinema verité* to lure viewers. Despite a respectable run between 1989 and 1996, it never obtained the ubiquity and pop cultural presence of its rival (indeed, after eighteen years *Cops* continues to be produced and consistently wins its time slot).

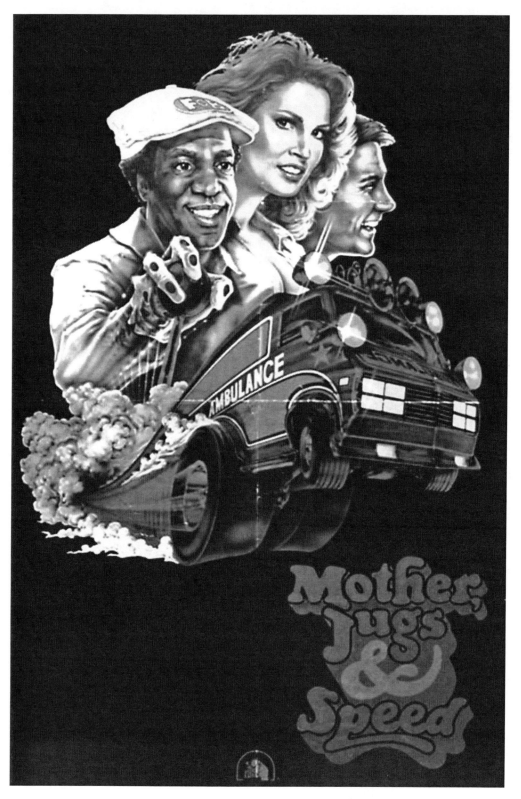

While critics were unimpressed, *Mother, Jugs, and Speed* (1978), starring Bill Cosby, Raquel Welch and Harvey Keitel, was a box office success and remains a cult favorite for many EMTs (Twentieth Century–Fox, all rights reserved).

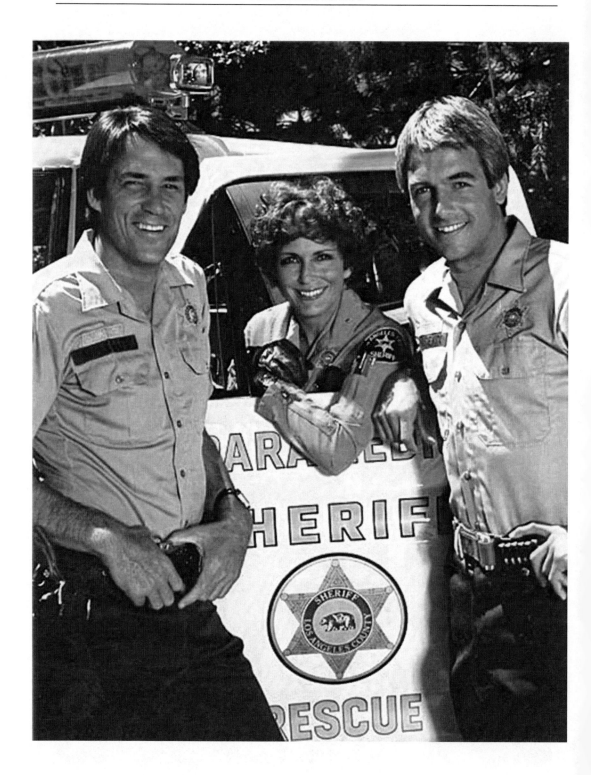

John Perry, Johanna Cassidy, and Mark Harmon starred as three search and rescue paramedics in the short lived series *240-Robert*. The title came from the call sign used by the Los Angeles Sheriff's Emergency Services Detail, on which the program was based (ABC, Inc., all rights reserved).

By the end of the 1990s the ambulance service had settled into a respectable period: the great scandals of the 1960s and early 1970s were not repeated, but neither was the enormous investment at the federal and state level. The public was largely satisfied with the quality of service, at least that portion of it that voted and sent letters to the editor, and the relative quietude of the intervening years called to mind the wisdom of John Waters, director of Jacksonville, Florida's successful paramedic program, who had given this advice to would be reformers in the early 1970s: "It seems we must kill someone before we get action [on ambulance service].... If you don't have a crisis and wish to get rolling, you had best manufacture one."[61] As it turned out, manufacturing a crisis wasn't going to be necessary. One would be delivered.

• 15 •

The Ambulance in the 21st Century

After decades of planning, studies, reports, and recommendations, by 2001 the nation's ambulance services were, largely, where they had been in the late 1960s: regulated at the state level for certification of crew members and equipment, including communications, with largely federal guidelines for vehicle construction and nationally set reimbursement schedules for the entitlement programs. Public attention to the emergency medical services was slight, but on September 11, 2001, the nation was forcibly reminded of their essential service when terrorists succeeded in using jet airliners to destroy the World Trade Center towers in New York and damaging the Pentagon (the fourth aircraft crashed in rural Pennsylvania after passengers fought back, averting a likely catastrophic attack on Washington, D.C.).

While the damage at the Pentagon was for the greater part confined to a single section and quickly contained, the collapse of the Trade Center Towers unfolded over approximately an hour and a half, providing ample time for the full resources of New York City's emergency responders to reach the scene and, ultimately, to be placed in harm's way when the buildings collapsed. The disintegration of the buildings claimed the lives of 411 first responders: the emergency medical service fatalities included two New York City Fire Department paramedics, fourteen New York City Police Department Emergency Service Unit officers (all of whom were cross-trained as emergency medical technicians), and eight privately employed paramedics and emergency medical technicians. Among the horrors of the day was the helplessness of on scene commanders who could see the imminent collapse of the buildings—especially after the first tower fell and it was clear the second must inevitably follow—but who found themselves unable to coordinate withdrawal and evacuation due to the mismatched array of radio equipment relied on by crews from different agencies. Many rescuers were caught unawares as they climbed smoke filled stairwells towards a descending avalanche of steel and masonry, others were caught in basements and at the base of the buildings. While the ESU command post was able to maintain coherent radio contact with its personnel, the Fire Department and the Port Authority experienced considerable difficulty in establishing radio contact with their personnel, making effective evacuation all but impossible: in all, the 9/11 Commission Report concluded that communication failure was a decisive factor in the fate of at least 121 of the 343 firefighters who died that day as well as an unknown number of the Port Authority police officers who were killed.[1]

In response the FCC developed an "interoperability" agency, to create a nationwide call channel for emergency responders of all stripes, but its most optimistic projections do not foresee achieving its aims before 2012, and the Department of Homeland Security has estimated it may take until 2024 to complete the process.[2] In the meantime, a 2005 survey conducted by the Public Safety Wireless Network Program found that three years after the communications failures on 9/11 over half of all ambulance and emergency medical service agencies reported having been limited in their ability to respond to emergencies due to an inability to commu-

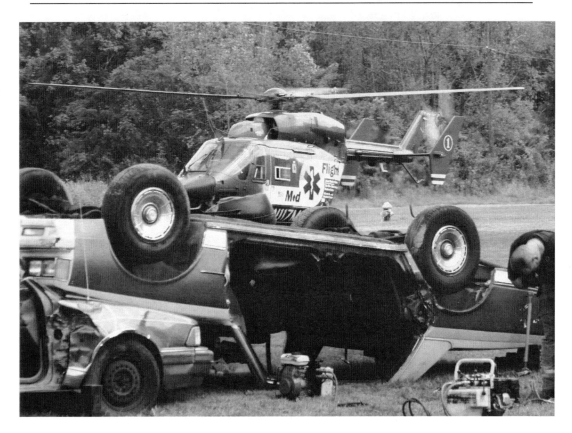

Medevac operations have become a standard of care since their introduction in 1970. Here, a contemporary helicopter ambulance responds to a car crash outside Columbus, Ohio (photograph by Kenn Kiser).

nicate with co-responders within their own jurisdiction, while approximately forty percent reported a lack of interoperability had limited their ability to coordinate with neighboring jurisdictions in a crisis.[3] The difficulties facing agencies are the same as those confronted by their predecessors in trying to start central call centers or to develop regional networks dependent on coordinated dispatch in the 1970s. Forty percent of agencies reported that local jurisdictional issues hampered their efforts, and all face the hurdle of absent universal communication standards and lack of funds to acquire upgraded equipment.[4] Politics aside, there are some things that can only be accomplished by central action: as the GAO reported in 2004, federal leadership is necessary so long as local authorities thrash about in a welter of jurisdictional squabbling and debate which standards to adopt in each locality.

Despite the widespread attention these catastrophic failures directed towards critical areas of weakness in emergency medical response, the response from all levels of government has been generally inadequate. The most detailed analysis of the issues raised by the 9/11 attacks and the official response appeared in *Emergency Medical Services, The Forgotten First Responder: A Report on the Critical Gaps in Organization and Deficits in Resources for America's Medical First Responders,* issued by New York University's Center for Catastrophe Preparedness and Response.[5] The paper notes that the government response to the attacks was to increase funding for law enforcement and fire fighters, but without a similar investment in EMS. It is here that the comparative absence of EMS from pop culture may actually be more than a moderately interesting fact for those looking for a term paper for their American Studies class.

This invisibility has a real and invidious counterpart in how scarce resources are allocated: EMTs and paramedics make up at approximately 25 percent of all United States emergency first responders, and yet they received only 4 percent of Homeland Security's $3.4 billion dollars in emergency preparedness in 2002, with similar percentages in recent years.[6] When the Department of Health and Human Services distributed a multimillion dollar Bioterrorism Grant the emergency medical services received a paltry 5 percent, despite the fact that ambulance crews would not only represent a significant proportion of those at the scene, but would also be the ones in the closest proximity to the victims—and thus at greatest risk for secondary exposure.[7] The consequence of this paucity of funding has been predictable: in the years since the attacks of September 11, when the federal government has made national security its overwhelming priority in name if not always in effect, twenty percent of EMTs and paramedics have received no training in how to respond to unconventional terrorist attacks, such as biological and chemical assault, and the majority of those who got training received less than sixty minutes of instruction—a percentage of time that the overwhelming number of experts consider so minimal as to approach worthlessness.[8] As these examples show, being invisible isn't just annoying—it's apt to be fatal.

Questions of Access, Questions of Payment

In 2007 the Institute of Medicine characterized, one more time, American's ambulance services as "fragmented and disorganized" and observed that the quality of emergency medical aid continues to be of variable quality across the country.[9] From a policy standpoint, this is particularly worrisome because the emergency medical service is the only source of care for 47 million uninsured Americans and tens of millions more whose inadequate insurance curtails their access to preventive care—indeed, in recent years the largest increase in ER visits has been among those who *have* private insurance, not the uninsured or those on government benefits.[10] The reliance on the ER was unintentionally highlighted by President Bush when he deflected criticism over health care access by opining "People have access to health care in America. After all, you just go to an emergency room."[11] And so they do—with the foreseeable result that the most expensive primary care clinics in the world are America's overcrowded emergency rooms: by mid decade the average was 114 million ER visits a year, with 16 million arriving in an ambulance.[12] In the absence of reliable preventive care, they show up sicker and the number of otherwise avoidable hospitalizations continues to climb.

The predictable result of this crisis was that in 2006 over half a million ambulances were diverted from their destination hospital because there were no beds: this delay in care could only have had an adverse impact on patients, since the critically ill don't get better while they are waiting for definitive care, but since no one has studied the issue neither the magnitude of the problem nor its urgency are known.[13] Crowded ERs also take longer to receive and admit patients while rooms are being cleared or space made in a hallway, and this waiting time results in delayed turnaround time for the ambulance idling in the driveway and decreases the number of units available for service.

While the financial impact of overcrowded emergency rooms and inadequate primary care has primarily been borne by hospitals and third party payers, the collateral effects of this excess spending has had a direct impact on ambulance reimbursements. When Medicare (federal health insurance for the elderly) and Medicaid (providing limited health benefits to certain categories of the indigent and funded by a combination of state and federal dollars) were created in 1965 they initially did not include a benefit that covered paramedic services, but swiftly were amended to provide reimbursement for the entire range of pre-hospital emergency medical

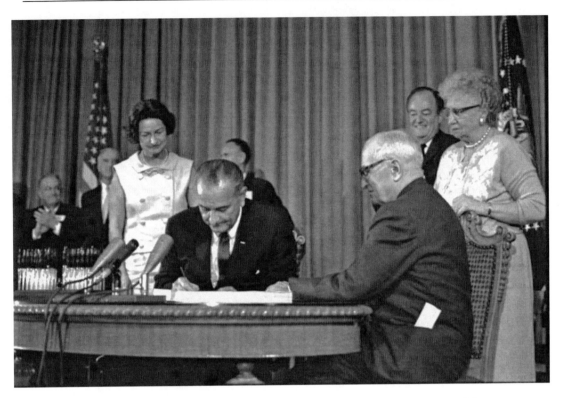

President Lyndon Johnson signs legislation authorizing Medicare. After the ceremony Johnson personally enrolled former President Truman (seen here on the right side of the desk) as the first Medicare beneficiary (Social Security Administration).

services. Forty years later these two programs represent fully 70 percent of the typical ambulance provider's total billing—55 percent from Medicare, and 15 percent from Medicaid.[14] Additionally, Medicare's statutory reimbursement rates directly influence the allowable rates of most private insurance plans as well, demonstrating the overwhelming influence the federal programs have on the viability of ambulance services in the United States. As the costs of these programs has risen dramatically (Medicare's expenditures for ambulance service alone went from $1.8 billion in 1997 to $3 billion in 2002) there has been enormous pressure to reduce costs by scaling back payments.[15] The problem has been especially acute in Medicaid, since the federal government has been steadily decreasing its share of payments and states have struggled to make up the shortfall. As a result, Medicaid ambulance payments in many jurisdictions have sunk to levels that look like typographical errors: in some states, Medicaid pays $25 for an ambulance, regardless of services provided.[16] This sum is close to what a typical funeral director was charging for an aid car in the late 1950s—which means that, adjusted for inflation, a modern ambulance operator providing paramedic service is being paid *86 percent less* in real dollars than a mortician with a hearse and first-aid card got in 1959. Further, in many areas Medicaid pays nothing unless the patient is transported, further diminishing reimbursement levels.

Reflective of the escalating funding crisis, on April 1, 2002, the Centers for Medicare and Medicaid Services (CMS) imposed a fee schedule for Medicare ambulance reimbursement, as required by the Balanced Budget Act of 1997, with the new repayment schedule to be uniform across the country after a five year phase-in period (slight deviations were permitted for areas with exceedingly high or extremely low costs). Under the terms of the act, the total amount that Medicare paid for ambulance services nationwide could not be increased: with the inevitable increase in population and inflation, this meant that the actual reimbursement for each trip would constantly be adjusted downwards. According to the GAO, between 2001 and 2004 the average ambulance provider took a 6 percent loss on every run billed to Medicare, although the distribution of these losses was not uniform: in "super rural" areas the loss was actually 17 percent, in rural areas the loss was a mere 1 percent, and in urban markets the shortfall was 6 percent.[17] (The difference probably reflects the preponderance of volunteer ambulance services in moderately rural areas: since the majority of their employees are unpaid, their operating budget is obviously much lower, while in "super rural" areas the great distances involved increase costs significantly.)

Diminished Medicare margins are not the only drain on ambulance providers: as far back as the days of the funeral home, collecting ambulance fees has been difficult for providers, a challenge that has not eased with time. The American Ambulance Association estimates that its members must write-off between 10 percent and 16 percent of their billable expenses, a burden not shared by other providers—for example, physicians typically write off an average of 4.3 percent of their charges, while the national average for hospitals is 5.6 percent unreimbursed care.[18] The GAO estimates that by 2010 the average ambulance provider will be taking a 6 percent loss for each Medicare ambulance transport (although the statistical range was large, varying from a potential loss of 35 percent for "super rural providers" to a potential net profit of 12 percent for rural services).[19] The difference will either be taken as a loss by the provider or will have to be made up by cutting salaries, reducing overhead by eliminating some service, charging patients more, or through increased subsidies from local government. Alternatively, they will go out of business. For example, by early 2007 twenty-four ambulance providers in Oklahoma had recently ceased operation, saying the insurance cuts crippled them financially: the effect on similarly largely rural operators is expected to be appreciable, since they have the smallest local reserves from which to draw supplemental income.[20] Stop-gap measures by Congress, including the Medicare Prescription Drug, Improvement and Modernization Act of 2003, have provided temporary upward adjustments to certain classes of providers but fail to address the long term trend.

The Contemporary Ambulance

After centuries of development where is the ambulance service today? The idea has been adopted by every industrialized nation on the planet, in one form or another, but in the United States, where the modern ambulance service was born in Dalton's image of a service responding to any medical emergency, centrally dispatched, and integrated with local government resources, in the society where so much promise was generated, the emergency medical service remains embroiled in controversies that would have been familiar to any 19th century ambulance surgeon clutching their black bag in the back of a wooden wagon. Measured by scale, Dalton's ideas have triumphed. In 2006 it was estimated that in the United States there were 12,000 ambulance services operating a combined fleet of 23,575 ground vehicles and at least 650 medevac helicopters, along with a smaller number of fixed wing aircraft.[21] Legislatively, however, the canopy of federal licensing regulations was never realized despite the aspirations of reformers active in the 1960s and 1970s, and currently individual states set their own standards for vehicles, equipment, and training of personnel, although the role of national accrediting boards and multi-state associations has contributed to some uniformity. Generally speaking ambulances are divided between Basic Life Support and Advanced Life Support services. A BLS unit is staffed by EMTs and equipped with oxygen, splints, suction devices to clear airways, ventilators, first aid supplies, medications, litters, back boards, and usually an automatic defibrillator. ALS rigs are staffed with at least one certified paramedic and carry a broader array of medications, supplies for intravenous access, a greater variety of devices to open and maintain an airway, and more advanced cardiac equipment, including manually adjusted defibrillators and instruments to monitor and display heart activity. A combination medical and rescue unit would, of course, include an array of tools to extricate victims from tangled vehicle wreckage and other dangerous situations.

The vehicles themselves are almost invariably built to at least meet the federal government's KKK-A-1822 specifications, which are mandatory for any ambulance purchased by a federal agency or by any local group receiving federal financing for its operations. (In addition, many states have adopted local rules incorporating the federal standards and a number of manufacturers exceed the federal specifications in at least some areas.) An area of growing concern, however, is that the regulations pay insufficient attention to the safety of the working environment inside the ambulance: as one example, a recent study concluded that at least forty percent of the most common tasks performed by ambulance crew members (checking blood pressure, administering oxygen, and so on) exposure providers to clinically significant musculoskeletal strain.[22] Whether more ergonomic designs could reduce the incidence of work-related injury while preserving optimal patient care is an area that has received comparatively little attention.

Perhaps the greatest problem confronting the ambulance services is the paucity of evidence about what works and what does not. While the enormous variation in quality and serv-

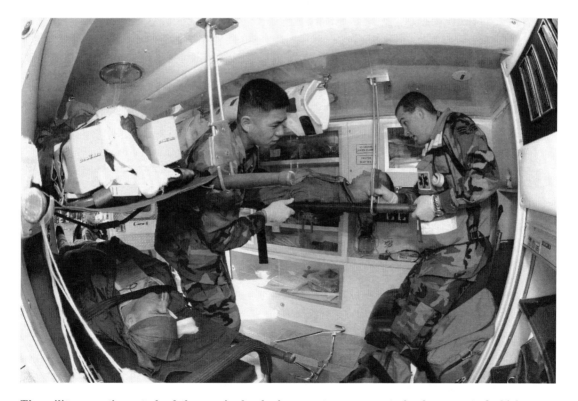

The military continues to lead the way in developing new trauma care technology, most of which eventually finds its way into civilian ambulances. Here, USAF firefighters with the 374th Medical Group, in Yokota, Japan, participate in a "Major Accident Response Exercise" in 2004 (Val Gempis, DefenseLINK/DOD).

ice that epitomized ambulance service only thirty years ago has largely been sanded down by more rigorous oversight and prescriptive legislation, unless there is some mechanism to evaluate results we risk fossilizing inadequate procedures that seemed optimal only because they had been insufficiently tested—or which have been superseded by better policies, or challenged by new theories. As the authors of the 2007 *EMS at the Crossroads* ruefully noted, we have

> a fragmented and sometimes balkanized network of underfunded EMS systems that often lack strong quality controls, cannot or do not collect data to evaluate and improve system performance, fail to communicate effectively within and across jurisdictions, [and] allocate limited resources inefficiently.[23]

Consider the most symbolic ambulance emergency: the heart attack. America's most prestigious paramedic services were built around this single event, and to this day cardiac care is considered the *sine qua non* of ambulance service. Despite this, there are no comprehensive means for jurisdictions to compare how they are handling this staple emergency relative to their peers. The evidence that has leaked out suggests a startling amount of variation continues to exist between services despite thirty years of improved training and the trend to comparable standards across states. For example, investigative research by *USA Today* found the percentage of persons experiencing ventricular fibrillation who arrive at the hospital in an ambulance and are later discharged with good brain function ranges from an abysmal 3 percent (Omaha) to a comparatively respectable 45 percent (Seattle)—and 42 percent of the cities contacted either refused to divulge their statistics, or had never bothered to collect the information in the first place.[24] Since these differences could not be attributed to differences between hospitals in the same city, either Seattleites are fifteen times as robust as the puny Nebraskans in Omaha or some critical difference exists between treatments by pre-hospital responders in various American cities. (The example of British Columbia, which saw a twenty-percent improvement in heart attack survival rates after changing how CPR was taught to its provincial ambulance service members, suggests that dramatic change can be achieved by comparatively slight modifications in training.) Without ongoing efforts to collect outcome information and comparing the practices of the best performers with the worst, further improvement in ambulance services will depend on chance, with delayed dissemination, unequal distribution, and irregular implementation. To obtain the most reliable and informative results these studies must be done on a national scale, and America's resolute insistence that emergency medical services remain a local institution limits our opportunities to close the chasm between what is possible in ambulance services and what the majority of our citizens receive.

Conclusion

At the end of all the centuries in which men and women have ridden towards help in the backs of ambulances, today's modern problems would be instantly recognizable to the earliest pioneers. The ratcheting down of reimbursement in the age of Medicare and Medicaid would elicit a rueful smile from a Texas mortician in the 1940s, looking down at the pile of unpaid bills for emergency calls. Emergency medical technicians grumbling over turning out for yet another frivolous call echo the groans of countless 19th century interns called out in the dead of night to pick up a "toper" from the gutter and then carry the inebriate back to the alcoholic ward to sleep it off. Reformers still wonder why the best practices aren't identified and exported to all, government officials at the federal, state, and local level argue over their relative share of the costly burden, and the public all too often blithely ignores this essential public utility, confident that should they ever require the service, an ambulance can be had for the time it takes to dial 911.

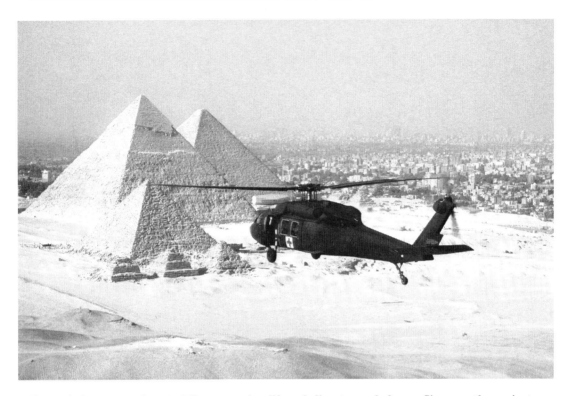

Humanity's most modern tool for preserving life, a helicopter ambulance, flies over the ancient world's most enduring monuments to death—the pyramids at Giza—during a training exercise in 1983 (Joint Service Audiovisual Team, DefenseLINK/DOD).

And, of course, for virtually anyone in the country an ambulance *will* be in the offing when they call, bolting out of the fire station down the street or the volunteer rescue squad's garage in the next valley over. The ambulance service endures because the whipping wind of a fast car fans some spark in our substance that burns brighter when much is asked of us in the name of sympathy and courage. There will always be someone to work the rotating shifts, take the chaff that comes with having the skills of an emergency room nurse but the salary of a health aide, and who will take home in pride what they don't get in pay. But if the ambulance service is to continue to improve and develop, it requires the community to understand the intensity of the resources required. The men and women of the emergency medical service will always be well armed with compassion and dedication, and when the call comes they will do what they have always done—serving with whatever tools they have, pouring out whatever they have left to give. The only limit to their ability is the investment the community is willing to make in the training, the research, and the equipment with which we arm them as we send them into lop-sided battle with mortality and morbidity. In the long history of the ambulance it has overcome many obstacles, but how much more might be achieved if these services were repaid with the tenth part of what they give to us in dedication, compassion, and professionalism?

Appendix I.

In Search of the Origins of the Misericordia

While the most widely circulated origin of the Misericordia remains the one recounted in Landini's *Istoria della venerabile arciconfraternita di santa maria del misericordia,* written in 1779 and citing source material of uncertain vintage, this story of 13th century wool porters organizing a crude ambulance service while huddled in a cellar drinking wine has had many detractors. In its defense Landini's version is plausible as to the date of origin in 1240, since the Misericordia's oldest extant record is a property deed from 1321 when the society was sufficiently well established, and endowed, to acquire part of a small building to serve as a meeting place and to house its effects. Certainly eighty years was ample time for the group to have progressed from a cellar full of blaspheming porters financed by pocket change to a charitable company with sufficient resources to buy property.[1] Also, the account upon which Landini said he relied on was written in Gothic script, a style arriving in Italy sometime in the mid to late 13th century, just after the time the Misericordia was reportedly founded: by the late 1500s the common Italian script had evolved and Italian Gothic was largely confined to formal liturgical works, explaining why a document in the archaic hand would require translation when Father Fici reproduced the old manuscript in 1605. Against this story is the unfortunate absence of any source materials buttressing Landini's reproduction of a paraphrase of a translation of a lost book.

Counter histories for the origins of the Misericordia are plentiful, and these alternative histories bring with them documentary evidence susceptible to proof—or more precisely, disproving: an inconvenience from which the historically incorporeal Pietro Borsi enjoys immunity. For example, St. Antonius alleged that the Misericordia evolved from the Laudesi Brotherhood of Or San Michele. (The Laudesi had formed in 1291 to perform public hymns called "lauds" in veneration of a portrait of the Virgin Mary hanging in the loggia of Florence's grain market, an image credited with miraculous healing powers.)[2] According to the saint, when a plague enveloped the city in 1363 the Laudesi began gathering the dead for burial and carried some of the afflicted to local hospitals when there was no one else to care for them.[3] The dates given are not compatible with what we know of the Misericordia, however, since a deed of purchase proves the fraternity had acquired the use of part of a building for meetings in 1321, fully forty years before Antonius' inspirational plague arrived in Florence.

Of course, it is entirely possible, even probable, that a group like the Laudesi imitated the efforts of the Misericordia during this legendary pestilence, especially since the Misericordia was a "closed shop" excluding members of any profession save its own until the 15th century: thus, like-minded volunteers would have had to form their own ambulance militias. A 19th century sketch (which may incorporate elements of earlier work) speaks to this issue in its representation of the 1348 plague. In a view of a large piazza, three groups are shown carrying off

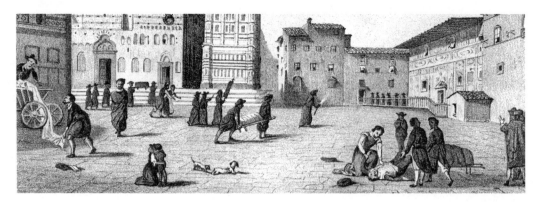

In this 19th century sketch three groups engage in gathering up the ailing and the dead as the plague lays waste to Florence. While the figures in the left rear clearly represent the Misericordia, with their distinctive shoulder borne litter and traditional procession, the other groups are varied in costume and equipment and likely represent other lay groups active in the same field. (C. Gastognola, in Landini's "Istoria della misericordia," 1843)

the sick and the dead: the figures of the Misericordia are clearly seen in the far corner, with their distinctive robes and carrying the stretcher on their shoulders. In contrast, in the center of the piece two men, in similar robes but without the hoods of the Misericordia, are carrying a conventional stretcher without the procession always associated with the Misericordia; and, lastly, in the right foreground two men supervise the loading of a body onto a stretcher. These two figures wear breeches and what appear to be simple dark masks over their faces, without hats. While engaged in the same work, the three groups are clearly dissimilar, and given the evidentiary record that in 1432 there was a unification of at least two groups under the banner of the ancient order, it appears that the Misericordia was an inspiration before it was a monopoly.[4]

Another persistent belief is that the Misericordia was established by the papal inquisitor and Florentine folk-hero, Peter of Verona (later St. Peter the Martyr after earning his celestial elevation the hard way, being stabbed and hacked to death by Cathar heretics who had survived his militant efforts to suppress them). The cleric arrived in Florence in 1244, sent by the Holy See to exterminate an increasingly successful heresy that was claiming converts in northern Italy. Peter was a mesmerizing orator and achieved celebrity status in the city, using his charisma to organize a "Society of Faith" that, in the manner of most organizations built around a cult of personality, enforced doctrine through example, informing on non-believers, and ultimately mob violence—in this case, two pitched battles in the streets of Florence that sent the surviving non-conformists into hiding (from which two would emerge, eight years later, just long enough to assassinate Peter on the road to Milan).[5]

After Peter moved on to other ecclesiastical battlefields in 1245 his Society of Faith carried on, but from the scanty historical record it appears to have devolved into factions that adopted different charitable purposes. One recipient of their attention was the pre-existing Bigallo Hospital, which had begun life many years before as a wayside inn whose emblem, in those preliterate days, had been a board decorated with a white rooster (hence "bianco gallo").[6] In time, the hostelry became a refuge for the ill pilgrim en route to Florence, and later a proper hospital with an organized charity to support it. In 1389 a remnant of Peter's Society of Faith took over its administration, but later attempts to claim Peter as the actual founder of the Bigallo are obviously spurious, given its ancient origins. Similarly, at some point it was alleged that Peter had not only personally founded the Bigallo, but also the Misericordia. (This attempt to appropriate the popular saint was hardly novel, as he was also supposed to have founded the

Servites of Mary, although in reality he only recommended them to the Pope for formal recognition, the order having been extant for decades prior to his arrival in Florence.)

The strongest evidence for the claim that Peter founded the Misericordia are four ledgers in their archives, volumes dating from 1361 and listing the members of "the great company of our Lady the glorious Virgin Saint Mary of the city of Florence [*i quali sono della compagnia magiore della detta nostra Donna Vergine gloriosa Santa Maria della cittade di Firenze*]." While not mentioning the Misericordia by name, the quoted phrase at least alludes to the company's formal name at the time: *Compagnia Maggiore di Santa Maria della Misericordia*. It must be admitted, however, that this is hardly dispositive, since this generic language was also incorporated into the formal title of the Bigallo, properly known as *Compagnia Maggiore di Santa Maria del Bigallo*. In their introductions each ledger claims that this company was formed by Peter the Martyr in 1240, which cannot be the case since Peter didn't reach Florence until four years later.[7] It is much more likely that, as with the Servites, this ambiguously styled organization was attempting to yoke itself to a popular historical figure for the attendant prestige. As to its actual identity, it might have been the Misericordia itself, or it might have been a corporate condominium enfolding both the Misericordia and the Bigallo, even prior to their formal merger in 1425 at the behest of Coismo Medici.

Ultimately, any claim to unite the Misericordia with Peter the Martyr founders on the undisputed fact that the company has never claimed Peter as a patron saint—in stark contrast to other organizations, like the Bigallo, which have claimed Peter for special veneration from the earliest times. Instead, the two patrons of the Misericordia have always been the Virgin Mary and St. Tobit (or Tobias), a figure in the Apocrypha who defied edicts suppressing Jewish religious rituals during the Assyrian exile in Nineveh, risking his life to secretly ensure that the dead were buried with the proper rites. Obviously this story clearly relates to the Misericordia's mission of gathering the impoverished dead and ensuring that they were given a proper Christian burial, a task forming one of their core missions at inception, and just as obviously it would be bizarre for a charity founded by Peter the Martyr to ignore a figure who was canonized in 1253, only nine years after he supposedly founded the group, while his name and activities were still widely revered in Florence. Given his prominence in associations whose relationship to him is much better supported by the historical evidence, this omission suggests a different origin for the Misericordia, despite subsequent efforts to link them to the name of the saint.

As mentioned, the history of the Misericordia is rich in speculation, but short on substantiation. Whatever the truth, it is appears indisputable that the company did not have its origin in the Bigallo, the Laudesi of Or San Michele, or at the instigation of Peter the Martyr, and so the name of Pietro Borsi remains as a place-holder in the otherwise abandoned historical niche reserved for the genius behind the world's oldest continuously operated ambulance service.

Appendix II.

Barber Surgeons

While the inadequacies of the barber surgeons following the early armies certainly played a role in the reluctance of military planners to invest heavily in ambulance operations, how had barber surgery evolved? As it turns out, the Sweeney Todds of trauma medicine were created by a quirk of medieval theology and flourished under a guild system that gave them a longevity unrelated to their utility.

It began with the intellectual rubble of medieval Europe after the fall of Rome: those medical treatises surviving the post-imperial implosion of learning and education were protected behind mossy monastery walls and the tonsured craniums of the clergy— the last literate caste on the continent. This, plus the inevitable medicinal herb garden, made monasteries popular with medieval peasants seeking intelligent, if not necessarily accurate, medical attention, including simple surgery. Monasteries were also attractive destinations for the village barber as Church tradition considered flowing beards suitable only for the patriarchs and long hair symbolic of the sin of pride. What had been custom became canon law in 1177 when an edict from Pope Alexander III man-

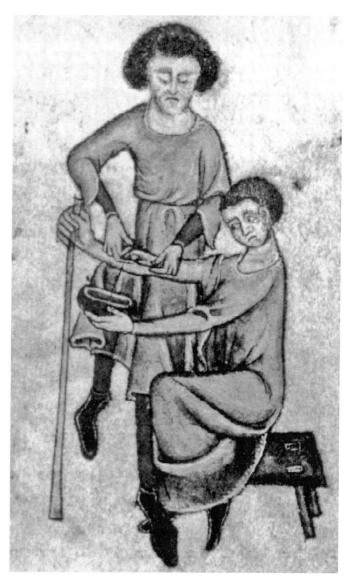

A medieval barber surgeon bleeds a patient. (Courtesy National Library of Medicine)

dated extreme modesty in facial hair, with archdeacons empowered to shear disobedient clergy by force, if necessary: one result was that barbers became even more indispensable to a well-run monastery.[1] The next, defining, step in the evolution of the barber surgeon came with the Fourth Lateran Council of 1215, when the Church's aversion to the reality of our earthly bodies was expressed in Canon XVIII, declaring the shedding of blood, even for medical purposes, incompatible with holy office.

The need for surgery having outlived the monks' ability to operate, the brothers cast about for successors. Naturally, they turned to the razor toting barbers, and as the clergy laid aside their lancets and scalpels they instructed their attending barbers in how to employ them, and the barber-surgeon was born.[2] Illiterate and lacking a tradition of scholarship, barber-surgery was passed down father to son and master to apprentice, the ancient techniques protected by a guild monopoly. Thus mortality rates that had been enviable in 1215 when a forgotten ancestor first learned the technique from a diligent monk had, by 1600, made barber-surgeons the butt of macabre jest, ultimately blunting the incentive to provide comprehensive military ambulance services to supply them.

Appendix III.

Dalton: A Life of Service

Edward Barry Dalton was born in Lowell, Massachusetts in 1834. Although contemporaries described him as a slight man whose "physical organization had an appearance of extreme delicacy," he served in the field almost without cease throughout the Civil War, at one point resigning a comfortable administrative post in order to rejoin his regiment.[1] Malaria contracted during a siege in the Chickahominy swamps weakened his constitution, and as early as 1867 it was clear his health was failing. Perhaps fearing his span would be too brief to waste in rest, Dalton pursued a number of professional projects: in addition to serving as Superintendent of the Board of Health for New York City, he was an Associate Physician to the municipal Lunatic Asylum and, in 1868, was secretary to a select committee tasked with reforming New York City's asylums. (An unfriendly minority of his overseers at the Board of Health felt he was overextending himself and unsuccessfully attempted to pass a rule that no officer could be employed in "any service, except that of the Board.")[2]

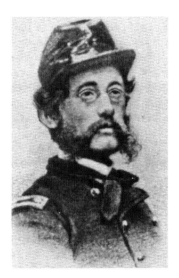

Edward Barry Dalton, pioneer of the modern civilian ambulance, circa 1863, while he was serving as a regimental surgeon in the Army of the Potomac.

At the same time he was beset by terrible personal tragedies: first, the loss of his only child, a young daughter, in 1868, and almost exactly one year later the death of his wife and their infant in childbirth. He was also subject to debilitating pleuritic chest pain, probably related to underlying tuberculosis. Increasingly poor health, as well as frustration with the political machinations of Tammany New York, led him to resign his municipal posts by the summer of 1869. After submitting his design for the Bellevue ambulance, a holiday in Switzerland and the south of France brought him some relief from his respiratory distress and distraction from the recent loss of his wife and child.[3] Rejuvenated, he joined his brother's medical practice in Boston, but the next year a stifling New England summer triggered relentless, suffocating coughing spells. That fall he formed a desperate resolution to take up farming in southern California, hoping that vigorous exercise in a favorable climate would strengthen his failing lungs. Giving up all he had known, Dalton left for California in October, 1871, ultimately settling outside Santa Barbara in the tiny hamlet of Montecito—but it was too late to stem the inexorable advance of his tuberculosis. Death found him the night of May 13, 1872, while he was staying at the hacienda of Major W.A. Hayne, a former Confederate officer who had befriended the Union physician. Dr. Dalton, pioneer of civilian ambulance services, was only 37 years old.[4]

Appendix IV.

Shock of Life: The Portable Defibrillator

In 1926 John W. Lieb, vice president of the New York Edison Company, couldn't help but notice that, modern miracle though it was, the increased use of electrical power in homes and business was resulting in more and more of his customers and employees being electrocuted.[1] At the time the Rockefeller Institute, also in Manhattan, was the nation's preeminent center for medical research, making it natural that Lieb turn to its director, the noted pathologist Simon Flexner, for help. With Flexner's guidance, and Lieb's financial backing, several physician committees were assembled to tackle various aspects of the biological and practical mechanisms of electrocution, with the hope that from such basic research better therapies and preventive measures could be derived.[2]

In a canny move, research on the cardiac effect of electric shock was assigned to parallel labs, one at Case Western Reserve in Cleveland, the other at Johns Hopkins, not only increasing the odds that a significant discovery would be made, but ensuring that a breakthrough by one group would be subject to replication and confirmation by the other before it would be accepted by the corporate office.[3] At Hopkins one of the principal investigators, and the one for whom this topic would become his life's work, was William Kouwenhoven. (His opposite number at Case Western was Carl Wiggers.) In 1931, shortly after research had begun, a colleague showed Kouwenhoven a scientific paper from 1889 describing how direct electrical stimulation of the heart muscle could reverse ventricular fibrillation (the ventricles are the largest chambers in the heart, and in fibrillation the muscle cells no longer fire in synch: instead of steadily pulsing like a massive, clenching fist, the heart ineffectually quivers and writhes and the blood fails to circulate).

Since it was understood that the cause of death in electrocution was generally heart failure, and further that the form this failure took was frequently ventricular fibrillation, the thought that a controlled dose of the lethal agent would actually be curative was fascinating (although not especially novel to anyone who had been to see one of the year's hit films, *Frankenstein*, whose monster was reanimated by a massive infusion of electricity). Taking their lead from the dusty manuscript the researchers set up shop to verify the claim that a shock of electric current could reverse fibrillation, choosing to use Rhesus monkeys in their research. Curiously (and fortunately for Maryland's monkey population) the little primates proved wholly unsatisfactory—no matter how hard the experimenters tried to induce ventricular fibrillation, the monkeys' possessed some physiologic quirk that snapped the cardiac muscle into syncopation without any intervention from the technicians.[4] In the end they abandoned the obnoxiously robust primates and worked on dogs instead, whose hearts proved every bit as fallible as our own. By the late 1940s the research was broadened to include artificial respiration, since it was not uncommon for those receiving electrical shock to experience paralysis of the muscles of respiration even as their hearts continued to beat. However, as the only known way to restore circulation was to literally open the chest, seize the heart in your hands, and squeeze (from the bottom up, like "milking a cow backwards," in the words of one surgeon) the need to find some less drastic treatment for fibrillation presented the most pressing challenge in the rescue of the electrocuted.[5]

Then the war came, of course, and the team was broken up to pursue research related to defeating the Axis, and when it was over they went back to their labs and at Johns Hopkins, at least, the question of ventricular fibrillation became just one of many to be considered. In the laboratories of the Midwest the topic of fibrillation was not so easily eclipsed, however, and by 1947 C.S. Beck, at Case Western, had demonstrated that an irregular heart beat could be abolished by opening the chest and applying electric current directly to the exposed cardiac muscle, but the limits of this intervention were obvious, and this therapy wasn't going to do much for an electrocuted lineman laying on the side of a road in Wichita.[6] By 1950 experiments had evolved to the point of applying electricity to the chests of dogs and measuring its cardiac effect, thus avoiding the messy detail of opening the thorax and clamping conductors directly to the heart: in this the researchers were, at last, prefiguring practical "external" defibrillation. Things picked up speed in 1951 when Kouwenhoven was contacted by the Edison Electric Institute, a private trade group, with a request that he develop a portable external defibrillator, something that could be used by lineman crews to restart the heart of a crewmember who had sustained a life threatening shock.[7] They were not only interested, they were willing to pay for the research, and so work on a clinically useful defibrillation device entered a new and more urgent stage.

Electrode "paddles" were developed and the optimal placement on the chest worked out: additionally, the use of the device by laypersons in the field made it imperative that the device not be harmful to someone who only *appeared* to be in cardiac arrest but who was, in fact, merely stunned and sustaining a normal heart beat. How to test this in human beings presented a bit of a problem, for the obvious reason that if the experiment went the wrong way it might kill the subject. The difficulty was overcome in the usual way—a convenient accident that exposed a random and unsuspecting person to the full force of the device. In this case it was Kouwenhoven himself who was the unwitting guinea pig: he was getting the paddles ready to shock a lab dog when an overeager assistant threw the switch prematurely—instead of delivering 9 amps of electricity for two-thirds of a second to an anesthetized dog, the current passed through a wide-awake Kouwenhoven. The jolt was powerful enough to crumple him like wax under a blowtorch, but after a moment or two his muscles stiffened up again and he declared himself fit for duty and the defibrillation device safe for use on a normally functioning heart.[8] (The next day the unit was rigged to include a new foot-pedal so the person holding the paddles was now the one who turned on the current, as well.)

While they had established their "proof of concept" that external electric shock could be used instead of open defibrillation, they were not destined to be the first to attempt it in human beings. That honor went to Paul Zoll, a superficially stern, somewhat forbidding cardiologist whose taciturn qualities seem to have concealed a certain fundamental shyness and even awkwardness around strangers (he had originally considered pursuing exclusively lab work, feeling his interpersonal skills were too feeble to make him successful as a clinician). It was Zoll who, in 1952, successfully paced a human heart by threading electrodes under the skin—the first working "pacemaker." Building from this success, in 1955 he rigged up an external defibrillator and used its paddles to "counter shock" four patients out of ventricular fibrillation caused by a heart attack, tachycardia, digoxin overdose, and recurrent heart block.[9] Three of the patients had experienced circulatory collapse for at least seven minutes, and their debilitated systems were too weak to sustain life, but the fourth was converted within two minutes on several occasions, and went on to be discharged from the hospital. This remarkable outcome was widely heralded and marked the official debut of clinical defibrillation.

Almost simultaneously the efforts in Baltimore to create a portable defibrillator continued apace, and the initial result of their efforts was a 280 pound defibrillator that was portable in the sense that a steel I-beam is portable once you load it onto a flatbed truck. The Hopkins Defibrillator was built into a sturdy table mounted on casters and buttressed by side panels: obviously limited to hospital use, this was the first "crash cart," a name the top-heavy object earned with its tendency to tip over when excitable interns tried to rush around corners too quickly. Still, the hospital supervisors would not approve the device for use on human beings, requesting yet more tests on animal subjects. As part of these studies it was necessary not only to monitor the electrical activity of the heart but also to have some standardized way of comparing circulation, which in this case included measuring blood flow through the femoral artery in the thigh. As suggested by the nearly three-hundred pound weight of the defibrillator unit, the parts of this machine were scaled up relative to what is standard in today's micro-sized world, and this included the paddles themselves, which were comparatively thick and heavy — especially relative to the chest of a medium sized dog.

So it happened that on May 6, 1956, someone noticed, and jotted down, the curious observation that when the paddles were held down on a dog's chest the pressure in the femoral artery increased, even prior to the administration of the shock itself.[10] This passing observation was quickly seized on, and someone wondered if perhaps it were possible that merely by applying external pressure to the chest the heart muscle could be sufficiently compressed to sustain circulation. Back to the lab Kouwenhoven and his colleagues went, and for some time they pushed and punched the chests of anesthetized dogs with induced ventricular fibrillation to see if they could sustain life: in the end, they discovered that simply by applying vertical pressure to the lower half of the sternum they could create enough circulation to keep an animal alive — up to twenty-one minutes, after which they applied counter-shock and brought the heart into a normal rhythm.

Suddenly, the need for a portable defibrillator became much less acute, since cardiac compression could keep the patient alive long enough to deliver them to a hospital where a three hundred pound resuscitator on wheels could be rolled up to zap their heart back in synch. Still, for almost two years they conducted additional research on animal subjects, and it was not until 1958 that manual compression was attempted on human beings, with Hopkins making their first successful resuscitation in February 1959 on a surgical patient. By 1960 the application of the technique to laypeople was considered viable, and the Baltimore Fire Department was shown the technique using anesthetized dogs (after thirty years of similar research, one suspects that the city was not a healthy one for strays). Dubious as they were, they obviously paid attention because on January 6, 1960, a fire department ambulance was called to the home of a man who had suffered a heart attack while resting on his couch. When they arrived he had no pulse and wasn't breathing, and, with nothing to lose, the ambulance crew launched into a combination of mouth to mouth resuscitation and cardiac compression: after a few moments they were stunned to see their patient breathing spontaneously as color suffused his face. He was transported to the hospital, defibrillated with the "crash cart," and discharged whole and sound six weeks later: nine years passed, and he still called the hospital on the anniversary of his discharge to let them know that he was very much alive and very grateful.[11]

Of course, profound as the creation of CPR had been, it was not the ultimate solution for the power companies, since it was quite common for two men crews to be working on high tension wires and, particularly in a rural area, there would be no way for one man to both deliver CPR to an injured coworker and drive to the hospital at the same time. So in 1959 the Mine Safety Appliance Company came to Dr. Kouwenhoven's group and asked, once again, for a

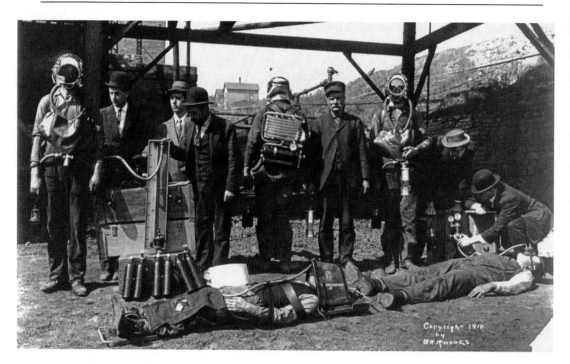

Prior to the development of external cardiac compression and electrical defibrillation, resuscitation techniques were limited to respiratory support and warming the body. Here, coal miners in LaSalle demonstrate a variety of oxygen apparatus, including Draeger smoke helmets and, at right, a pulmotor. The hazards of mining had long made it a laboratory for emergency medicine, and in 1959 the Mine Safety Appliance Company sponsored the final research leading to a portable defibrillator. (B.H. Rhodes, 1910. Library of Congress Prints and Photographs Division, LC-USZ62-61734)

truly portable defibrillator, something they could market to power companies for use on their trucks.[12] By now the technical aspects had been sufficiently well marked out that it was possible to compress the "crash cart" behemoth into something that could actually be carried. Working with Mine Safety the Hopkins group (which by now included G.G. Knickerbocker and James Jude) was able, by May 1959, to fabricate a prototype portable defibrillator, a forty-five pound bit of luggage fashioned out of a twenty by fifteen inch fiberglass case.[13] In light of its intended market, it was designed to operate off any of several power sources, such as the kind of 6 volt battery that powered an electric fence, the auto battery of a power company work truck (or an ambulance), or a standard 115 volt AC plug if the emergency occurred indoors. Rather than being deployed on Con Edison trucks right away, it was given some experimental airing at the Hopkins labs, and only in August 1961 was the first unit shipped out to Medford, Oregon, in care of Claude Haggard, a power company safety director and member of the Edison Electric Institute's subcommittee on resuscitation.[14] Meanwhile, additional units were constructed and distributed to other sites—one naturally stayed at Hopkins, and by early 1962 the Baltimore team had used their portable defibrillator on ten patients in the Emergency Room. Of this pilot group, who were treated between 1959 and early 1962, all were successfully defibrillated, with varying results: two died despite defibrillation when their hearts could not be induced to beat with sufficient force to sustain life; five survived for brief periods lasting from four hours to six days, before succumbing to their underlying disease; and the remaining three were still alive when the authors published their findings, representing recoveries lasting from two and a half years to six months and counting.[15]

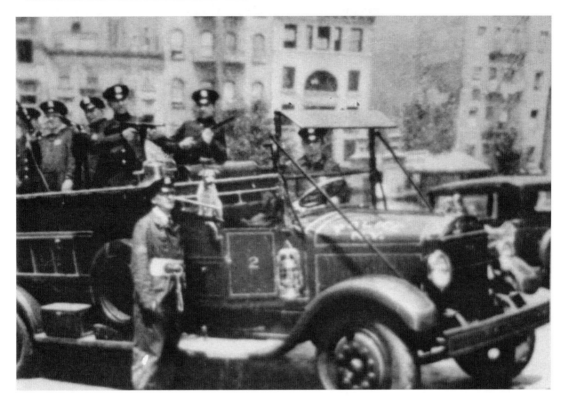

This Emergency Services Division truck dates to the re-organization of the unit in 1930, when the original two rig squad was expanded to a fleet of six and the crews were given additional training in rescue and first aid. (Courtesy Kevin Reynolds. Copyright 2001, New York City Police Department, all rights reserved. Used with permission)

The portable defibrillator was finally a reality (and along the way it had led to the re-discovery of external cardiac compression), and one of the defining elements of the modern ambulance crew was at hand. Today such devices are de rigueur on ambulances of all descriptions and automated versions are increasingly being stationed in public places such as airports, where they can be instantly put to use by a bystander, who has only to place the paddles on the chest and press a button to deliver the shock of life.

Chapter Notes

Chapter 1

1. Mauriticius, *Ars Militaris*, vol. 2, trans. Joh. Scheffero (Uppsala, Sweden, 1664), 64, quoted in Johann Beckmann, *Beckmann's History of Inventions, Discoveries, and Origins*, trans. William Johnston (London: Richard and John Taylor, 1846), 440 (for description of stirrups).
2. F.H. Garrison, *Notes on Military Medicine* (Washington, D.C.: Association of Military Surgeons, 1922), 79. See also E.T. Withington, *Medical History from the Earliest Times* (London: Scientific Press, 1894), 118.
3. Placido Landini, *Istoria dell'oratorio e della Venerabile Arciconfraternita di Santa Maria della Misericordia della città di Firenze* (Florence: Cartoleria Peratoner, 1843).
4. Ibid., 52.
5. Ibid., 53.
6. Walter Scaife, *Florentine Life during the Renaissance* (Baltimore: Johns Hopkins University Press, 1893), 185.
7. "Fratelli Della Misericordia—The Brotherhood of Mercy," *New Monthly Magazine* 17, no. 72 (December 1826): 503, 506.
8. Ibid. The controversy over who originated the Misericordia is discussed in the appendix of the present book, and is mentioned in Howard Saalman's *The Bigallo* (New York: New York University Press, 1969), n.8.
9. "Fratelli Della Misericordia," 508.
10. Saalman, 7.
11. Susan Horner and Joanna Horner, *Walks in Florence*, Vol. 1 (London: Strahan & Co., 1873), 98.
12. "Fratelli Della Misericordia," 507.

Chapter 2

1. Garrison, 95.
2. Pedro Bosca, *Oratio Romae habita XI Kal. Novembris ad Sacrum, etc.*, 1487 (Rome), quoted in Garrison, 96.
3. See, generally, Miller J. Stewart, *Moving the Wounded: Litters, Carolets and Ambulance Wagons* (Ft. Collins, Colo.: Old Army Press, 1979).
4. David Riesman, *The Story of Medicine in the Middle Ages* (New York: Paul B. Hoeber, 1936), 314.
5. A medical field chest carried by the Bavarian artillery against the Turks in 1688 tells the tale: it weighed 320 pounds and contained thirty-seven instruments and one-hundred-ninety-seven different compounds, including pulvis ad casum, a combination of rhubarb, powdered red clay, palm juice, spermaceti, and mummy dust, and the simpler remedies of rainworm oil and a plaster of frog-spawn and mercury. See, generally, J. Schuster, *Deutsche militar arztliche Ztschr.* 45 (1916): 123–31, quoted in Garrison, 119.
6. Stephen Brandwell, *Helps* (London: Thomas Purfoot, 1633).
7. "A true report of the great costs and charges of the foure hospitals, in the city of London: in the maintenance of their great number of poore, this present yeare, 1644, as followeth" (London: n.p., 1644); see also "A true Report of the great Costs and Charges of the five Hospitals in the city of London under the Care of the Lord Mayor, Commonalty and Citizens of London, in the maintaining of a very great Number of poore the yeare last past [dated] 11th day of Aprill, 1653" (London, 1653).
8. Harold W. Hart, "The Conveyance of Patients to and from Hospital, 1720–1850," *Medical History* 22, no. 4 (1978): 404.
9. Hart, 397.
10. Katherine Traver Barkley, *Ambulance* (Hicksville, N.Y.: Exposition Press, 1978).
11. Dr. Steedman, *The History and Statutes of the Royal Infirmary of Edinburgh* (Edinburgh: Balfour and Smellie, 1778).
12. See, generally, Ray Porter, "Accidents in the 18th Century," in *Accidents in History: Injuries, Fatalities, and Social Relations*, ed. Roger Cooter (Atlanta, Ga.: Ridopi, 1997).
13. Middlesex Hospital Board minutes of October 28, 1777, cited in Hart, 400.
14. *Memorials of John Flint South* (London: Murray, 1884), cited in Porter 98, 106.
15. Thomas Bernard, *An account of the House of Recovery, established by the board of health at Manchester, from The Reports of the Society for Bettering the Condition and Increasing the Comforts of the Poor*, Vol. l, Section 13 (Manchester, England, 1798), 98.
16. Reginald Harrison, *The Use of the Ambulance in Civil Practice: Portions of the Inaugural Address at the Liverpool Medical Institution* (Liverpool: Holden, 1881).

Chapter 3

1. Dominique Larrey, *Memoirs of Military Surgery and Campaigns of the French Armies*, Vol. 1, trans. Richard Wilmott Hall (Baltimore: Joseph Cushing/University Press of Sergeant Hall, 1814), 23. In the quoted text, Larrey uses the term "ambulance" in its military sense of a mobile field hospital rather than a particular vehicle.
2. Ibid., 28.
3. Ibid., 81.
4. Ibid., 81.
5. Ibid., 80.
6. Ibid., 81.

7. Ibid., 79.
8. Robert L. Pearce, "War and Medicine in the 19th Century," *ADF Health* 3, no. 1 (2002): 88–92.
9. *Times*, "London," October 18, 1854, 6.
10. *Times*, "Turkey," October 13, 1854, 8.
11. *Times*, "To the Editor," October 23, 1854, 9.
12. Christopher Hibbert, *The Destruction of Lord Raglan* (Boston: Little, Brown, 1962).
13. John Haller, *Farmcarts to Fords—A History of the Military Ambulance from 1790–1925* (Carbondale: Southern Illinois University Press, 1992).
14. *Times*, "London," December 30, 1854, 6.
15. Henry Bowditch, "The Ambulance System," *Medical and Surgical Reporter* 9, no. 2 (October 11, 1862): 50.
16. Otto Bettman, *Pictorial History of Medicine* (Springfield, Ill.: Charles C. Thomas, 1956), 236.
17. "Street Cabs and Contagious Diseases," *The Lancet*, April 12, 1856, 409.
18. Charles Creighton, *A History of Epidemics in Britain*, Vol. 2 (Cambridge: Cambridge University Press, 1894), 816.
19. Ken Smith, "The Ambulance Service Past, Present and Future," *Practitioner*, August 1988, 879.
20. Hart, 1978.
21. "Street Cabs," 409.
22. "City Sewers: Sanitary Condition of the City," *Times*, April 2, 1856, 11.
23. "City Commission of Sewers," *Times*, June 25, 1863, 7.
24. Horace Jefferson, "London Fever and London Cabs," *Times*, March 5, 1866, 10.
25. Jefferson, "London Fever," 10.
26. Horace Jefferson, "Propagation of Disease by Public Vehicles," *Times*, January 21, 1869, 7 (failure of the Sanitary Act); *London Illustrated News*, February 24, 1867, 190 (carriage fund).
27. *London Illustrated News*, February 24, 1867, 190.
28. James H. Crossman, "Ambulances," *Times*, December 1, 1881, 10.

Chapter 4

1. John D. Morgan, *A Vindication of His Public Character in the Station of Director General of the Military Hospitals and Physician-in-Chief to the American Army* (Boston: Powers and Willis, 1777), quoted by R.K. Wilbur, *Revolutionary Medicine* (n.p., 1976), 28.
2. John Bemrose, *Reminiscences of the Second Seminole War*, ed. John Mahon (Gainesville: University of Florida Press, 1966); J. Mann, *Medical Sketches of the Campaign of 1812–13–14*, (Dedham, England, 1816), 250.
3. William Hernsley Emory, *Lieutenant Emory Reports*, ed. Ross Calvin (Albuquerque: University of New Mexico Press, 1951), 171; see also, generally, Arthur Woodward, *Lances at San Pascual* (San Francisco: California Historical Society, 1948).
4. U.S. House of Representatives, *House Journal*, February 8, 1859, 359.
5. P.M. Ashburn, *A History of the Medical Department of the United States Army* (New York: Houghton Mifflin, 1929), 63.
6. Office of the Surgeon General, United States Army, *Medical and Surgical History of the War of the Rebellion*, Part 3, Vol. 2, *Surgical History* (Washington, D.C.: Government Printing Office, 1883), 931 et seq.
7. Russell, "The Civil War in America," *Philadelphia Inquirer*, July 30, 1861, 5.
8. "The French Ambulance System," *New York Times*, May 30, 1861, 8.
9. "Army Supplies [request for bids]," *Philadelphia Inquirer*, July 27, 1861, 5.
10. Peter N. Purcell and Robert P. Hummel, "Samuel Preston Moore: Surgeon General of the Confederacy," *American Journal of Surgery* 164, no. 4 (October 1992): 361, 362.
11. *Medical and Surgical History of the War of Rebellion*, Vol. 2, 931 et seq.
12. *The Ambulance System* (Boston: Crosby and Nichols, 1864).
13. "Ambulances," *Macon Daily Telegraph*, August 31, 1861, 3.
14. Alfred J. Bloor, *Letters from the Army of the Potomac* (Washington, D.C.: McGill, Witherow, Printers and Stereotypes, 1864), 19.
15. Ibid., 23.
16. Ibid., 24.
17. Ibid.
18. Ibid.
19. Vincent Bowditch, ed., *Life and Correspondence of Henry Ingersoll Bowditch*, Vol. 2 (Cambridge: Riverside Press, 1902), 10.
20. Ibid.
21. Edward Munson, "Transportation of Federal Sick and Wounded," in *Prisons and Hospitals*, Vol. 7 of *Photographic History of the Civil War*, ed. Holland Thompson (New York: Review of Reviews Co., 1911), 304, 306.
22. Gideon Welles, July 26, 1863, in *Diary of Gideon Welles*, Vol. 1 (Boston: Houghton, Mifflin, 1911), 384.
23. Bowditch, 5, 14.
24. Bowditch, 15.
25. Bowditch, 7, 9, 15.
26. A. Leahy, "Field Hospital Equipments—Class 37," *Illustrated London News*, August 31, 1867, 247.
27. United States Surgeon General's Office, "Ambulance Corps," in *Medical and Surgical History of the War of the Rebellion*, Part 3, Vol. 2 (Washington, D.C.: GPO, 1883), 935.
28. S.P. Moore to S.H. Stout, "Regarding the Ambulance Corps," Oct. 25, 1863, cited by Purcell.
29. Paul Slezdik, "Medicine and Surgery during the Civil War" (paper presented at the United States and Canadian Academy of Pathology 2003 Annual Meeting, Forensic Pathology Specialty Conference), www.uscap.org.
30. Deering Roberts, "Field and Temporary Hospitals," in *Prisons and Hospitals*, Vol. 7 of *Photographic History of the Civil War*, ed. Holland Thompson (New York: Review of Reviews Co., 1911), 258, 260.
31. Ibid.
32. *Georgia Weekly Telegraph*, June 13, 1862, 4.
33. Purcell, 1992.
34. *MacMillan's Magazine* 19, no. 87 (November 1868): 90.
35. See Bloor, 21, and "Jubilee," *New York Times*, October 17, 1865, 1.
36. Teresa Lehr and Phillip Maples, *To Serve the Community: A Celebration of Rochester General Hospital 1847–1997* (Virginia Beach: Donning Company, 1997).
37. "Philadelphia and the Soldiers," *Medical and Surgical Reporter* 9, no. 3 (December 27, 1862), 296.
38. *The Philadelphia Inquirer*, "A Beautiful Ambulance," January 26, 1863, 4.
39. "In Commemoration of The Great Parade of the Philadelphia Fire Department October 16th, 1865, Broad Street, under portrait of Chief Engineer D. M. Lyle," lithograph, James Queen, after a design by Schell (P. S. Duval & Son, 1865).
40 "Devoted to a New Purpose," *Philadelphia Inquirer*, July 31, 1865, 3 (orphanages); "Arm and Leg Bro-

ken," July 17, 1865, 2; "Accident at a Fire," August 21, 1865, 3. Reports of their use for emergency work continue to appear for the rest of the decade, as well.

41. "The Fire Department," *Philadelphia Inquirer,* January 27, 1868 (Globe sale); "Local Summary," April 24, 1871, 3 (Good Will Fire Company, sold ambulance to private party in Germantown).

42. "Annual Report of the Chief Engineer of the Fire Department," *The Philadelphia Inquirer,* February 18, 1870, 3; Fireman's Hall Museum (Philadelphia), "Historical Timeline: 1865," *Who We Are,* www.firemanshall.org.

43. "Ambulances for Washington," *Philadelphia Inquirer,* July 24, 1861, 8.

44. Benjamin Howard, "Hospital and Accident Ambulance Service for London," *The Lancet,* February 4, 1882, 174.

45. O.O. Howard, Preface, *Prisoners of Russia,* by Benjamin Howard (New York: Appleton and Co., 1902), v.

46. Ibid., vi.

47. Ibid., viii, and "Obituary," *Medical News* 77, no. 1 (July 7, 1900), 39.

48. O.O. Howard, viii.

49. Ibid.

50. Ibid., ix.

51. Ibid., x.

52. *New York Observer and Chronicle,* May 5, 1868, 150.

53. "A Humane Society," *New York Times,* May 15, 1873, 8.

54. *Literary World,* 1902, 117, and O.O. Howard, 1902, xii et seq. The latter suggests that Howard's proposal was immediately implemented in Paris, but this is not the case: even as late as 1883 advocates were still trying to establish an ambulance service in the capital, see "Dr. Henri Nachtel," *New York Times,* March 5, 1883, 4.

55. "A Hospital and Accident Ambulance Service," *The Lancet,* January 28, 1882, 155.

56. B. Howard, "Hospital," 174; *Times,* "Hospital Ambulance," December 21, 1881, 8.

57. B. Howard, 174.

58. Harrison.

59. Peter Alexander Young, "City Ambulance Associations," *Edinburgh Medical Journal* 30, no. 4 (October 1884): 297, 299.

60. *Literary World,* 1902, 117.

61. "Died," *New York Times,* June 23, 1900, 7. See also *Literary World,* 117 (cancer), and O.O. Howard, xviii.

Chapter 5

1. S.B. Nelson and J.M. Runk, *History of Cincinnati and Hamilton County* (Cincinnati, Ohio: S.B. Nelson & Co. Publishers, 1894), 361.

2. *Ordinance, Rules and Regulations for the Management of the City Infirmary and the Relief of the Out-Door Poor* (Cincinnati, Ohio: John D. Thorpe, Publisher, 1864). The hospital had been sharply criticized five years earlier in *Laws and Regulations for the Management of the City Infirmary, Commercial Hospital, Pest House, City Burying Ground and the Granting of Out-Door Relief to the Poor* (Cincinnati: Marshall and Hefley, 1859), after which the Commercial Hospital began publishing annual trustee reports, the better for city officials to keep track of its works.

3. *The Physicians and Surgeons of the United States,* ed. William Atkinson (Philadelphia: Charles Robson, 1878), 145; see also "Hospital History 1850–1880," *College of Medicine, University of Cincinnati: About COM* (2001), www.med.uc.edu/about/history/htmlversion/page 14.cfm (accessed May 2005).

4. *Board of Trustees, Sixth Annual Report of the Commercial Hospital of the City of Cincinnati* (Cincinnati, Ohio: Gazette Steam Book and Job Printing Establishment, 1867); "Accounts of the Commercial Hospital of Cincinnati, 1864 through 1865," holographic ledger, Cincinnati Medical Heritage Center, University of Cincinnati, uncatalogued.

5. *Board of Trustees, 12th Annual Report of the Cincinnati Hospital, for the 10 months ending December 31, 1872* (Cincinnati, Ohio: Gazette Steam Book and Job Printing Establishment, 1873).

6. University of Cincinnati, "College of Medicine History: 1850–1880."

7. B. Howard, 174.

8. "Brutal Inhumanity by a Woman," *The National Police Gazette* 22, no. 1113 (December 29, 1866): 4.

9. "Hand Ambulances for the Injured," *Brooklyn Eagle,* January 5, 1872, 3.

10. "Annual Report," *New York Times,* January 26, 1870, 6.

11. Edwin M. Knights, Jr., "Bellevue Hospital," *History Magazine,* no. 2 (Dec./Jan. 2000).

12. *Minutes of the Common Council, December 1734 and March 1736,* quoted in "Bellevue History/History of Bellevue Hospital," *Bellevue Literary Review Online,* 2001, www.blreview.org/bellevuehistory.htm.

13. "Warden's Report," *Board of Governors, First Annual Report, Board of Governors of the Alms House* (New York: Geo. F. Nesbitt, 1849), 32; *Fifth Annual Report, Governors of the Alms House* (New York: Jos. Harrison, 1854), 19.

14. John White, "Bellevue," *Fourth Annual Report of the Commissioners of Public Charities and Corrections* (New York: Frank McElroy, 1864), for quotation; Daniel Connolly, "Among the Inebriates," *Appleton's Journal of Literature, Science, and Art* 5, no. 117 (June 24, 1871): 738, for appearance of the street.

15. John Call Dalton, *Memorial of Edward B. Dalton, M.D.* (New York: n.p., 1872), 4.

16. Bliss Perry, *Life and Letters of Henry Lee Higginson* (Boston: Atlantic Monthly Press, 1921), 533.

17. "Board of Health," *New York Times,* January 3, 1867, 8.

18. B. Howard, 175.

19. *Memorial of Edward B. Dalton,* 42; Edward B. Dalton, "Annual Report of the Metropolitan Board of Health of New York, 1866," *North American Review* 106 (April 1868): 369.

20. George Leonard, "Ambulances for Civil Services," in *A Reference Handbook of the Medical Sciences,* ed. Albert H. Buck (New York: William Wood, 1885). While the handbook dates this event to 1868 (without attribution), Schultz said the incident occurred while he was president of the board, a position he resigned in early January 1868. Notably, on April 19th, 1867 (when Schultz was still president), the *New York Times* reported that a first mate was carried into New York Hospital with peritonitis after being shot by his captain, and it is likely that this was the actual event triggering Dalton's remark. Even though fifteen years later Schultz remembered the patient as being a captain, not a first mate, he is unlikely to have been mistaken about his own position at the time of the event, and the coincidence seems too great to ignore. See "The Ottawa Homicide," *New York Times,* April 19, 1867, 5; also "Board of Health," *New York Times,* January 10, 1868, 8 (Schultz's resignation).

21. Commissioners of Public Charities, New York City, "May 27: Reception Hospital," *Minutes of the Com-*

missioners of Public Charities and Corrections, Vol. 10 (New York: N.P., 1869).

22. Letter from James Beekman to Commissioner of Charities and Corrections, dated April 17, 1869, *Minutes*, Vol. 10, 240.

23. Ibid.

24. Ibid.

25. "May 27," *Minutes*, Vol. 10, 287.

26. Ibid., *Minutes*, Vol. 10, 288, 290.

27. "Commissioners of Charities and Corrections," *New York Times*, June 25, 1869, 2.

28. "June 19," *Minutes*, Vol. 10. In October they were replaced by G.R. Phillips and H.C. Gorham, in accordance with a schedule designed to seat new surgeons after the May and October graduations; see Thomas Brennan, "Bellevue Hospital, Annual Report," *Tenth Annual Report of the Commissioners of Public Charities and Correction* (Albany, N.Y.: Argus Co., 1870), 42.

29. "June 17," *Minutes*, Vol. 10.

30. "Communications," October 13, *Minutes*, Vol. 10.

31. Brennan, *Tenth Annual Report*, 38.

32. "City Ambulances," *New York Times*, July 24, 1869, 2.

33. "Rules for Casualty Cases," *Minutes*, Vol. 10, 293.

34. Ibid., 291.

35. Robert Carlisle, ed., *An Account of Bellevue Hospital* (New York: Society of the Alumni of Bellevue Hospital, 1893), 71.

36. *Tenth Annual Report*, 42; "September 22," *Minutes*, Vol. 10.

37. "At Bellevue," *Time*, November 7, 1927.

38. "Bellevue and Potter's Field," *New York Times*, April 7, 1872, 1.

39. Ibid.

40. In a macabre irony, these dogs were known to "do themselves what they will not allow others to do. The light covering of earth over the coffins is no protection, and these fierce quadrupeds dig down, and tearing open the frail coffins, every now and then enjoy a horrible banquet." Ibid.

41. Commissioners of Public Charities, *Eleventh Annual Report of the Commissioners of Public Charities and Corrections* (New York: New York Printing Co., 1871), 52.

42. Rochester City Hospital (New York), "The Ambulance Service of New York," *The Hospital Review* 28, no. 18 (January 16, 1893), 297.

43. *Tenth Annual Report*, 23.

44. "Report of the Warden," *Eleventh Annual Report*, 51.

45. "Report of the Medical Board of Bellevue Hospital," ibid., 72.

46. From *New York Times*: "Attempted Suicides," May 24, 1870, 2; "Crimes and Casualties," July 6, 1870, 3; "Serious Explosion," October 4, 1870, 5; "A Man Thrown Out of a Window by his Wife," October 5, 1870, 5.

47. Rochester City Hospital (New York), "With an Ambulance," *The Hospital Review*, 23, no. 8 (March 15, 1887).

48. Account based on eyewitness reports published in the *New York Times*: "Bloody Riot," July 13, 1870, 1, and "The Riot," July 14, 1870, 8.

49. "Bloody Riot."

50. "Report of the Warden," *Eleventh Annual Report*, 52.

51. Carlisle, 70.

52. *Eleventh Annual Report*, 52 et seq.

53. "Reception Hospitals," *New York Times*, March 18, 1874, 4.

54. "The Heat in New York," *Times*, August 12, 1870, 10. The paper described the infirmary as "the new Sunstroke and Accident Hospital in Centre-Street."

55. "Report of the Medical Board of Bellevue Hospital," *Eleventh Annual Report*, 71; see also "The Centre-Street Hospital," *New York Times*, January 6, 1873, 2.

56. Eli Ginzberg, "Philanthropy and Nonprofit Organizations in U.S. Healthcare," *Inquiry* 28, no. 2 (1991): 179.

57. B. Howard, 176.

58. "The Ambulance Service of New York," 297.

59. Warfield Firor, "Lord Lister," *Bulletin of the American College of Surgeons*, Jan./Feb. 1968, 26.

60. "In and About City Hall," *Brooklyn Daily Eagle*, September 24, 1870, 4.

61. "The Relapsing Fever District," *Philadelphia Inquirer*, May 16, 1870, 2.

62. "Philadelphia and Suburbs," *Philadelphia Inquirer*, September 3, 1872, 3.

63. *Philadelphia Inquirer*, August 26, 1874, 2.

64. Myron Metzenbaum, "Cleveland's Present Ambulance Service," *The Cleveland Medical Journal* 7, no. 7 (1908): 7.

65. David Andelman, "Ambulance Aid Found Deficient," *New York Times*, Aug. 19, 1973, 33.

66. Metzenbaum, 10.

67. Case Western Reserve University, Encyclopedia of Cleveland History, s.v. "Ambulance Services," www.ech.cwru.edu (accessed March 2004).

68. Metzenbaum, 9.

69. Ibid.

70. "Survey of Ambulance Service."

71. Raymond Van Zandt, "What 316 Patients Paid in Five Rochester Hospitals," *The Modern Hospital* 38, no. 6 (June 1932): 83.

72. "Editorial," *New York Times*, March 4, 1880, 4.

73. Ibid.

74. "The Night Medical Service in New York City," *The Medical and Surgical Reporter*, 44, no. 6 (February 5, 1881): 166.

75. For example, the *New York Times*:"Editorial," March 4, 1880, 4, and "Medical Night Calls," March 24, 1880, 8.

76. *New York Times*: "A Night Medical Service," July 1, 1880, 2, and "The Night Medical Service," September 5, 1880, 12.

77. "A Night Medical Service," July 1, 1880; see also "Night Medical Service," *New York Times*, August 26, 1880, 8 (hours available).

78. *New York Times*, March 5, 1883, 4.

79. "Night Medical Service," *New York Times*, February 1, 1882, 8.

80. "The Night Call Fund Exhausted," *New York Times*, July 19, 1892, 9.

81. *New York Times*, August 7, 1883, 4, blaming "French conservatism" for the delay.

82. *Brooklyn Eagle*, December 20, 1871, 4.

83. Brooklyn Board of Aldermen, "January 29," *Proceedings of the Board of Aldermen of the City of Brooklyn* (Brooklyn, 1872).

84. Brooklyn Board of Aldermen, "February 5," *Proceedings of the Board of Aldermen of the City of Brooklyn* (Brooklyn, 1872).

85. DeForest Willard, *Ambulance Service in Philadelphia* (Philadelphia: n.p., 1883).

86. Howard Sprogle, *The Philadelphia Police, Past and Present* (Philadelphia: n.p., 1887), 74.

87. Rochester City Hospital (New York), no title, *The Hospital Review* 25, no. 3 (October 15, 1888), 41.

88. Grover Sampson, "Reminiscences," January 8, 1940. ViaHealth Archives Consortium, Genesee Hospital Collection, Rochester, New York, TGH Series I: History, folder marked "Reminiscences."
89. Walt Bogdanich, "Death on the Tracks: How Railroads Sidestep Blame," *New York Times*, July 11, 2004, 1.

Chapter 6

1. Rochester Town Watch (New York), *Watch Book, No. 5* (Rochester: 1837); Rush Rhees Library, University of Rochester, Rochester, N.Y., Manuscript Collection (CX.126).
2. Ibid.
3. "The Mayor's Police Surgeons," *New York Times*, July 13, 1855, 3.
4. Ibid.
5. Ibid.
6. "The Police Surgeons," *New York Times*, July 30, 1855, 8. For details on Dr. Hasbrouck's political career, see James Brooks, *History of the Court of Common Pleas* (New York: Werner, Sanford & Co., 1896), 52, and, generally, F. Byrdsall, *The History of the Loco-Foco, or Equal Rights Party* (New York: Clement and Packard, 1842).
7. "Police Commissioners, Duties of Police Surgeons," *New York Times*, December 31, 1857, 3.
8. "The Ambulance Orders," *New York Times*, June 12, 1869, 2.
9. Ibid.
10. "The Ambulance System—Instructions to the Police," *New York Times*, June 18, 1869, 2.
11. "The Police Surgeons—Secret Meeting Held by Them Yesterday," *New York Times*, June 16, 1869, 8.
12. "How to Save Public Funds," *New York Times*, November 18, 1880, 3.
13. "Would Have Police Surgeon's Aid: Hospital Representatives Urge Co-operation to Relieve the Ambulance Service," *New York Times*, September 28, 1895, 13.
14. "Doctors for Emergency," *New York Times*, July 27, 1917, 10.
15. Based on estimate of 200,000 telephones nationwide. Russell Naughton, "2500 Years of Communication History: 1887," in *Adventures in Cybersound*, www.acmi.net.au/AIC/phd8400.html (accessed April 2004).
16. Sprogle, 212.
17. "The Weather," *The New York Times*, July 4, 1878, 5.
18. "Police Ambulance Class," *Times*, August 14, 1878, 10; also Sprogle, 74.
19. George Matsell, *Rules and Regulations for Day and Night Police of the City of New York* (New York: Casper Childs, 1846), Sections 96–98.
20. For example, John Bonfield, Pat. No. 379,266, March 13, 1888, and Edward Hutchinson, Pat. No. 546,855, April 24, 1895.
21. Emily Dunning Barringer, *Bowery to Bellevue* (New York: Norton, 1950), 158. In *Office Hours: Day and Night,* Dr. Janet Travell recalled that during her New York ambulance service in 1927, she held the rank of acting police lieutenant (New York: New American Library, 1968).
22. "Proposed Ambulance Service for London," *Times*, February 3, 1882, 7.
23. Ibid.
24. "A Horse Ambulance Service," *Times*, July 8, 1882, 5.
25. A.H. Haggard, "London Ambulance Service," *Times*, October 18, 1882, 4; see also Young, 289 (police stations).
26. Jeffrey Williamson, "The Structure of Pay in Britain: 1710–1911," *Research in Economic History* 7 (1982).
27. G.J.H. Evatt, *Ambulance Organization, Equipment, and Transport* (London: William Clowes and Sons, 1884).
28. London Metropolitan Police, "Timeline, 1850–1869," in *History of the Metropolitan Police*, www.met.police.uk/history/timeline1850–1869 (accessed November 2007).
29. "New Police Ambulance Litter," *Times*, August 15, 1878, 6.
30. City of London Police, "Police Ambulances," in *Museum,* www.cityoflondon.police.uk/history/history (accessed November 2007).
31. William F. Peck, *History of the Rochester Police Force* (Rochester, N.Y.: Police Benevolent Association, 1903), 210.
32. George W. Adams, *Doctors in Blue* (New York: Henry Schuman, 1952), 50–52.
33. Blake McKelvey, *Rochester Police Bureau, 1819–1969* (Rochester, N.Y.: Bureau of Police, 1969), and Peck, 210.
34. *Union Advertiser* (Rochester, N.Y.), December 10, 1890, 6.
35. Rochester (New York) Common Council, "Annual Report of Police Committee, Thursday, March 26," *Proceedings of the Common Council, 1890–91* (Rochester: Democrat and Chronicle Press, 1891).
36. Rochester (New York) Common Council, "Superintendent of Police Report, March 31 and August 23," *Proceedings of the Common Council 1891–92* (Rochester: Democrat and Chronicle Press, 1892).
37. Peck, 1903.
38. Rochester (New York) Common Council, "Police Clerk Report, September 7," *Proceedings of the Common Council Common Council, 1892* (Rochester: Democrat and Chronicle Press, 1893).
39. *Manufacturer and Builder,* "Average Wages," 24, no. 6 (1892), 124.
40. Rochester (New York) Common Council, "Annual Report of Police Committee, March 30," *Proceedings of the Common Council 1893* (Rochester: Democrat and Chronicle Press, 1894).
41. Rochester (New York) Common Council, *Proceedings of the Common Council, 1896* (Rochester, NY: Democrat and Chronicle Press, 1897).
42. Rochester (New York) Common Council, *Proceedings of the Common Council 1895* (Rochester: Democrat and Chronicle Press, 1896).
43. "Poor Committee," *Proceedings 1895*, February 27.
44. "December 29," *Proceedings 1896.*
45. Judy Thomson, Manager, Seattle Metropolitan Police Museum, email to author, January 27, 2004.
46. Francis D. Donohughe, "The Patrol Ambulance: An Adjunct to the Ambulance Service in Cities; A Substitute Therefore in Towns," *Boston Medical and Surgical Journal* 146, no. 19 (May 8, 1902): 481–84.
47. Ibid.
48. Cincinnati Police Department, "Honoring Our Heroes," www.cincinnati-oh.gov (accessed February 2003).
49. "Nassau Will Speed Heart Attacks Care," *New York Times*, May 18, 1970, 33.
50. "Heart Monitors Will Be Installed in Nassau Police Ambulances," *New York Times*, February 14, 1971, BQ86.
51. Rochester (New York) City Hospital, no title, *The Hospital Review* 35, no. 6 (January 16, 1899), 54.
52. "Ambulance Log, 1900" (holographic notebook), ViaHealth Archives Consortium (uncatalogued).

53. Metzenbaum, 12.
54. Charles Mackay, *Life and Liberty in America* (New York: Harper and Bros., 1859), 37.
55. C.M., "American Firemen," *Illustrated London News* 32, no. 899 (January 23, 1858), 94.
56. M.W. Thomas, *Police Communications* (Springfield, Ill.: C.C. Thomas, 1974).

Chapter 7

1. National Resident Matching Program, *Save the Match*, "What It Was Like before the Match," www.savethematch.org/history/before (accessed February 2004).
2. "City Ambulance Service: An Examination of the System, Which Admits Certain Imperfections in It and Asserts for It Manifold Merits," March 28, 1892, 9.
3. Early examples: "The Roosevelt Hospital Surgeons," *New York Times*, March 19, 1880: Police Surgeon alleges instances of ambulance surgeons refusing to accept seriously ill patients (lung hemorrhage; man who impaled thigh on chisel; woman in labor); "Someone to Blame," *New York Times*, November 24, 1880: ambulance late, surgeon refused to dress head wound of intoxicated prisoner.
4. "City Ambulance Service," 9.
5. Morton Galdston, "Ambulance Notes of Bellevue Hospital Intern," *Journal of Urban Health* 76, no. 4 (1999): 509.
6. "Wages for Internes," *Time*, September 30, 1935, online at www.time.com (accessed October 2006).
7. "Like a Bird," interview by Clarence Weinstock with unnamed ambulance driver, May 23, 1939, Library of Congress Online, "American Memory," American Life Histories: Manuscripts from the Federal Writer's Project, 1936–1940, http://memory.loc.gov/cgi-bin/query/D?wpa:2:./temp/~ammem_Ik2j (accessed November 2007).
8. Galdston, 509.
9. Ibid.
10. "City Takes Doctors from Ambulances—Hospital Attendants Replace Them as Ranks of Internes Are Depleted by War," *New York Times*, February 16, 1942, 13.
11. "City Ambulance Service ... Manifold Merits," *New York Times*, 9.
12. Rochester (New York) City Hospital, no title, *The Hospital Review* 26, no. 8 (March 15, 1900).
13. "Attendants to Continue on City's Ambulances," *New York Times*, January 25, 1948, 49.
14. Strouse, SM16.
15. Ibid.
16. United States Census Bureau, Decennial Census Abstracts 1940 and 1950 (population 1,889,924 in 1940 and 1,960,101 in 1950, exclusive of the Bronx and Queens).
17. Strouse, SM16.
18. Robert Brown, "What's the Matter with Internships?" *The Modern Hospital* 74, no. 3 (March 1950).
19. Ibid.
20. See, for example, 1950 Genesee Hospital (Rochester, N.Y.) Ambulance Protocol (interns to collect ambulance bag from surgery office and travel by taxi or ambulance to scene), ViaHealth Consortium Archives, Rochester, New York (uncatalogued); see also S.P. Lehman and K.H. Hollingsworth, "Ambulance Service in Seattle," *Public Health Reports* 75, no. 4 (1960): 343 (interns from Seattle City Hospital sent on emergency cases with ambulance).
21. "Physicians Dropped: Newark City Ambulances Will Have First Aid Attendants," *New York Times*, July 16, 1960, 17.
22. "A Brave Woman," *The Christian Recorder*, June 9, 1887.
23. "A Heroine," *The Christian Recorder*, August 20, 1864.
24. Barringer, 79.
25. Ibid., 99.
26. "Woman Ambulance Surgeon," *New York Times*, June 30, 1903, 2.
27. Ibid.
28. Barringer, 142
29. "Woman Surgeon Has First Call," *New York Evening World*, July 1, 1903 (Night Edition), 4.
30. Ibid.
31. "Doctor Emily on the Bus," *Sun*, July 2, 1903, 9.
32. Ibid.
33. "Dr. Dunning's Busy Day," *New-York Daily Tribune*, July 2, 1903, 7.
34. "Woman on the Ambulance," *New York Times*, April 24, 1902, 7.
35. "Won't Serve a Woman Doctor," *Evening World*, June 28, 1902, quoted in Barringer, 112.
36. Barringer, 133.
37. "Big Tenement Caves In," *New York Times*, September 18, 1903, 14.
38. "Cop Quinn Gets a Medal," *Sun*, August 6, 1903, 10.
39. Ibid.
40. Ibid.
41. "The Man in the Street," *New York Times*, July 26, 1903, SM1.
42. "Dr. Emily Dunning Surprised," *Sun*, December 20, 1904, 1.
43. "Good Wishes for Dr. Dunning," *Sun*, December 25, 1904, 6 (second edition).
44. Ibid.
45. David Lam, "Marie Marvingt and the Development of Aeromedical Evacuation," *Aviation, Space, and Environmental Medicine* 74, no. 8 (August 2003), 863.
46. "Marie Marvingt, Early Aviator, 88," *New York Times*, December 16, 1963, 33.
47. Lam, 866.
48. "Alice M'Lean, 82, of A.W.V.S. Is Dead," *New York Times*, October 27, 1968, 82.
49. "Women Drivers Needed," *New York Times*, August 24, 1942, 11; Shirley Alexander, "Riding to Trouble," *Colliers*, October 1942, 17.
50. Alexander, 17.
51. Ibid.
52. "Women Drivers Sought," *New York Times*, February 22, 1943, 14 (twelve hospitals served), and "Alice M'Lean" (volunteers at war's end).
53. "That Woman in Ambulance Is Doctor," *Democrat and Chronicle*, April 2, 1947.
54. Patricia Franks et al. "Emergency Medical Technicians and Paramedics in California," The Center for Health Professions, University of California, San Francisco, www.futurehealth.ucsf.edu/pdf_files/EMT14pfdoc.pdf (accessed August 2003).
55. Ibid.

Chapter 8

1. "News and Miscellaneous," *Medical and Surgical Reporter* 14, no. 8 (February 24, 1866): 159.
2. G.W.L. Nicholson, *The White Cross in Canada* (Ottawa: Runge Press, 1967).
3. "The Monastic Knights," *Littell's Living Age*, May 10, 1884, 324.
4. Quoted by Edgar E. Hume, "Medical Work of the Knights Hospitallers," *Bulletin of the Institute of the History of Medicine* 6, no. 4 (1938): 399.

5. Ibid.
6. Hume, 426.
7. E. J. King, *The Knights of St. John in the British Empire* (Bristol, England: John Wright and Sons, 1934), 177; see also John Pearn, "The Earliest Days of First Aid," *British Medical Journal* 309 (December 24, 1994): 1718.
8. King, 177.
9. Ibid. 178; see also Pearn, 1719 (description of litters), and Francis Duncan, "Hospitaller Work at St. John's Gate in 1880," *The Gentleman's Magazine* 247, no. 1798 (October 1880): 459 (distribution of hand ambulances).
10. Pearn, 1719; John E. Ransom, "Civilian Ambulance Service," *Ciba Symposia,* February 1947, 560. For the debate within the National Aid Society, see the remarks of Col. Brackenbury in "Proceedings of a Public Meeting Held on Wednesday Evening, February 6th, 1878, at the Pall Mall Restaurant," ed. Sir Edmund A.H. Lechemere (Woolwich, England: A.W. and A.P. Jackson, 1878).
11. Francis Duncan, quoted in "Proceedings of a Public Meeting." While Duncan does not give a precise date for the meeting, he says it occurred shortly before a dreadful bridge collapse in Bath—apparently referring to the Widcombe Bridge catastrophe of June 6, 1877, and placing the meeting in the late spring. See "Fall of a Bridge," *Times,* June 7, 1877, 10.
12. "Shocking Accident at Woolwich," *Daily Telegraph,* March 14, 1878, 1.
13. Francis Duncan, "The St. John Ambulance Association," *Times,* September 5, 1878, 6.
14. Young, 298; "St. John Ambulance Association," *Times,* February 17, 1881, 11.
15. "The St. John Ambulance Association," *The Gentleman's Magazine* 245, no. 1895 (November 1888): 435.
16. Ibid.
17. Sir John Furley, *In Peace and War* (London: Smith, Eden & Co., 1905), 280.
18. Sir John Furley, "A Horse Ambulance Service," *Times,* July 12, 1882, 4.
19. Ibid; see also O.O. Howard, xv.
20. Hume, 401. The idea of a horse ambulance service had first been proposed to the St. John Society around 1878 by Dr. Benjamin Howard, but nothing had come of it. See "A Hospital and Accident Ambulance Service," *The Lancet,* January 28, 1882.
21. Hume, 399.
22. Pearn, 1721.
23. "St. John Ambulance Association," *Times,* May 3, 1886, 11.
24. Ibid.
25. "Glasgow," *The Lancet,* May 6, 1882, 763. Similar complaints in Australia reached the highest levels of government, and threatened to derail the incipient Queensland ambulance service in the 1890s: see J. Pearn and M. Wales, "Dr. John Thompson," *The Medical Journal of Australia,* no. 1157 (7 December 1992): 774.
26. "The St. John Ambulance Association," *The Gentleman's Magazine* 245, no. 1895 (November 1888): 435, 441.
27. John F. Hutchinson, "Civilian Ambulances and Lifesaving Societies," in *Accidents in History: Injuries, Fatalities, and Social Relations,* ed. Roger Cooter and Bill Luckin (Atlanta, Ga.: Ridopi, 1997).
28. Charles S. Young, *Clara Barton, A Centenary Tribute* (Boston: Gorham Press, 1922), 255 et seq.
29. "A Practical and Simple Ambulance Service," *Daily Charlotte* (North Carolina) *Observer,* September 3, 1895, 4.

30. "Need for Emergency Hospital Again Forcibly Illustrated," *Oregon Journal,* April 12, 1907, 10.
31. "Emergency Hospital," *Oregonian,* December 19, 1913, 16.
32. "A Night in the Port of Broken Heads," *San Francisco Call,* May 1, 1910, 16.
33. Paul Scholten, "The San Francisco Emergency Ambulance Service," *San Francisco Medicine* 71, no. 9 (October 1998), http://www.sfms.org/sfm/sfm1098.htm (accessed September 2003).
34. Ibid.
35. James Fifield, ed., *American and Canadian Hospitals* (Minneapolis: Midwest Publishers Co., 1933).
36. Frank Cameron, "They Race Death Every Night," *The Saturday Evening Post,* January 3, 1953.
37. Ibid.
38. "Killed Four of His Relatives," *New York Times,* July 27, 1894, 9.
39. *Los Angeles Record,* August 18, 1906; Los Angeles Police Historical Society, "Transportation of the Sick and Injured," *The Link,* February 2001, www.laphs.com (accessed November 2003).
40. *Los Angeles Times,* "New Receiving Hospital Ready," August 29, 1927, A8; Joan A. Dektar, "Time Running Out for Landmark, Once Central Emergency Hospital," *Los Angeles Times,* August 28, 1988, 1.
41. "Man Mountain Sends Rival to Hospital," *Los Angeles Examiner,* August 16, 1934.
42. Dektar, 1988; see also Fifield, 1933.
43. Los Angeles Police Historical Society.
44. "Need for Emergency Hospital," *Oregon Journal,* and "Emergency Hospital," *Oregonian.*
45. "Emergency Hospital."
46. Ibid.
47. "Hospital," *Oregon Journal,* February 15, 1914, sect. 2, 7, and "Need for Emergency Hospital."
48. Jay Weaver, "History of the Boston Emergency Medical Services, 1891–1900," *Boston EMS,* www.bostonems.com/history.html (accessed March 2004).
49. Ibid.
50. Fifield, 1933.
51. In some hospitals there were no physicians in the ER at all: typical in the late 1960s and early 1970s was Providence Hospital in Anchorage, where an overhead page for "Dr. Brown to Emergency" was used when a physician was needed. When the call came over the loudspeakers, nurses were instructed to run to the exit doors to keep scurrying physicians from hiding in the parking lot until the all-clear sounded (Karen S. Bell, R.N., personal communication, May 2005); see also, J. Wiegenstein, "The Need for Training Physicians in Emergency Medicine," *Journal of Trauma* 12, no. 5 (May 1972): 375.

Chapter 9

1. Mark Theobald, "Frederick Wood," *Coachbuilt,* www.coachbuilt.com/bui/w/wood/wood.htm (accessed March 3, 2008).
2. "St. Vincent's Ambulance," *New York Tribune,* February 25, 1900, 2.
3. Ibid.
4. Thomas Pearson, *American Funeral Cars and Ambulances* (Glenn Ellyn, Ill.: Crestline Publishing, 1973).
5. "First Auto Ambulance for an Army Hospital," *New York Daily Tribune,* August 26, 1905, 5.
6. "Army Hospital."
7. Ibid.
8. Edward Dean, "Caring for Emergency Cases," *The Modern Hospital* 32, no. 4 (April 1929): 46.

9. David Rosner, "Portrait of an Unhealthy City," in *The Living City/NYC*, http://156.145.78.54/htm/living_city/development_lab/develop.htm (accessed March 2004).
10. Norman Maul, "Systematic Ambulance Service for Metropolitan Hospitals," *The Modern Hospital* 4, no. 1 (January 1915): 32.
11. *The Modern Hospital* 5, no. 6 (December 1915).
12. Ibid.
13. Maul, 33.
14. Waldon Fawcett, "The Cost of Operating a Motor Ambulance," *The Modern Hospital* 8, no. 1 (January 1917): 21.
15. *Carriage Monthly* 44 (May 1909): 79.
16. Fawcett, 21.
17. *The Modern Hospital* 8 (March 1917): 3.
18. *The Modern Hospital* 4 (February 1915): 2.
19. Travell, 152.
20. *The Modern Hospital* 4 (February 1915): 2.
21. Fawcett, 23.
22. *The Modern Hospital*, "Hints About Buying a Modern Ambulance," 7 (1916).
23. "Twelve Can Ride," *The Modern Hospital* 79, no. 4 (October 1952): 10.
24. Lehman and Hollingsworth, 343.
25. *The Modern Hospital* 17, no. 2 (February 1934): 44.
26. "Buck Ambulance Celebrates Six Decades," *AID*, March 1973.
27. "Obituary," *New York Times*, October 28, 1951, 84; U.S. Patents 693,822 and 980,780.
28. Rochester (New York) City Hospital, no title, *The Hospital Review* 40, no.11 (August 15, 1904): 108.
29. Ibid.
30. Albert Truby, U.S.A., "The Airplane Ambulance," in "History of the Airplane Ambulance," unpaginated typescript, 1922, prepared for the Office of the Chief of Air Service (National Library of Medicine, National Institute of Health, Bethesda, Maryland).
31. *The Modern Hospital* 1, no. 1 (September 1913): 67.
32. T.M. Gibson, "Samuel Franklin Cody: Aviation and Aeromedical Evacuation Pioneer," *Aviation, Space and Environmental Medicine* 70, no. 6 (June 1999): 612.
33. Truby, 1922.
34. Ibid.; see also *Scientific American*, "Winged Ambulance of the United States Army," December 7, 1918. Historians remain skeptical of claims that the French used balloons to evacuate the wounded in the Franco-Prussian War of 1870.
35. Truby, 1922.
36. M.D. Scholl and C.L. Geschekter, "The Zed Expedition: The World's First Air Ambulance?" *Journal of the Royal Society of Medicine* 82, no. 11 (November 1989): 679.
37. Mrs. Walter Hardy, "The Ardmore Ambulance Plane," *The American Journal of Nursing* 23, no. 3 (December 1922): 182.
38. *The Modern Hospital* 20, no. 4 (April 1923): 364.
39. Royal Flying Doctor Service of Australia, "The Birth of an Idea," in *Our History*, www.flyingdoctor.net/birth.htm (accessed January 21, 2007).
40. Royal Flying Doctor Service of Australia, "Aviation," in *Our History*, www.flyingdoctor.net/aviation.htm (accessed January 21, 2007).
41. Royal Flying Doctor Service of Australia, "Medicine," in *Our History*, www.flyingdoctor.net/medicine.htm (accessed January 21, 2007).
42. Royal Flying Doctor Service of Australia, "Facts at a Glance," in *Annual Report*, www.flyingdoctor.net/pastannual.htm (accessed February 24, 2008).
43. Don Paonessa, "The New Ambulance That Flies," *Better Homes and Gardens* 34, no. 1 (January 1956): 24.
44. Ibid.
45. "Drug Company Fits Helicopter for Emergency," *Los Angeles Times*, April 18, 1946, A1; see also an N.W. Ayer & Sonpress release ("First Helicopter Mercy Ship") typed on back of a photograph, Library of Congress Prints and Photographs Division, "Bell Aircraft Corporation,'" Lot 6010.
46. Paonessa, 27.
47. Ibid., 32.
48. Ibid., 28.
49. Carole Cooper and Mel Powell, "Chicago," in *Description and Analysis of Eighteen Proven Ambulance Service Systems,* Vol.1, National Association of Counties Research Foundation, 1968, 196.
50. Ibid., 199.
51. Ibid., 207.
52. Ibid., 196.
53. Robert Coleman, "Pennsylvania's Helicopter Ambulance Study," *Highway Research Record,* no. 272 (1969): 50–64, 50.
54. Ibid., 62, 64.
55. Ibid., 60.
56. James Hegarty, "AMES—Air Medical Evacuation System," *Police Chief*, June 1970, 22.
57. Ibid.
58. Aerospace Industries Association, *Directory of Hospital Heliports in the United States* (Washington, D.C.: Aerospace Industries Association, 1968).
59. University of Maryland Medical Center, "History," in *R Adams Cowley Shock Trauma Center,* www.umm.edu/shocktrauma/history.htm (accessed January 23, 2008).
60. Blaine Taylor, "Close Encounters of the Cowley Kind," *Maryland State Medical Journal* 27, no. 6 (1978): 35–49.
61. R Cowley et al. "An Economical and Proved Helicopter Program for Transporting the Emergency Critically Ill and Injured Patient in Maryland," *Journal of Trauma* 13, no. 12 (1973): 1029–38, 1032–35.
62. Ibid., 1035.
63. "On Using Swords as Plowshares," *Family* (Supplement to the *Army Times*), October 18, 1972.
64. Dustoff Association, "History," www.dustoff.org/newsletter (accessed April 2004).
65. Ibid.
66. Ibid.
67. Ibid.
68. Steven Acai and Herbert Proctor, "First Year of the North Carolina MAST Program," *Emergency Medical Services* 5, no. 6 (Nov./Dec. 1976): 15–25 (data collected from 1973–74).
69. Association of Air Medical Services, "Frequently Asked Questions about AAMS and Air Evacuation/Medevac," www.aams.org/Content/NavigationMenu/AboutAAMS/FrequentlyAskedQuestions/default.htm (accessed September 2007).
70. Jim Dowling, "Concord Coaches," Downing Family Historical Society, www.downingfamily.org/AbbotDowning (accessed September 2003).
71. MGH Hotline/Online, "First Horse Drawn Ambulance," Jan. 2001, www.mgh.harvard.edu/DEPTS/pubaffairs/Issues/01120lambulance (accessed September 2003).
72. Harrison.

Chapter 10

1. W. Schroeder, "History of the Ambulance System in Brooklyn, New York," *Brooklyn Medical Journal* 16 (1902): 381–95.

2. Michael Warren, "A Chronology of State Medicine, Public Health, Welfare and Related Services in Britain: 1066–1999," www.chronology.ndo.co.uk/1500-1699.htm (accessed September 2007).

3. John C. Sherman, "The Ambulance," *Munsey's Magazine* 18, no. 1 (October 1897):157

4. "A Board of Ambulances," *New York Times*, April 13, 1909, 8. See also, Nathan Bijur, "Social Significance of Ambulance Control," *The Survey* 22 (June 12, 1909): 404.

5. "Miller Wants City Owned Ambulances," *New York Times*, April 14, 1909, 7.

6. Maul, 33.

7. Shroeder.

8. Travell, 153.

9. Ibid., 143, 157.

10. "Are Ambulances Emergency Vehicles?" *Oregon Journal*, April 13, 1945.

11. Ibid.

12. "Death Heightens Controversy over Rein on Ambulance Operation," *Oregonian*, August 7, 1959, 19.

13. Ibid.

14. Ibid.

15. *The Modern Hospital* 27, no. 6 (December 1926): 101.

16. *The Modern Hospital* 29, no. 3 (September 1927): 60.

17. *The Modern Hospital* 27, no. 8 (February 1927): 75.

18. Ibid.

19. "Survey of Ambulance Service Shows ... It's Awful," *The Modern Hospital* 85, no. 2 (August 1955).

20. Dan Gowings, *Ambulance Attendant Training Manual* (Harrisburg: Penna. Dept. of Health, 1965)

21. George Curry and Sydney Lyttle, "The Speeding Ambulance," *American Journal of Surgery* 95 (April 1958): 507.

22. Irma West et al., "Study of Emergency Ambulance Operations—A Preliminary Report," typescript, 1964, prepared for the California State Department of Health and California State Highway Patrol (National Library of Medicine, National Institute of Health, Bethesda, Maryland).

23. John Erich, "Road Trauma," *Emergency Medical Services* 32, no. 6 (June 2003): 55; Bryan Bledsoe, "EMS Mythology, Part 4," *Emergency Medical Services* 32, no. 6 (June 2003): 72 (number of accidents); SL Proudfoot et al., "Ambulance Crash-Related Injuries among Emergency Medical Services Workers—United States, 1991–2002," *Journal of the American Medical Association* 289, no. 13 (April 2003): 1628 (number of deaths in ambulance crashes).

24. Centers for Disease Control and Prevention, "Ambulance Crash-Related Injuries among Emergency Service Workers—United States, 1991–2002," *Morbidity and Mortality Weekly Report* 52, no. 154 (2003): 154–55.

25. Proudfoot et al., 1630.

26. "LifeCare Emphasizes Safe Driving," *Emergency Medical Services* 32, no. 6 (June 2003): 68.

27. *Regulations Governing the Ambulance Service of all Hospitals in the City of New York* (New York: Board of Ambulance Services, 1919); "Manual Containing the Rules and Regulations of the Police Department of the City of Portland" (Portland, OR: Executive Board, 1903).

Chapter 11

1. *Scientific American Supplement*, Sept. 19, 1914.

2. "The Last Word in Motor Ambulances," *The Modern Hospital* 9, no. 5 (November 1917): 369.

3. "Telephones in Mine Rescue Work," *The Modern Hospital* 4, no. 6 (June 15, 1915): 451.

4. Ibid.

5. "Firemen Poisoned by Arsenic Fumes," *New York Times*, April 23, 1915, 6.

6. "Pulmotor Fire Squad Now," *New York Times*, January 19, 1915, 5.

7. "First Year's Record of the Fire Department's Rescue Squad," *New York Times*, March 5, 1916, X-5.

8. "Pulmotor Fire Squad Now" (crew size, gloves); "First Year's Record of the Fire Department's Rescue Squad."

9. "Ammonia Explodes," *New York Times*, April 27, 1915, 8; "War Gas Empties Rubber Laboratory," *New York Times*, September 8, 1915, 6; "Poisoned by Arsenic Fumes."

10. "Honors Eight Fire Heroes At Firemen's Parade," *New York Times*, June 13, 1915, 11.

11. J. Raymond Burger, "Meeting of Firemen's First Aid and Safety Squad (Minutes)," January 29, 1928 (referring to prior meeting, apparently January 22, when the squad chose its name, according to Prostem, below); see also William Evans, "Send Help ... Quick!" *Los Angeles Times*, February 23, 1941, J-8.

12. Evans, J-9.

13. David Prostem, "First Aid Squad Sets Events," *Newark Sunday News*, Section 1, 1967.

14. Secretary, First Aid and Safety Squad, March 19, 1928 (letter to commissioner of motor vehicles to request free automobile licensing for new ambulance); Grace Roper, *The Borough of Belmar in Retrospect* (Belmar, N.J.: Hoffman Press, 1978).

15. Asbury Park Press, "Shore First Aid Squad Organized," August 20, 1929; Evans, J-8.

16. Matt Chittum, "New Jersey Town Challenges Roanoke as Birthplace of the Volunteer Rescue Squad," *Roanoke Times*, February 10, 2002.

17. Roanoke E.M.S., "History," www.roanokeems.org/history.shtml (accessed April 2004).

18. Jack Kelly, "Rescue Squad," *American Heritage* 47, no. 3 (May/June 1996).

19. State of Delaware, Public Archives, "Historical Markers," in *First In the World: VFW Ambulance Service in Smyrna*, http://archives.delaware.gov/markers/kc/KC-67.shtml (accessed October 2007).

20. The sheer number of fire departments active in the late 19th century makes it nearly impossible to identify which has maintained the longest continuous ambulance service, but a likely contender is the Fame Volunteer Fire Department in Lewiston County, Pennsylvania, which purchased its first ambulance wagon in 1894. Fame Emergency Services, "History of Fame EMS," www.fameems.org/history.htm (accessed November 2007).

21. Stefan Timmermans, "Hearts Too Good to Die," *Journal of Historical Sociology* 14, no. 1 (March 2001), 111.

22. "Disaster Car Fund," *Oregonian*, March 29, 1963, 2.

23. "Committee Orders Baker Car," *Oregonian*, June 14, 1933; "First Aid Car Here Tuesday for Exhibit," clipping from Newberg, Oregon, newspaper, June 1935.

24. *News Telegram*, June 21, 1933.

25. Unidentified Oregon news clipping, "Demonstration of 1st Aid Here," June 1935.

26. "Gresham to Have First Aid Truck," unidentified newspaper clipping, circa August 29, 1935.

27. Personal Correspondence, Guy C. Weed (Member of the Portland Accident Prevention Committee) to the Officers and Members of the Townsend Old Age Pension Clubs, July 20, 1936 (Multnomah County Central Library, Portland, Oregon).

28. "Elks to Sponsor First Aid Car," unidentified newspaper clipping, Baker, Oregon, 1935; "First Aid Car Proposal Is Backed by Council Group," unidentified newspaper clipping, Salem, Oregon, 1935.
29. "Aaron Frank: Lawyer, Merchant, Engineer," *Lewis and Clark Chronicle* 8, no. 3 (Fall 1999).
30. Bureau of Fire (Portland, Oregon), "The Jay W. Stevens Disaster Unit," March 1939.
31. Don Porth, personal communication to author, March 11, 2008.
32. "Portland's 'Coffee Wagon' Comes of Age," *Oregonian*, March 10, 1940, Supp. 2; Edward Boatright, "A Municipal Truck for All Emergencies," *The American City*, June 1939, 108.
33. "Coffee Wagon."
34. Bureau of Fire.
35. *Mt. Adams Sun*, November 27, 1952.
36. D. Anderson, Warehouse Receipt, Office of the City Auditor, Property Control Division, May 9, 1972; see also Apparatus Service Record, unnumbered, March 11, 1971.
37. "Super Truck Is Added to Police Department's Fleet," *New York Times*, April 29, 1941, 21.
38. Ibid.
39. "Nothing Surprises Emergency Squads," *New York Times*, Feb. 6, 1949, 3.
40. "Emergency Services Squad," *Spring 3100*, April 1930.
41. Ibid.
42. "2 New Police Trucks Ready with Squads," *New York Times*, July 6, 1925, 1.
43. Ibid.
44. "Walter Klotzback, 88; Led Emergency Squad," *New York Times*, March 25, 1989, 11.
45. "Klotzback."
46. "Puts in 20 Hour Day," *New York Times*, December 22, 1929, 3.
47. Ibid.
48. S.J. Woolf, "A New Hand Guides the Police Force," *New York Times*, January 29, 1929, SM2.
49. "Whalen Abolishes Homicide Squad," *New York Times*, December 22, 1928, 1; Karl E. Smith, "Emergency Service Unit: A Historical Perspective," typescript, 1999 (New York City Police Museum); see also James J. McGuire, "New York City Police Department Emergency Service Division," typescript, n.d. (New York City Police Museum). Deputy Chief Inspector McGuire was the head of the ESD from 1928 until 1967. He died in 1988.
50. See K. Smith, McGuire.
51. "Less Violent Crime Recorded by Police," *New York Times*, April 13, 1931, 12; "Unusual Emergencies Find the Police Ready," *New York Times*, Dec. 25, 1932, 22.
52. Police Commissioner Mulrooney, "Report of Police Work of the Year 1931," as quoted by K. Smith.
53. "Nothing Surprises."
54. Emmanuel Perlmutter, review of *Emergency!* by Norman Lobsenz, *New York Times*, Dec. 7, 1958; "Nothing Surprises."
55. "Unusual Emergencies."
56. Ibid.
57. Ibid.
58. Ibid.
59. "Nothing Surprises."
60. "New Emergency Patrol Cars," *New York Times*, Oct. 25, 1961, 29.
61. John P. Shanley, "Real-Life Adventures of 2 Patrolmen," *New York Times*, Feb. 19, 1962, 49; "Dupont Show of the Week," *TV Tome*, http://www.tvtome.com (accessed April 2004).
62. Shanley.
63. Kevin Reynolds, interview by author, November 29, 2006.
64. Larry Shapiro, *Special Police Vehicles* (Osceola, Wis.: MBI Publishing, 1999).
65. Leahy.
66. Ibid.
67. Thomas Evans, "A Report on Class XI, Group II, Paris Exposition 1867" (Paris: E. Briere, 1867).
68. Albert Shaw, "Notes on City Government in St. Louis," *Century Illustrated Magazine* 52, no. 2 (1896): 253.
69. *Hub*, March 1895, 876.
70. Walter McCall, *The American Ambulance, 1900–2001* (Hudson, WI: Iconografix, 2002), 40.
71. Rolland Jerry, "Cunningham Firm Set Its Sights on the Gun-Shy Carriage Trade," in *The Best of Old Cars*, Vol. 1 (Iola, Wis.: Krause, 1978), 222.
72. Cooper, "Baltimore," 5.
73. Mike Margerum, interview by author, December 4, 2005.
74. Ibid.
75. Ibid.
76. Ibid.
77. Cooper, 15.
78. Ibid.
79. "Specialty Ambulance for the Obese," *Oregonian*, February 5, 2003.

Chapter 12

1. C. Rufus Rorem, "Why Hospital Costs Have Risen" (Washington, D.C.: Chamber of Commerce, 1950), reprint of article from *American Economic Security*, August-September 1950.
2. Virginia Association of Volunteer Rescue Squads, "Members," www.vavrs.com (accessed September 2003).
3. "How Good Is Your Emergency Room?" *The Modern Hospital* 83, no. 6 (December 1954): 61.
4. "Ambulance Services," *The Modern Hospital* 85, no. 5 (November 1955): 47; "Hospitals Report Ownership and Operation of Trucks, Ambulances, Passenger Cars," *The Modern Hospital* 88, no. 3 (March 1957): 160.
5. "Moss Funeral Home Celebrates 50 Years," *Breese Journal*, Feb. 6, 2003.
6. "Survey of Ambulance Service Shows ... It's Awful," *The Modern Hospital* 85, no. 2 (August 1955).
7. Ibid.
8. "Committee Proposes Public Ambulance Service," *The Modern Hospital* 51, no. 5 (Nov. 5, 1938): 106.
9. King County Hospital Trustees, "Emergency Department," *Annual Report of Harborview Hospital, 1933* (Seattle, Wash., 1934).
10. Sheppard Remington, "What Is Due the Accident Patient?" *The Modern Hospital* 47, no. 1 (July 1936): 75.
11. "Survey of Ambulance Services."
12. Ibid.
13. "One Agency Urged for Ambulances," *New York Times*, Nov 28, 1950, 50.
14. "Survey of Ambulance Services."
15. Ibid.
16. Ibid.
17. Ibid.
18. "One Agency Urged."
19. Ibid.
20. Alan G. Hevesi, "Where Do 911 System Ambulances Take Their Patients? Differences between Voluntary Hospital Ambulances and Fire Department Ambulances" (City of New York, Office of the Comptroller, June 2001); Sharon Lerner, "Ambulance Wars: How Private Ambulance Crews Steer Patients away From Public Hospitals," *Village Voice*, June 27, 2001.

21. "Don't Overlook the Ambulance as a Public Relations Tool," *The Modern Hospital* 79, no. 9 (September 1950).
22. "64 Hospitals Seek Immediate Aid," *New York Times*, December 8, 1952, 43.
23. Murray Illson, "4 Hospitals Plan New Ambulance Runs," *New York Times*, January 31, 1964, 39.
24. "Don't Overlook the Ambulance."
25. "Hospitals of Nation Facing Huge 3-Fold Task in Crisis," *New York Times*, Jan 29, 1951, 1.
26. Rochester Common Council (New York), *Proceedings of the Common Council* (1953): Rochester City Ordinances 52-257 and 52-253.
27. "White Car to the Rescue," *The Modern Hospital* 83, no. 5 (November 1954): 10.
28. "Operation Ostrich: Is Mass Evacuation Strictly for the Birds?" *The Modern Hospital* 87, no. 3 (September 1956): 74.
29. *The New York Times:* "30 Die" and "Scenes at Los Angeles," January 23, 1956, 1.
30. Robert J. Cole, "Cost of Ambulance Service Is Rising across Country (Personal Finance)," *New York Times*, June 26, 1969, 55.
31. Richard Weingroff, "President Dwight D. Eisenhower and the Federal Role in Highway Safety, Chapter One," in Federal Highway Administration, *Highway History*, www.fhwa.dot.gov/infrastructure/safety01.htm (accessed January 2007).

Chapter 13

1. Geoffrey Gibson, "Emergency Medical Services," in "Health Services: The Local Perspective," special issue of *Proceedings of the Academy of Political Science* 32, no. 3 (1977): 121–35. Somewhat confusingly, in 1969 the Public Health Service took the vintage Cold War "Division of Health Mobilization" (whose mission included teaching a first aid course similar to the Red Cross program, but intended to be used by survivors of a nuclear attack in the absence of organized facilities) and renamed it the Division of Emergency Health Services. While broadly consistent with its previous efforts to disseminate first aid education, its new mandate overlapped that of sister agencies in the Department of Transportation and Health, Education and Welfare and is emblematic of the bureaucratic confusion plaguing early federal efforts in the field.
2. Julian Waller, "Reflections on Half a Century of Injury Control," *American Journal of Public Health* 84, no. 4 (April 1994): 664, 666.
3. President's Committee for Traffic Safety, *Health, Medical Care and Transportation of the Injured* (Washington, D.C.: U.S. GPO, 1965).
4. Alexander Kuehl, ed. *Prehospital Systems and Medical Oversight* (Dubuque, Ia.: Kendall Hunt, 2002), 10.
5. Lyndon Johnson, "State of the Union," January 12, 1966. "Speeches and Messages," Lyndon Baines Johnson Library and Museum, www.lbjlib.utexas.edu (accessed February 18, 2008).
6. Highway Safety Act, 1966. Public Law 89-564 (23 USC Chapter 4, Section 401 et seq.)
7. National Academy of Sciences, National Research Council, *Accidental Death and Disability: The Neglected Disease of Modern Society* (Washington D.C.: National Academy Press, 1966).
8. "Ambulance Operation," *Mortuary Management*, October 1958, 16.
9. Department of Health, Education and Welfare, *Ambulance Services and Hospital Emergency Departments,* DHEW Publication No. (HSM) 72-2022. Data collected 1968–71 (Washington, D.C.: United States Printing Office, 1972).
10. California Ambulance Association, *National Ambulance Directory* (Chicago: Albert Carriere, 1962).
11. Department of Health, Education and Welfare.
12. Cooper, 50.
13. Committees on Trauma and Shock, National Academy of Sciences/National Research Council, *Accidental Death and Disability: The Neglected Disease of Modern Society* (Washington, D.C.: National Academy of Sciences, 1966).
14. "Texas Cities Take Over Ambulance Services as Undertakers Quit," *The Modern Hospital* 109, no. 1 (July 1967): 174.
15. "Texas Ambulance Crisis Growing," *The Modern Hospital* 113, no. 5 (November 1969): 38.
16. Ibid.
17. "Survey Shows Decrease in Private Ambulances," *The Modern Hospital* 109, no. 4 (October 1967): 216.
18. Geoffrey Gibson, 123. See also 23 Code of Federal Regulations 204 (1966), Standard 11.
19. *Bulletin of the American College of Surgeons* 52, no. 92 (1967): 131; U.S. Dept. Health, Education and Welfare: Division of Emergency Health Services, *Compendium of State Statutes on the Regulation of Ambulance Services, Operation of Emergency Vehicles and Good Samaritan Laws*, Pub. 1071-A11 (Washington, D.C.: U.S. GPO, June 1969).
20. Norman McSwain et al. "Deke," *The EMT Journal* 2, no. 4 (December 1976): 41–44, 43.
21. McSwain, 42.
22. J.D. Farrington, "Death in a Ditch," *Bulletin of the American College of Surgeons* 5, no. 3 (May/June 1967): 121–30, 121; see also Cooper, 198.
23. Ibid., 121.
24. Ibid., 123.
25. "Community Training Program," *Bulletin of the American College of Surgeons*, July/Aug. 1968, 178.
26. Farrington, 1967, 126.
27. J.D. Farrington and Oscar Hampton, "A Curriculum for Training Emergency Medical Technicians," *Bulletin of the American College of Surgeons*, Sept./Oct. 1969, 273–75.
28. J.F. Pantridge and J.S. Geddes, "A Mobile Intensive Care Unit in the Management of Myocardial Infarction," *Lancet* 2, no. 7510 (August 5, 1967): 271.
29. Phillip Hallen, interview by author, October 18, 2005.
30. Ibid.
31. John Capitman, "Emergency Care Challenged," *Pittsburgh News*, May 1, 1973.
32. Phil Hallen, "Preliminary Thoughts on the Development of a Private Ambulance Service in the Hill District," February 21, 1967, typescript (records of the Maurice Falk Medical Fund, 1960–1994, MSS 204, Historical Society of Western Pennsylvania).
33. Richard Long, "Ambulance Service Comes to the Inner City," Office of Economic Opportunity, July 1971 (two non-profits, the Hill House Emergency Lift Program and the Adult Day Care Program, used vans and cars to transfer 2,600 residents annually to medical appointments and scheduled hospital admissions). See also Freedom House Enterprises Ambulance Service Committee, "Background Material: Need for Services," typescript, circa 1967 (Freedom House material from the records of the Maurice Falk Medical Fund, 1960–1994, MSS 204, Historical Society of Western Pennsylvania).
34. Hallen, "Preliminary Thoughts."
35. Ibid. See also "Community Concern Sparks Am-

bulance Service," *The Modern Hospital*, 113, no. 2 (August 1969): 93.

36. Hallen, interview by author, December 4, 2007.

37. Freedom House Ambulance Committee, "Minutes," typescript, June 3, 1967 (records of the Maurice Falk Medical Fund, 1960–1994, Western Pennsylvania Historical Society).

38. Freedom House Ambulance Committee, "Meeting with Dr. Safar," typescript, June 15, 1967 (records of the Maurice Falk Medical Fund, 1960–1994, Western Pennsylvania Historical Society).

39. Ibid.

40. Freedom House Ambulance Service Committee, "Minutes," typescript, June 17, 1967 (records of the Maurice Falk Medical Fund, 1960–1994, Western Pennsylvania Historical Society).

41. Freedom House Ambulance Service, "Establishment Proposal," typescript, 1967 (Maurice Falk Medical Fund, 1960–1994, Western Pennsylvania Historical Society); *Pittsburgh Post-Gazette*, "Full Ambulance Service," July 2, 1968 (city contribution).

42. James O. Page, *The Paramedics* (Morristown, N.J.: Backdraft Publications, 1979).

43. "Community Concern."

44. George Cheever, "Freedom House Ambulance Service," *University Times*, July 23, 1970, 7; see also D. Benson and G. Esposito, "Mobile Intensive Care by 'Unemployable' Blacks Trained as Emergency Medical Technicians in 1967–69," *Journal of Trauma* 12, no. 5 (May 1972): 408.

45. Roger Stuart, "Ex-Jobless Rushing to Rescue," *Pittsburgh Press*, November 11, 1968.

46. Benson and Esposito.

47. Ibid.

48. Ibid.

49. Ibid.

50. Hallen, 2005 interview.

51. Cheever.

52. Roger Stuart, "Ambulance Score," *Pittsburgh Press*, January 11, 1970.

53. Dolores Frederick, "Telemetry Keeps Doctor, Emergency Unit in Touch," *Pittsburgh Press*, July 25, 1972.

54. Dolores Frederick, "Doctor Can Write Book on Ambulance Emergencies," *Pittsburgh Press*, August 17, 1975.

55. Roger Stuart, "Ex-Jobless to the Rescue," *Pittsburgh Press*, November 17, 1968.

56. Ibid.

57. Ibid.

58. Long.

59. Cheever.

60. "Begin OEO Program for Ambulance Drivers," *Pittsburgh Courier*, March 8, 1969; Dale McFeatters, "Super Ambulances Make Debut Here," *Pittsburgh Press*, April 8, 1969 (Safar quote); "Unemployables Provide Service," *Pittsburgh Post-Gazette*, April 9, 1969; Cheever.

61. Stuart.

62. Dolores Frederick, "Ambulance Training Setup OK with FOP," *Pittsburgh Press*, May 3, 1973.

63. Dolores Frederick, "Too Often Distress Call Brings Ride to Eternity," *Pittsburgh Press*, July 23, 1972.

64. Cheever.

65. Ibid.

66. Dolores Frederick, "District Lets Medical Service Funds Slip Away," *Pittsburgh Press*, July 27, 1972.

67. "Hunt, Pitt Doctor Trade Views in City Ambulance Battle," *Pittsburgh Press*, May 6, 1973, A-22.

68. Dolores Frederick, "City's 5 'Super Ambulances' Ready for Road, but Await Plan," *Pittsburgh Press*, August 18, 1975.

69. Aki Mukaili, "Freedom House—Mobile Medicine's Best," *Pittsburgh Courier*, December 1, 1973.

70. Ibid.

71. Thomas Hritz, "Flaherty Calls Pitt Blast on Ambulances Political," *Pittsburgh Post-Gazette*, April 28, 1973.

72. Ibid.

73. Ibid.

74. "Hunt, Pitt Doctor Trade Views," 1973.

75. Dolores Frederick, "City Easing Its Ambulance Stand," *Pittsburgh Press*, May 30, 1973; Henry Pierce, "Colville Okays 3 Steps to Improve Ambulances," *Pittsburgh Post-Gazette*, May 30, 1973; *Pittsburgh Post-Gazette*, "Ambulance Radio Net Gets County Support," July 27, 1973.

76. Karolyn Schuster, "Freedom House Tells Staffers of Phase-Out," *Pittsburgh Post-Gazette*, May 30, 1974.

77. Ibid.

78. Ibid.

79. Robert Flipping, Jr., "City Policemen to Assume Freedom House Tasks," *Pittsburgh Courier*, June 8, 1974.

80. Frederick, "5 Super Ambulances;" *Pittsburgh Post-Gazette*, "Emergency Care at Last," September 5, 1975.

81. Al Donaldson, "Superambulance Police Image Said to Lack Warmth," *Pittsburgh Press*, October 24, 1975.

82. "Born in Freedom," *Facets* (University of Pittsburgh School of Health and Rehabilitation), Fall 2003.

83. Hallen, 2005 interview.

84. Nancy L. Caroline, *Emergency Care in the Streets* (Boston: Little, Brown, 1979).

85. Ibid.

86. Anita Srikameswaran, "Obituary," *Pittsburgh Post-Gazette*, December 21, 2002.

87. Hallen, 2005 interview.

88. Ayward Clontz, interview by author, October 8, 2007; Charlene Howell, interview by author, September 12, 2007.

89. Marty Stamey, interview by author, September 10, 2007.

90. U.S. Bureau of the Census, *Census of the Population: 1960*, Vol. 1, Part 35, North Carolina (Washington, D.C.: U.S. GPO, 1963).

91. Stamey.

92. Clontz.

93. Howell.

94. E.B. Goodwin, interview by author, September 21, 2007.

95. Stamey.

96. Goodwin.

97. Page.

98. Stamey, Goodwin.

99. Goodwin.

100. Page.

101. Clontz.

102. Stamey.

103. Page.

104. Goodwin.

105. Clontz.

106. Page.

107. Howell.

108. Walter Brooks, Captain, Haywood County Rescue Society, interviewed by author, October 9, 2007.

109. Page; Jim Hirshmann and Eugene Nagel, "Prehospital Emergency Care in Miami, Florida, A Historical Commentary," *Journal of the Florida Medical Association* 68, no. 8 (August 1981): 624.

110. Ibid.
111. E.L. Nagel et al., "Telemetry of Physiologic Data," *Southern Medical Journal* 61, no. 6 (June 1968): 598; Page.
112. Ibid.
113. Mickey Eisenberg, *Life in the Balance* (New York: Oxford University Press, 1997), 227.
114. Clontz.
115. Nagel et al.
116. Hirschman and Nagel.
117. Ibid.
118. Ibid.
119. Digby Diehl, "The Emergency Medical Services Program," in *To Improve Health and Health Care 2000*, ed. Stephen Issacs and James Knickman (San Francisco: Jossey-Bass, 2000), www.rwjf.org/files/publications/books/2000/chapter_10.htm (accessed February 2004).
120. Hirschmann and Nagel.
121. Eisenberg, 242.
122. Ibid., 239
123. Ibid., 239.
124. Ibid., 240.
125. Cooper, 178.
126. Ibid.
127. Cooper, 177.
128. Ibid.
129. Eisenberg, 235.
130. Ibid., 236.
131. Ibid., 238.
132. Cooper, 178.
133. Eisenberg, 243.
134. Lou Gomolak, "Hot Wheels: New York Hospital's Mobile ICU," *The Modern Hospital* 120, no. 6 (June 1973): 95.
135. Ibid.
136. Richard Keller, "EMS in the United States," *Journal of Emergency Medical Services*, 1989, 74–85, 75.
137. Nancy Caroline, "Will the Real Paramedic Please Stand Up?" *Emergency Medical Services* 6, no. 2 (March/April 1977): 16.
138. Ibid., 16 et seq.
139. Ibid., 85.
140. Committee on Trauma and Shock, 15.
141. Division of Medical Services, National Academy of Sciences–National Research Council, *Summary Report of the Task Force on Ambulance Services* (Washington, D.C., 1967), 3.
142. John Baerwald, "The Interdisciplinary Development of Ambulance Design Criteria," *Highway Research Record* 332 (1970): 54–62, 55.
143. Ibid., 59.
144. Ibid., 57.
145. John Collins, M.B., "Organization and Function of an Accident Flying Squad," *British Medical Journal* 2, no. 513 (September 3, 1966): 578–80; R. Snook, "Accident Flying Squad," *British Medical Journal* 3, no. 826 (September 2, 1972): 569, 571.

Chapter 14

1. Merlin DuVal, "The Federal Role in E.M.S." *Emergency Medical Services* 2, no. 1 (January/February 1973): 12.
2. Richard Lepper et al. "An Overview of Rural EMS," *Emergency Medical Services* 4, no. 5 (September/October 1975): 27.
3. Andelman, 33.
4. The Robert Wood Johnson Foundation, "Neglected for Years, Emergency Medical Services Now Seem to Be Catching on in the U.S.," in *To Improve Health and Health Care*, Vol. 3 (November 1977): 7.
5. Cooper, Vol. 1, "Chicago."
6. William Jones, "Men of Mercy? Profit in Pain," *Chicago Tribune*, June 7, 1970, 1, 2.
7. William Jones, "Ambulances' Crews Pilfer Hospital Goods for Supplies," June 12, 1970, 1, 2.
8. Jones, "Crews Pilfer," 2.
9. Jones, "How Ambulances Pay Off the Police," *Chicago Tribune*, June 10, 1970, 2.
10. Jones, "Profit in Pain," 2.
11. Jones, "Pay Off Police," 2.
12. Jones, William Jones, "Sadism Rides the Ambulance," *Chicago Tribune*, June 8, 1970, 2.
13. Jones, "Heart Victim Left in Flat," *Chicago Tribune*, June 9, 1970, 1.
14. Jones, "Sadism," 2.
15. Ibid.
16. Ibid.
17. William Jones, "Ex-State Official Inflates Costs for Ambulances' Welfare Clients," *Chicago Tribune*, June 11, 1970, 1.
18. Jones, "Inflates Costs," 2.
19. Ibid.
20. William Jones, "3 Ambulance Firms Banned in Aid Cases," June 11, 1970, 2.
21. Gomolak, 95.
22. California Fire Chiefs Association, "The Foundations of Emergency Medical Services," www.calchiefs.org/items/Foundations_of_EMS.doc (accessed March 22, 2008).
23. Jim Page, "One of the Boys," *Journal of Emergency Medical Services,* January 1983, 110.
24. Ibid.
25. Ibid.
26. "On Using Swords as Plowshares."
27. John Perkins, "Commentary," *Emergency Medical Services* 6, no. 1 (Jan./Feb. 1977), 80.
28. Richard Lepper, et al. "An Overview of Rural EMS," *Emergency Medical Services* 4, no. 5 (Sept./Oct.): 26.
29. University of California, Santa Barbara. The American Presidency Project, Documents: Document Archive, State of the Union Messages, Nixon, 1972. www.presidency.ucsb.edu/sou.php
30. J.M. Chaiken and R. J. Gladstone, *Some Trends in the Delivery of Ambulance Service* (Santa Monica, Calif.: Rand Corporation, 1974).
31. Chaiken and Gladstone.
32. Margaret O'Leary, *A Historical Overview of EMS System Development in the U.S.: The 1960s and 1970s,* Suburban Emergency Management Project, Biot 246, August 6, 2005, www.semp.us/publications/biot_reader.php?BiotID=246IOT (accessed January 23, 2008).
33. Gerald Looney, "Getting What We Pay For," *Journal of Emergency Medical Services* 6, no. 6 (1973: 14.
34. Patrick Storey, "The Challenge of the Skoraya," *Journal of Trauma* 13, no. 5 (1973): 482–83.
35. Ibid., 252.
36. David Boyd, "A Systems Approach to EMS," *Emergency Medical Services* 6, no. 6 (1977): 93–104, 93.
37. 1974 NBC Press Release, from Emergencyfans.com, Show Info, "About the Production," www.emergencyfans.com/general_info/show_info.htm (accessed March 22, 2008).
38. O'Leary.
39. Linda Leddy. "The Quality of EMS," *Emergency Medical Services* 6, no. 3 (1977): 8, 13.
40. Ronald Hollaway and Linda Orzeck, "The Changing Focus of Pre-Hospital Care," *Emergency Medical Services* 6, no. 3 (1977): 36.

41. O'Leary.
42. Ibid.
43. Alan Cranston, "The Emergency Medical Services Systems Act—What to Expect in 1978," *Emergency Medical Services* 6, no. 6 (1977): 91.
44. O'Leary, 2005.
45. Fred Vogt, "Open Memorandum: Standards," *Emergency Medical Services* 4, no. 1 (1975): 12.
46. Kuehl, 11.
47. LeRoy Pope, "Federal Aid to the Rescue of Ambulances," *Chicago Daily Defender*, March 31, 1975, 7.
48. Donald Buchholz, "An Individualized Approach to EMS," *Emergency Medical Services* 4, no. 1 (1975): 46.
49. Teresa Romano et al. "Nationwide Paramedic Clearinghouse," *Emergency Medical Services* 6, no. 5 (1977): 41.
50. British Columbia Ambulance Service, "Brief History," www.healthservices.gov.bc.ca (accessed March 12, 2008).
51. British Columbia Ambulance Service, "Paramedics Help Increase Cardiac Arrest Survival Rates," *News*, www.health.gov.bc.ca/bcas/news/2007/1214_cardiac.pdf (accessed March 23, 2008).
52. Kuehl, 11.
53. Government Accounting Office, *States Assume Leadership Role in Providing Emergency Medical Services*, GAO/HRD-86-132, 1986.
54. Gerald Looney, "Getting What We Pay For," *Journal of Emergency Services* 6, no. 6 (1977): 14, 30.
55. Lynn Cooper and Alisdair Conn, "Regionalization and Designation of Medical Facilities," in *Prehospital Systems and Oversight*, ed. Alexander Kuehl (Dubuque, Ia.: Kendall Hunt, 2002).
56. American Medical Response, "Corporate Profile," www.amr.net/company/profile.asp (accessed March 9, 2008).
57. National Highway Traffic Safety Administration, *EMS Agenda for the Future* (Department of Transportation: 1996), 23.
58. Charles Champlin, "Mother, Jugs a Basket Case," *Los Angeles Times*, May 26, 1976, G-14, G-15.
59. "Bringing Out the Dead: Daily Chart Record," *The Numbers*, www.the-numbers.com/movies/1999/BRING.php (accessed March 12, 2008)
60. "Episodes," *240-Robert*, www.240-robert.com (accessed March 12, 2008).
61. John Waters, "Am I My Brother's Keeper?" *Journal of Emergency Services* 6, no. 6 (1973): 24.

Chapter 15

1. Representative Bart Stupak, "9-11 Tapes Reveal Communication Chaos, Stupak Stresses Need for First Responder Interoperability," August 15, 2005, www.house.gov/list/press/mi01_stupak/081505interop.html (accessed February 12, 2008). For more specifics, see 9/11 Commission, *9/11 Commission Report*, Chapter 9, "Analysis," Section 4.9: *Radio Communication Difficulties* (Washington, D.C.: U.S. GPO: 2004).
2. Department of Homeland Security, SAFECOM, *About SAFECOM*, "Frequently Asked Questions," www.safecomprogram.gov/SAFECOM/about/default.htm (accessed February 12, 2008).
3. Public Safety Wireless Network Program Survey (2005), quoted in Institute of Medicine, Committee on the Future of Emergency Care in the United States Health System, *Emergency Medical Services: At the Crossroads* (Washington, D.C.: National Academies Press, 2007), 164.
4. Wireless Survey, 164.
5. Champion, et al. *Emergency Medical Services, The Forgotten First Responder: A Report on the Critical Gaps in Organization and Deficits in Resources for America's Medical First Responders* (New York: Center for Catastrophe Preparedness and Response, New York University, 2005).
6. Bureau of Labor Statistics for 2006 report 293,000 firefighters (exclusive of administrative staff), 861,000 police and detectives (including first line supervisors), and 201,000 paid paramedics and EMTs. During the same year there were an estimated 500,000 volunteer EMTs and paramedics and approximately 800,000 volunteer firefighters. It is reasonable to assume that a number of volunteer firefighters are cross-trained as EMTs, and with a conservative estimate of 10 percent overlap between the two volunteer groups, the total percentage of EMT first responders is approximately 27 percent, with the actual number probably higher. In urban areas, where volunteers are unlikely to represent a significant percentage, the medical first responder percentage would be closer to 16 percent. EMT/Paramedic Volunteers: National Association of Emergency Medical Technicians, *EMS Week Planning Guide*, 2005; volunteer firefighter estimate from the Center for Disease Control, *Morbidity and Mortality Weekly Report* 55, no. 16 (April 28, 2006): 453–55.
7. Institute of Medicine, 12.
8. Ibid., 43.
9. Ibid., xiii (Preface).
10. Ibid., xv (Preface).
11. News/More News/News by Date, *The White House*, July 2007, "President Bush Visits Cleveland, Ohio (July 10, 2007)," www.whitehouse.gov/news/releases/2007/07/20070710-6.html (accessed March 23, 2008).
12. Institute of Medicine, xiv (Preface).
13. Ibid., 40.
14. Todd Hatley and Daniel Patterson, "Management and Financing of Emergency Medical Services," *North Carolina Medical Journal* 68, no. 4 (July/August 2007): 259–61, 259.
15. Hatley and Patterson; Office of the Inspector General, Department of Health and Human Services, "Medicare Payments for Ambulance Transports," January 2006 (OEI-05-02-00590).
16. Institute of Medicine, 41.
17. Government Accountability Office, "Ambulance Providers: Costs and Expected Medicare Margins Vary Greatly," GAO-07-383 (Washington, D.C.: May 23, 2007), 24.
18. Testimony Robert E. O'Connor, House Committee on Oversight and Government Reform, June 22, 2007, www.oversight.house.gov/documents/20070622135412.pdf (accessed March 2, 2008).
19. Government Accountability Office, 24.
20. Ashland (Oregon) Fire and Rescue, "Ambulance Services Program Review," January 14, 2008, City of Ashland, *Ambulance Funding*, www.ashland.or.us/Page.asp?NavID=10725 (accessed March 2, 2008).
21. American Ambulance Association, *Ambulance Facts*, www.the-aaa.org/media/Ambulance-Facts.htm (accessed February 16, 2008). See also Institute of Medicine, 11.
22. Institute of Medicine, 159.
23. Ibid., 18.
24. Davis R. Coddington, and J. West, *The State of Emergency Medical Services across the USA: How 50 Major Cities Stack Up*, 2003, www.usatoday.com/graphics/life/gra/ems/flash.htm (accessed January 1, 2008).

Appendix I

1. Florence, Archivo di Stato, Carte Strozziane, Magliabecchiana, cl. xxxvii, cod. 300, c. 132, cited by Howard Saalman, *The Bigallo*. (New York: New York University Press: 1989).
2. Blake Wilson, *Music and Merchants: The Laudesi Companies of Republican Florence* (Oxford: Oxford University Press, 1992): 74.
3. Antoninus, *Summa Historialis, sive Chronica, Tribus Partibus distincte, ab Orbe, condito ad Annum 1459*, vol. III (Florence, 1586): 233.
4. Another putative founder of the Misericordia was the Bigallo franchise Spedale dei Portatori, a small neighborhood hospice. There is scant evidence for the hypothesis, but it is certainly possible that the infirmary operated a similar transportation service. R. Davidson, *Geschichte von Florenz IV*, pt. 3 (Berlin, 1927), 55.
5. Horner, 96.
6. Ibid., 97.
7. The actual passage reads: "In the name of our Lord, Jesus Christ, and his venerable saint mother, The Virgin Saint Maria, queen of heaven and the world: In this book will be written the names and last names of men and women [who] belong to the great company of our Lady the glorious Virgin Saint Mary of the city of Florence, begun by blessed Saint Peter Martyr, of the Order of the Preaching Priests, in the year 1240 of the incarnation of our Lord Jesus Christ ... and these books were renewed [rinnuati] in the year of Our Lord 1361, in the month of May." Of passing note, the Misericordia had historically divided the city into six sections for its labors, while these volumes divided Florence into quarters, adding some additional weight to the theory that the "compagnia" described was not equivalent to the Misericordia itself.

Appendix II

1. Local customs and rules against elaborate beards, or any at all, dated to at least the Fourth Council of Carthage in 419 and its Canon XLIV. The bearded clergy were threatened with excommunication by the Council of Latrouse in 1119, but the proscription did not enter canon law until Pope Gregory III (1227-41). See Herbert Thurston, "Beard," in *The Catholic Encyclopedia*, Vol. 2 (New York: Appleton, 1907).
2. Ira Rutkow, *Surgery: An Illustrated History* (St. Louis: Mosby-Yearbook, 1993), 5.

Appendix III

1. J. Dalton, "Memorial," 3.
2. "Metropolitan Board of Health Minutes," January 11, 1869, holographic ledger at 115 (microfilm holding, New York City Archives, Surrogate's Court Building).
3. "Minutes," January 12, 1870 (resignation); *Commissioners of Charities, Ninth Annual Report of the Commissioners of Public Charities and Correction* (Albany, N.Y.: Charles Von Benthuysen & Sons, 1869): 22 (lunatic asylum); *Commissioners of Charities, Tenth Annual Report of the Commissioners of Public Charities and Correction* (Albany, N.Y.: Argus Co., 1870): 162.
4. *Santa Barbara Times*, "Death Notices," May 18, 1872, 2; Stella H. Rouse, "Olden Days," *Santa Barbara News-Press*, July 15, 1984, H-5 (biography of Major Hayne).

Appendix IV

1. W.B. Kouwenhoven, *Annals of Internal Medicine* 71, no. 3 (September 1969): 449–458, 449. In the article, Kouwenhoven mistakenly describes Lieb as the president of Consolidated Edison: in fact, he was vice president of the New York Edison Company, a predecessor to Con Ed. See "Edison Co. Gives Prizes," *New York Times*, June 22, 1927, 38.
2. Ibid., 449.
3. Stefan Timmermans, "Hearts Too Good to Die: Claude S. Beck's Contributions to Life-Saving," *Journal of Historical Sociology* 14, no. 1 (March 2001).
4. Kouwenhoven, 450.
5. "Back to Life," *Time*, April 23, 1951 (quoting Cuthbert Owens).
6. C. S. Beck et al. "Ventricular Fibrillation of Long Duration Abolished by Electric Shock," *Journal of the American Medical Association* 135 (1947): 985.
7. Kouwenhoven, 452.
8. Ibid., 453.
9. Paul Zoll et al. "Termination of Ventricular Fibrillation in Man by Externally Applied Electric Counter Shock," *The New England Journal of Medicine* 254, no. 16 (1956): 727–31, 730.
10. Kouwenhoven, 454.
11. Ibid., 455.
12. Ibid., 456.
13. Roger White, "Shocking History," *Journal of Emergency Medical Services*, October 1995, 41–45, 42.
14. Ibid., 42, 44.
15. J.R. Jude et al., "An Experimental and Clinical Study of a Portable External Cardiac Defibrillator," *Surgical Forum* 13 (Chicago, American College of Surgeons, 1962): 185–87, 186.

Bibliography

"Aaron Frank: Lawyer, Merchant, Engineer." *Lewis and Clark Chronicle* 8, no. 3 (Fall 1999).

Acai, Steven and Herbert Proctor. "First Year of the North Carolina MAST Program." *Emergency Medical Services* 5, no. 6 (Nov./Dec. 1976).

Adams, George. *Doctors in Blue*. New York: Henry Schuman, 1952.

Alexander, Shirley. "Riding to Trouble." *Colliers*, October 1942.

"Ambulance Operation." *Mortuary Management*, October 1958.

"Ambulance Services." *The Modern Hospital* 85, no. 5 (November 1955).

The Ambulance System. Boston: Crosby and Nichols, 1864.

American College of Surgeons. "Minimal Equipment List for Ambulances." *Bulletin of the American College of Surgeons* 52, no. 92 (1967).

Andelman, David. "Ambulance Aid Found Deficient." *New York Times*, Aug. 19, 1973.

Anderson, D. Warehouse Receipt, Office of the City Auditor, Property Control Division, May 9, 1972.

"Annual Report." *New York Times*, January 26, 1870.

Anonymous, interviewed by Clarence Weinstock. "Like a Bird." Library of Congress. http://memory.loc.gov/cgi-bin/query/D?wpa:2:./temp/~ammem_Ik2j.

Antoninus. *Summa Historialis, sive Chronica, Tribus Partibus distincte, ab Orbe, condito ad Annum 1459*. Florence, 1586.

Ashburn, P.M. *A History of the Medical Department of the United States Army*. New York: Houghton Mifflin, 1929.

"At Bellevue." *Time*, November 7, 1927.

Atkinson, William, ed. *The Physicians and Surgeons of the United States*. Philadelphia: Charles Robson, 1878.

"Attempted Suicides." *New York Times*, May 24, 1870.

"Average Wages." *Manufacturer and Builder* 24, no. 6 (1892).

Baerwald, John. "The Interdisciplinary Development of Ambulance Design Criteria." *Highway Research Record* 332 (1970).

Barkley, Katherine Traver. *Ambulance!* Hicksville, N.Y.: Exposition Press, 1978.

Barringer, Emily. *Bowery to Bellevue*. New York: Norton, 1950.

Beck, C.S., et al. "Ventricular Fibrillation of Long Duration Abolished by Electric Shock." *Journal of the American Medical Association* 135, no. 985 (1947).

Beckmann, Johann. *Beckmann's History of Inventions, Discoveries, and Origins*. Trans. William Johnston. London: Richard and John Taylor, 1846.

Bell, Karen. Personal communication, May 2005.

"Bellevue and Potter's Field." *New York Times*, April 7, 1872.

Bellevue Literary Review Online. "Bellevue History/History of Bellevue Hospital." www.blreview.org/bellevuehistory.htm.

Bemrose, John. *Reminiscences of the Second Seminole War*. Edited by John Mahon. Gainesville: University of Florida Press, 1966.

Benson, D. and G. Esposito. "Mobile Intensive Care by 'Unemployable' Blacks Trained as Emergency Medical Technicians in 1967–69." *Journal of Trauma* 12, no. 5 (1972).

Bernard, Thomas. *An account of the House of Recovery, established by the board of health at Manchester, from The Reports of the Society for Bettering the Condition and Increasing the Comforts of the Poor*. Vol. 1. Manchester, 1798.

Bettman, Otto. *Pictorial History of Medicine*. Springfield, Ill.: Charles C. Thomas, 1956.

Bijur, Nathan. "Social Significance of Ambulance Control." *The Survey* 22 (1909).

Bledsoe, Bryan. "EMS Mythology, Part 4." *Emergency Medical Services* 32, no. 6 (2003).

"Bloody Riot." *New York Times*, July 13, 1870.

Bloor, Alfred. *Letters from the Army of the Potomac*. Washington, D.C.: McGill, Witherow, Printers and Stereotypes, 1864.

Board of Ambulance Services. *Regulations Governing the Ambulance Service of All Hospitals in the City of New York*. New York: Board of Ambulance Services, 1919.

"Board of Health." *New York Times*, January 10, 1868.

"Board of Health." *New York Times*, January 3, 1867.

Boatright, Edward. "A Municipal Truck for All Emergencies." *The American City*, June 1939.

Bogdanich, Walt. "Death on the Tracks: How Railroads Sidestep Blame." *New York Times*, July 11, 2004.

Bosca, Pedro. *Oratio Romae habita XI Kal. Novembris ad Sacrum, etc*. Rome, 1487.

Bowditch, Henry. "The Ambulance System." *Medical and Surgical Reporter* 9, no. 2 (1862).

Bowditch, Vincent, ed. *Life and Correspondence of*

Henry Ingersoll Bowditch. Vol. 2. Cambridge: Riverside Press, 1902.

Brandwell, Stephen. *Helps for Suddain Accidents.* London: Thomas Purfoot, 1633.

Brennan, Thomas. "Bellevue Hospital, Annual Report." In *Tenth Annual Report of the Commissioners of Public Charities and Correction.* Albany, N.Y.: Argus, 1870.

Brooklyn Board of Aldermen. "February 5." In *Proceedings of the Board of Aldermen of the City of Brooklyn.* Brooklyn, 1872.

Brooklyn Board of Aldermen. "January 29." In *Proceedings of the Board of Aldermen of the City of Brooklyn.* Brooklyn: 1872.

Brooks, James. *History of the Court of Common Pleas.* New York: Werner, Sanford, 1896.

Brown, Robert. "What's the Matter with Internships?" *The Modern Hospital* 74, no. 3 (March 1950).

"Brutal Inhumanity by a Woman." *The National Police Gazette* 22, no. 1113 (1866).

Buchholz, Donald. "An Individualized Approach to EMS." *Emergency Medical Services* 4, no 1 (Jan./Feb. 1975).

Burger, J. Raymond. "Meeting of Firemen's First Aid and Safety Squad (Minutes)." Typescript. Belmar, N.J., 1928.

Burton, Alan. "History of 911." *Dispatch Monthly Magazine.* www.911dispatch.com/911/history.

Byrdsall, F. *The History of the Loco-Foco, or Equal Rights Party.* New York: Clement and Packard, 1842.

California Ambulance Association. *National Ambulance Directory.* Chicago: Albert Carriere, 1962.

Cameron, Frank. "They Race Death Every Night." *The Saturday Evening Post*, January 3, 1953.

Capitman, John. "Emergency Care Challenged." *Pittsburgh News,* May 1, 1973.

Carlisle, Robert, Ed. *An Account of Bellevue Hospital.* New York: Society of the Alumni of Bellevue Hospital, 1893.

Caroline, Nancy. *Emergency Care in the Streets.* Boston: Little, Brown, 1979.

———. "Will the Real Paramedic Please Stand Up?" *Emergency Medical Services* 6, no. 2 (March/April 1977).

Centers for Disease Control and Prevention. "Ambulance Crash-Related Injuries among Emergency Service Workers—United States, 1991–2002." *Morbidity and Mortality Weekly Report* 52, no. 154 (2003).

Chaiken, J.M. and R. J. Gladstone. *Some Trends in the Delivery of Ambulance Service.* Santa Monica, Calif.: Rand Corporation, 1974.

Champion, H., et al. *Emergency Medical Services, The Forgotten First Responder: A Report on the Critical Gaps in Organization and Deficits in Resources for America's Medical First Responders.* New York: New York University, Center for Catastrophe Preparedness and Response, 2005.

Chandler, Raymond. *The Little Sister.* New York: Houghton-Mifflin, 1948.

Cheever, George. "Freedom House Ambulance Service." *University Times,* July 23, 1970.

Chittum, Matt. "New Jersey Town Challenges Roanoke as Birthplace of the Volunteer Rescue Squad." *Roanoke Times,* February 10, 2002.

Cincinnati Police Department. "Honoring Our Heroes." www.cincinnati-oh.gov.

"City Ambulances." *New York Times,* July 24, 1869.

"City Commission of Sewers." *Times,* June 25, 1863.

City of Cincinnati. *Laws and Regulations for the Management of the City Infirmary, Commercial Hospital, Pest House, City Burying Ground and the Granting of Out-Door Relief to the Poor.* Cincinnati, Ohio: Marshall and Hefley, 1859.

City of Cincinnati. *Ordinance, Rules and Regulations for the Management of the City Infirmary and the Relief of the Out-Door Poor.* Cincinnati, Ohio: John D. Thorpe, 1864.

City of London Police. "Police Ambulances." www.cityoflondon.police.uk/history/history.

"City Sewers: Sanitary Condition of the City." *Times,* April 2, 1856.

Clune, Henry. "Seen and Heard." *Democrat and Chronicle,* January 28, 1936.

C.M. "American Firemen." *Illustrated London News* 32, no. 899 (1858).

Coddington, Davis and J. West. *The State of Emergency Medical Services across the USA: How 50 Major Cities Stack Up.* 2003. www.usatoday.com/graphics/life/gra/ems/flash.htm.

Cole, Robert. "Cost of Ambulance Service Is Rising across Country." *New York Times,* June 26, 1969.

Coleman, Robert. "Pennsylvania's Helicopter Ambulance Study." *Highway Research Record,* no. 272 (1969).

Collins, John. "Organization and Function of an Accident Flying Squad." *British Medical Journal* 2, no. 513 (1966).

Commercial Hospital of Cincinnati Trustees. *Accounts of the Commercial Hospital of Cincinnati, 1864 through 1865.* Handwritten ledger, 1865.

Commercial Hospital of Cincinnati Trustees. *Board of Trustees, 12th Annual Report of the Cincinnati Hospital, for the 10 Months Ending December 31, 1872.* Cincinnati, Ohio: Gazette Steam Book and Job Printing Establishment, 1873.

Commercial Hospital of Cincinnati Trustees. *Board of Trustees, Sixth Annual Report of the Commercial Hospital of the City of Cincinnati.* Cincinnati, Ohio: Gazette Steam Book and Job Printing Establishment, 1867.

Commissioners of Charities and Correction. *Commissioners of Charities, Ninth Annual Report of the Commissioners of Public Charities and Correction.* Albany, N.Y.: Charles Von Benthuysen & Sons, 1869.

"Commissioners of Charities and Corrections." *New York Times,* June 25, 1869.

"Committee Orders Baker Car." *Oregonian,* June 14, 1933.

"Committee Proposes Public Ambulance Service." *The Modern Hospital* 51, no. 5 (November 5, 1938).

"Community Concern Sparks Ambulance Service." *The Modern Hospital* 113, no. 2 (August 1969).

"Community Training Program." *Bulletin of the American College of Surgeons,* July/Aug. 1968.

Connolly, Daniel. "Among the Inebriates." *Appleton's Journal of Literature, Science, and Art* 5, no. 117 (1871).

Cooper, Carole, and Mel Powell. *Description and Analysis of Eighteen Proven Ambulance Service Systems.* Vol. 1. N.p.: National Association of Counties Research Foundation, 1968.

Cowley, R., et al. "An Economical and Proved Helicopter Program for Transporting the Emergency Critically Ill and Injured Patient in Maryland." *Journal of Trauma* 13, no. 12 (1973).

Cranston, Alan. "The Emergency Medical Services Systems Act—What to Expect in 1978." *Emergency Medical Services* 6, no. 6 (Nov./Dec. 1977).

Creighton, Charles. *A History of Epidemics in Britain.* Vol. 2. Cambridge: Cambridge University Press, 1894.

"Crimes and Casualties." *New York Times,* July 6, 1870.

Crossman, James. "Ambulances." *The Times,* December 1, 1881.

Curry, George and Sydney Lyttle. "The Speeding Ambulance." *American Journal of Surgery* 95 (1958).

Dalton, Edward B. "Annual Report of the Metropolitan Board of Health of New York, 1866." *North American Review* 106 (1868).

Dalton, John C. *Memorial of Edward B. Dalton, M.D.* New York, 1872.

Davidson, R. *Geschichte von Florenz IV.* Berlin, 1927.

Dean, Edward. "Caring for Emergency Cases." *The Modern Hospital* 32, no. 4 (1929).

Dektar, Joan. "Time Running Out for Landmark, Once Central Emergency Hospital." *Los Angeles Times,* August 28, 1988.

"Died." *New York Times,* June 23, 1900.

Diehl, Digby. "The Emergency Medical Services Program." In *To Improve Health and Health Care 2000.* Ed. Stephen Issacs and James Knickman. San Francisco: Jossey-Bass, 2000.

Division of Medical Services, National Academy of Sciences–National Research Council. *Summary Report of the Task Force on Ambulance Services.* Washington, D.C., 1967.

"Dr. Henri Nachtel." *New York Times,* March 5, 1883.

Donaldson, Al. "Superambulance Police Image Said to Lack Warmth." *Pittsburgh Press,* October 24, 1975.

Donohughe, Francis. "The Patrol Ambulance: An Adjunct to the Ambulance Service in Cities; A Substitute Therefore in Towns." *Boston Medical and Surgical Journal* 146, no. 19 (1902).

"Don't Overlook the Ambulance as a Public Relations Tool." *The Modern Hospital,* 79 no. 9 (September 1950).

Dowling, Jim. "Concord Coaches." Downing Family Historical Society. www.downingfamily.org/Abbot-Downing.

Duncan, Francis. "Hospitaller Work at St. John's Gate in 1880." *The Gentleman's Magazine* 247, no. 1798 (1880).

_____. "The St. John Ambulance Association." *The Times,* September 5, 1878.

Dustoff Association. "History." www.dustoff.org/newsletter.

DuVal, Merlin. "The Federal Role in E.M.S." *Emergency Medical Services* 2, no. 1, 1973.

Eisenberg, Mickey. *Life in the Balance.* New York: Oxford University Press, 1997.

Emory, William. *Lieutenant Emory Reports.* Ed. Ross Calvin. Albuquerque: University of New Mexico Press, 1951.

Evans, Thomas. *A Report on Class XI, Group II, Paris Exposition 1867.* Paris: E. Briere, 1867.

Evans, William. "Send Help ... Quick!" *Los Angeles Times,* February 23, 1941.

Evatt, G. *Ambulance Organization, Equipment, and Transport.* London: William Clowes and Sons, 1884.

Farrington, J.D. "Death in a Ditch." *Bulletin American College of Surgeons* 52, no. 3 (May/June 1967).

_____, and Oscar Hampton. "A Curriculum for Training Emergency Medical Technicians." *Bulletin of the American College of Surgeons,* Sept./Oct. 1969.

Fawcett, Waldon. "The Cost of Operating a Motor Ambulance." *The Modern Hospital* 8, no. 1 (1917).

Fifield, James, ed. *American and Canadian Hospitals.* Minneapolis: Midwest, 1933.

"First Auto Ambulance for an Army Hospital." *New York Daily Tribune,* August 26, 1905.

Flipping, Robert, Jr. "City Policemen to Assume Freedom House Tasks." *Pittsburgh Courier,* June 8, 1974.

Franks, Patricia. "Emergency Medical Technicians and Paramedics in California." University of California, Center for Health Professions, San Francisco. www.futurehealth.ucsf.edu/pdf_files/EMT14pfdoc.pdf.

"Fratelli Della Misericordia—The Brotherhood of Mercy." *New Monthly Magazine* 17, no. 72 (1826).

Frederick, Dolores. "Ambulance Training Setup OK with FOP." *Pittsburgh Press,* May 3, 1973.

_____. "City Easing Its Ambulance Stand." *Pittsburgh Press,* May 30, 1973.

_____. "City's 5 'Super Ambulances' Ready for Road, But Await Plan." *Pittsburgh Press,* August 18, 1975.

_____. "District Lets Medical Service Funds Slip Away." *Pittsburgh Press,* July 27, 1972.

_____. "Doctor Can Write Book on Ambulance Emergencies." *Pittsburgh Press,* August 17, 1975.

_____. "Telemetry Keeps Doctor, Emergency Unit in Touch." *Pittsburgh Press,* July 25, 1972.

_____. "Too Often Distress Call Brings Ride to Eternity." *Pittsburgh Press,* July 23, 1972.

Freedom House Ambulance Service Committee. "Establishment Proposal." Typescript, 1967.

Freedom House Ambulance Service Committee. "Meeting with Dr. Safar." Typescript, June 15, 1967.

Freedom House Ambulance Service Committee. "Minutes." Typescript, June 17, 1967.

Freedom House Enterprises Ambulance Service Committee. "Background Material: Need for Services." Typescript, n.d. (circa 1967).

Freedom House Enterprises Ambulance Service Committee. "Minutes." Typescript, April 15, 1967.

Freedom House Enterprises Ambulance Service Committee. "Minutes." Typescript, June 3, 1967.

"The French Ambulance System." *New York Times,* May 30, 1861.

Furely, John. "A Horse Ambulance Service." *Times,* July 12, 1882.

_____. *In Peace and War.* London: Smith, Eden, 1905.

Galdston, Morton. "Ambulance Notes of Bellevue Hospital Intern." *Journal of Urban Health* 76, no. 4 (1999).

Garrison, F.H. *Notes on Military Medicine.* Washington, D.C.: Association of Military Surgeons, 1922.

General Accounting Office. *States Assume Leadership Role in Providing Emergency Medical Services.* GAO/HRD-86-132. Washington, D.C.: U.S. GAO, 1986.

Genesee Hospital (Rochester, N.Y.). "Ambulance Protocol." Typescript, n.d. (circa 1958).

Gibson, Geoffrey. "Emergency Medical Services," in "Health Services: The Local Perspective," special issue of *Proceedings of the Academy of Political Science* 32, no. 3 (1977).

Gibson, T.M. "Samuel Franklin Cody: Aviation and Aeromedical Evacuation Pioneer." *Aviation, Space and Environmental Medicine* 70, no. 6 (1999).

Ginzberg, Eli. "Philanthropy and Nonprofit Organizations in U.S. Healthcare." *Inquiry* 28, no. 2 (1991).

Gomolak, Lou. "Hot Wheels: New York Hospital's Mobile ICU." *The Modern Hospital* 120, no. 6 (1973).

Government Accountability Office. *Ambulance Providers: Costs and Expected Medicare Margins Vary Greatly.* GAO-07-383. Washington, D.C.: U.S. GAO, May 23, 2007.

Gowings, Dan. *Ambulance Attendant Training Manual.* Harrisburg: Penna. Dept. of Health, 1965.

Haggard, A.H. "London Ambulance Service." *Times,* October 18, 1882.

Hallen, Phil. "Preliminary Thoughts on the Development of a Private Ambulance Service in the Hill District." Typescript, February 21, 1967.

Haller, John. *Farmcarts to Fords—A History of the Military Ambulance from 1790–1925.* Carbondale: Southern Illinois University Press, 1992.

"Hand Ambulances for the Injured." *Brooklyn Eagle,* January 5, 1872.

Hardy, Mrs. Walter. "The Ardmore Ambulance Plane." *The American Journal of Nursing* 23, no. 3 (1922).

Harrison, Reginald. *The Use of the Ambulance in Civil Practice: Portions of the Inaugural Address at the Liverpool Medical Institution.* Liverpool: Holden, 1881.

Hart, Harold. "The Conveyance of Patients to and from Hospital, 1720–1850." *Medical History* 22, no. 4 (1978).

Hatley, Todd and Daniel Patterson. "Management and Financing of Emergency Medical Services." *North Carolina Medical Journal* 68, no. 4 (July/August 2007).

Hevesi, Alan. *Where Do 911 System Ambulances Take Their Patients? Differences between Voluntary Hospital Ambulances and Fire Department Ambulances.* New York: Office of the Comptroller, 2001.

Hibbert, Christopher. *The Destruction of Lord Raglan.* Boston: Little, Brown, 1962.

Highway Safety Act, 1966 (Public Law 89-564). 23 USC Chapter 4, Section 401 et seq.

Hirshmann, Jim and Eugene Nagel. "Prehospital Emergency Care in Miami, Florida, A Historical Commentary." *Journal of the Florida Medical Association* 68, no. (1981).

Holloway, Ronald and Linda Orzeck. "The Changing Focus of Pre-Hospital Care." *Emergency Medical Services,* May/June 1977.

Horner, Susan and Joanna. *Walks in Florence.* Vol. 1. London: Strahan, 1873.

"Hospital." *Oregon Journal,* February 15, 1914

"Hospital Ambulance." *Times,* December 21, 1881.

"A Hospital and Accident Ambulance Service." *The Lancet,* January 28, 1882.

"Hospitals Report Ownership and Operation of Trucks, Ambulances, Passenger Cars." *The Modern Hospital* 88, no. 3 (March 1957).

"How Good Is Your Emergency Room?" *The Modern Hospital* 83, no. 6 (December 1954).

Howard, Benjamin. "Hospital and Accident Ambulance Service for London." *The Lancet,* February 4, 1882.

Howard, O. Preface. *Prisoners of Russia,* by Benjamin Howard. New York: Appleton, 1902.

Hritz, Thomas. "Flaherty Calls Pitt Blast on Ambulances Political." *Pittsburgh Post-Gazette,* April 28, 1973.

"A Humane Society." *New York Times,* May 15, 1873.

Hume, Edgar. "Medical Work of the Knights Hospitallers." *Bulletin of the Institute of the History of Medicine* 6, no. 4 (1938).

Hutchinson, John. "Civilian Ambulances and Lifesaving Societies." In *Accidents in History: Injuries, Fatalities, and Social Relations.* E. Roger Cooter and Bill Luckin. Atlanta, Ga.: Ridopi, 1997.

"Illinois' Trauma System: Problems are Planning and Communication." *The Modern Hospital* 120, no. 1 (1973).

Illson, Murray. "4 Hospitals Plan New Ambulance Runs." *New York Times,* January 31, 1964.

Institute of Medicine. Committee on the Future of Emergency Care in the United States Health System. *Emergency Medical Services: At the Crossroads.* Washington, D.C.: National Academies Press, 2007.

Jefferson, Horace. "London Fever and London Cabs," *Times,* March 5, 1866.

———. "Propagation of Disease by Public Vehicles." *Times,* January 21, 1869.

Jerry, Rolland. "Cunningham Firm Set Its Sights on the Gun-Shy Carriage Trade." In *The Best of Old Cars Weekly.* Vol. 1. Iola, Wis.: Krause, 1978.

Jones, William. "Ambulances' Crews Pilfer Hospital Goods for Supplies." *Chicago Tribune,* June 12, 1970.

———. "Heart Victim Left in Flat." *Chicago Tribune,* June 9, 1970.

———. "Men of Mercy? Profit in Pain." *Chicago Tribune,* June 7, 1970.

———. "Sadism Rides the Ambulance." *Chicago Tribune,* June 8, 1970.

"Jubilee." *New York Times,* October 17, 1865.

Jude, J.R. et al. "An Experimental and Clinical Study of a Portable External Cardiac Defibrillator." *Surgical Forum.* Vol. 13. Chicago: American College of Surgeons, 1962.

Kauffman, H. and J. Goodrich. "Byron Stookey." *Neurosurgery* 40, no. (1997).

Kelyy, Jack. "Rescue Squad." *American Heritage* 47 (May/June 1996).

King, E. J. *The Knights of St. John in the British Empire.* Bristol, England: Wright and Sons, 1934.

King County Hospital Trustees. *Annual Report of Harborview Hospital, 1933.* Seattle, Wash.: 1934.

Knights, Edwin, Jr. "Bellevue Hospital." *History Magazine* no. 2 (Dec./Jan. 2000).
Kouwenhoven, W.B. "The Development of. the Defibrillator," *Annals of Internal Medicine* 71, no. 3 (September 1969).
Kuehl, Alexander, Ed. *Prehospital Systems and Medical Oversight.* Dubuque, Ia.: Kendall Hunt, 2002.
Lam, David. "Marie Marvingt and the Development of Aeromedical Evacuation." *Aviation, Space, and Environmental Medicine* 74, no. 8 (August 2003).
Landini, Placido. *Istoria dell'oratorio e della Venerabile Arciconfraternita di Santa Maria della Misericordia della città di Firenze.* Florence: Cartoleria Peratoner, 1843.
Larrey, Dominique. *Memoirs of Military Surgery and Campaigns of the French Armies.* Vol. 1. Trans. Richard Wilmott Hall. Baltimore: Joseph Cushing/ University Press of Sergeant Hall, 1814.
"The Last Word In Motor Ambulances." *The Modern Hospital* 9, no. 5 (1917).
Leahy, A. "Field Hospital Equipments—Class 37." *Illustrated London News,* August 31, 1867.
Lechemer, A.H., Ed. "Proceedings of a Public Meeting Held on Wednesday Evening, February 6th, 1878, at the Pall Mall Restaurant." Woolwich, England: A.W. and A.P. Jackson, 1878.
Leddy, Linda. "The Quality of EMS." *Emergency Medical Services* 6, no. 3 (May/June 1977).
Lehman, S.P. and K.H. Hollingsworth. "Ambulance Service in Seattle." *Public Health Reports* 75, no. 4 (1960).
Lehr, Teresa and Phillip Maples. *To Serve the Community: A Celebration of Rochester General Hospital 1847–1997.* Virginia Beach: Donning Co., 1997.
Leonard, George. "Ambulances for Civil Services." In *A Reference Handbook of the Medical Sciences.* Ed. Albert Buck. New York: William Wood, 1885.
Lepper, Richard et al. "An Overview of Rural EMS." *Emergency Medical Services* 4, no. 5 (Sept./Oct. 1975).
Lerner, Sharon. "Ambulance Wars: How Private Ambulance Crews Steer Patients away from Public Hospitals." *Village Voice,* June 27, 2001.
"LifeCare Emphasizes Safe Driving." *Emergency Medical Services* 32, no. 6 (2003).
The Literary World 33, no. 8 (1902).
"London." *Times,* October 18, 1854.
"London." *Times,* December 30, 1854.
London Illustrated News, February 24, 1867.
London Metropolitan Police. "Timeline, 1850–1869." www.met.police.uk/history/timeline1850.
Mackay, Charles. *Life and Liberty in America.* New York: Harper, 1859.
MacMillan's Magazine 19, no. 87 (1868).
"A Man Thrown Out of a Window by His Wife." *New York Times,* October 5, 1870.
Mann, J. *Medical Sketches of the Campaign of 1812–13–14.* Dedham, England, 1816.
Matsell, George. *Rules and Regulations for Day and Night Police of the City of New York.* New York: Casper Childs, 1846.
Maul, Norman. "Systematic Ambulance Service For Metropolitan Hospitals." *The Modern Hospital* 4, no. 1 (1915).

Mauritius, *Ars Militaris.* Vol. 2. Trans. Joh. Scheffero. Uppsala, Sweden: 1664.
McCall, Walter. *The American Ambulance, 1900–2001.* Hudson, Wis.: Iconografix, 2002.
McFeatters, Dale. "Super Ambulances Make Debut Here." *Pittsburgh Press,* April 8, 1969.
McGuire, James. "New York City Police Department Emergency Service Division." Typescript, n.d. (pre–1988).
McKelvey, Blake. *Rochester Police Bureau, 1819–1969.* Rochester, N.Y.: Bureau of Police, 1969.
McSwain, Norman, et al. "Deke." *The EMT Journal* 2, no. 4 (December 1976).
"Medical-Care-On-Wheels Will Aid Hospitals and Patients." *The Modern Hospital* 114, no. 5 (1970).
Metropolitan Board of Health (New York City). "Metropolitan Board of Health Minutes, January 11, 1869." Holographic ledger.
Metzenbaum, Myron. "Cleveland's Present Ambulance Service." *The Cleveland Medical Journal* 7, no. 7 (1908).
The Modern Hospital 1, no. 1 (1913).
_____ 17, no. 2 (1934).
_____ 20, no. 4 (1923).
_____ 27, no. 6 (1926).
_____ 27, no. 8 (1927).
_____ 29, no. 3 (1927).
_____ 4, no. 7 (1915).
_____ 7 (1916).
_____ 8 (1917).
"The Monastic Knights." *Littell's Living Age,* May 10, 1884.
Mukaili, Aki. "Freedom House—Mobile Medicine's Best." *Pittsburgh Courier,* December 1, 1973.
Munson, Edward. "Transportation of Federal Sick and Wounded." In *Prisons and Hospitals.* Vol. 7 of *Photographic History of the Civil War.* Ed. Holland Thompson. New York: Review of Reviews Co., 1911.
Nagel, E., J. Hirschman et al. "Telemetry of Physiologic Data." *Southern Medical Journal* 61, no. 6 (1968).
National Academy of Sciences and National Research Council. *Accidental Death and Disability: The Neglected Disease of Modern Society.* Washington, D.C.: National Academy Press, 1966.
National Highway Traffic Safety Administration. *EMS Agenda for the Future.* U.S. Department of Transportation, 1996.
National Resident Matching Program. "What It Was Like before the Match." www.savethematch.org/history/before.
Naughton, Russell. "2500 Years of Communication History: 1887." www.acmi.net.au/AIC/phd8400.html.
Nelson, S.B. and J.M. Runk. *History of Cincinnati and Hamilton County.* Cincinnati, Ohio: S.B. Nelson, 1894.
New York City. Commission of Charities and Correction. *"Warden's Report." First Annual Report, Board of Governors of the Alms House.* New York: Geo. F. Nesbitt, 1849.
_____. *Fifth Annual Report, Governors of the Alms House.* New York: Jos. Harrison, 1854.
New York City. Commissioners of Public Charities and Corrections. *Eleventh Annual Report of the Com-*

missioners of Public Charities and Corrections. New York: New York Printing Co., 1871.

———. Minutes of the Commissioners of Public Charities and Corrections. Vol. 10. New York, 1869.

New York Observer and Chronicle, May 5, 1868.

"News and Miscellaneous." The Medical and Surgical Reporter 14, no. 8 (1866).

News Telegram (Portland, Oregon), June 21, 1933.

Nicholson, G. The White Cross in Canada. Ottawa: Runge Press, 1967.

"The Night Medical Service in New York City." The Medical and Surgical Reporter 44, no. 6 (1881).

9/11 Commission. 9/11 Commission Report. Washington, D.C.: U.S. Government Printing Office, 2004.

"Obituary." Medical News 77, no. 1 (1900).

O'Leary, Margaret. A Historical Overview of EMS System Development in the U.S.: The 1960s and 1970s. Suburban Emergency Management Project. Biot 246. August 6, 2005. www.semp.us/publications/biot_reader.php?BiotID=246IOT.

"Operation Ostrich: Is Mass Evacuation Strictly for the Birds?" The Modern Hospital 87 no. 3 (September 1956).

"The Ottawa Homicide." New York Times, April 19, 1867.

Page, James. "One of the Boys." Journal of Emergency Medical Services, January 1983.

———. The Paramedics. Morristown, N.J.: Backdraft Publications, 1979.

Pantridge, J.F. and J.S. Geddes. "A Mobile Intensive Care Unit in the Management of Myocardial Infarction." Lancet 2, no. 7510 (1967).

Paonessa, Don. "The New Ambulance That Flies." Better Homes and Gardens 34, no. 1 (1956).

Pearce, Robert. "War and Medicine in the 19th Century." ADF Health 3, no.1 (2002).

Pearn, John. "The Earliest Days of First Aid." British Medical Journal 309 (1994).

Pearn, J., and M. Wales. "Dr. John Thompson." The Medical Journal of Australia 1157 (1992).

Pearson, Thomas. American Funeral Cars and Ambulances. Glenn Ellyn, Ill.: Crestline, 1973.

Peck, William. History of the Rochester Police Force. Rochester, N.Y.: Police Benevolent Association, 1903.

Perkins, John. "Commentary." Emergency Medical Services 6, no. 1 (Jan./Feb. 1977).

Perlmutter, Emmanuel. "Review." New York Times, Dec. 7, 1958.

Perry, Bliss. Life and Letters of Henry Lee Higginson. Boston: Atlantic Monthly Press, 1921.

"Philadelphia and the Soldiers." The Medical and Surgical Reporter 9, no. 13 (1862).

Pierce, Henry. "Colville Okays 3 Steps to Improve Ambulances." Pittsburgh Post-Gazette, May 30, 1973.

Pope, LeRoy. "Federal Aid to the Rescue of Ambulances." Chicago Daily Defender, March 31, 1975.

Porter, Ray. "Accidents in the 18th Century." In Accidents in History: Injuries, Fatalities, and Social Relations. E. Roger Cooter. Atlanta, Ga.: Ridopi, 1997.

Portland (Oregon) Police Department. Manual Containing the Rules and Regulations of the Police Department of the City of Portland. Portland Executive Board, 1903.

President's Committee for Traffic Safety. Health, Medical Care and Transportation of the Injured. Washington, D.C.: U.S. GPO, 1965.

Prostem, David. "First Aid Squad Sets Events." Newark Sunday News, 1967.

Proudfoot, S.L. et al. "Ambulance Crash-Related Injuries among Emergency Medical Services Workers—United States, 1991–2002." Journal of the American Medical Association 289, no. 13 (2003).

Purcell, Peter and Robert P. Hummel, "Samuel Preston Moore: Surgeon General of the Confederacy." American Journal of Surgery 164, no. 4 (1992).

Queen, James. "In Commemoration of the Great Parade of the Philadelphia Fire Department October 16th, 1865, Broad Street, under portrait of Chief Engineer D. M. Lyle." Lithograph, after a design by Schell. P. S. Duval & Son, 1865.

Ransom, John. "Civilian Ambulance Service." Ciba Symposia, February 1947.

Remington, Sheppard. "What Is Due the Accident Patient?" The Modern Hospital 47, no. 1 (1936).

Riesman, David. The Story of Medicine in the Middle Ages. New York: Paul B. Hoeber, 1936.

"The Riot." New York Times, July 14, 1870.

Roberts, Deering. "Field and Temporary Hospitals." In Prisons and Hospitals. Vol. 7 of Photographic History of the Civil War. Ed. Holland Thompson. New York: Review of Reviews Co., 1911.

Rochester (New York) City Hospital. "Ambulance Log." Manuscript notebook, 1900.

———. No title. The Hospital Review 26, no. 8 (1900).

———. No title. The Hospital Review 35, no. 6 (1899).

———. No title. The Hospital Review 40, no.11 (1904).

Rochester (New York) Common Council. Proceedings of the Common Council, 1890–91. Rochester: Democrat and Chronicle Press, 1891.

———. Proceedings of the Common Council 1891–92. Rochester: Democrat and Chronicle Press, 1892.

———. Proceedings of the Common Council, 1892. Rochester: Democrat and Chronicle Press, 1893.

———. Proceedings of the Common Council 1895. Rochester: Democrat and Chronicle Press, 1896.

———. Proceedings of the Common Council, 1896. Rochester: Democrat and Chronicle Press, 1897.

———. Proceedings of the Common Council. Rochester, 1953.

Rochester City Hospital (New York). "The Ambulance Service of New York." The Hospital Review 28, no. 18 (1893).

———. No title. The Hospital Review 25, no. 3 (1888).

———. "With an Ambulance." The Hospital Review 23, no. 8 (1887).

Rochester Town Watch (New York). Watch Book, No. 5. Rochester, 1837.

Romano, Teresa et al. "Nationwide Paramedic Clearinghouse." Emergency Medical Services 6, no. 5 (Sept./Oct. 1977).

Roper, Grace. The Borough of Belmar in Retrospect. Belmar, N.J.: Hoffman Press, 1978.

Rorem, C. Rufus. Why Hospital Costs Have Risen. Washington, D.C.: Chamber of Commerce, 1950.

Rosner, David. "Portrait of an Unhealthy City." Columbia University, Mailman School of Public

Health. http://156.145.78.54/htm/living_city/development_lab/develop.htm.

Rouse, Stella. "Olden Days." *Santa Barbara News-Press,* July 15, 1984.

Rutkow, Ira. *Surgery: An Illustrated History.* St. Louis: Mosby-Yearbook, 1993.

Saalman, Howard. *The Bigallo.* New York: New York University Press, 1969.

Sampson, Grover. "Reminiscences." Manuscript, January 8, 1940.

San Francisco Call. "A Night in the Port of Broken Heads." May 1, 1910.

Scaife, Walter. *Florentine Life during the Renaissance.* Baltimore: Johns Hopkins University Press, 1893.

Scholl, M.D. and C.L. Geschekter. "The Zed Expedition: The World's First Air Ambulance?" *Journal of the Royal Society of Medicine* 82, no. 11 (1989).

Scholten, Paul. "The San Francisco Emergency Ambulance Service." *San Francisco Medicine* 71, no. 9 (1998).

Schroeder, William. "History of the Ambulance System in Brooklyn, New York." *Brooklyn Medical Journal* 16, no. 381 (1902).

Schuster, J. *Deutsche militar arztliche Ztschr* 45 (1916).

Schuster, Karolyn. "Freedom House Tells Staffers of Phase-Out." *Pittsburgh Post-Gazette,* May 30, 1974.

Scientific American Supplement, Sept. 19, 1914.

"Serious Explosion." *New York Times,* October 4, 1870.

Shanley, John. "Real-Life Adventures of 2 Patrolmen." *New York Times,* Feb. 19, 1962.

Shapiro, Larry. *Special Police Vehicles.* Osceola, Wis.: MBI, 1999.

Shaw, Albert. "Notes on City Government in St. Louis." *Century Illustrated Magazine* 52, no. 2 (1896).

Sheehy, Susan. "The Evolution of Air Medical Transport." *Journal of Emergency Nursing* 21, no. 2 (1995).

Sherman, John. "The Ambulance." *Munsey's Magazine* 18, no. 1 (1897).

Slezdick, Paul. "Medicine and Surgery during the Civil War." Paper presented at the United States and Canadian Academy of Pathology 2003 Annual Meeting. www.uscap.org.

Smith, Karl. "Emergency Service Unit: A Historical Perspective." Typescript, 1999.

Smith, Ken. "The Ambulance Service Past, Present and Future." *Practitioner,* August 1988.

Snook, R. "Accident Flying Squad." *British Medical Journal* 3, no. 826 (1972).

South, John. *Memorials of John Flint South.* London: Murray, 1884.

Sprogle, Howard. *The Philadelphia Police, Past and Present.* Philadelphia, 1887.

Srikameswaran, Anita. "Obituary." *Pittsburgh Post-Gazette,* December 21, 2002.

Steedman. *The History and Statutes of the Royal Infirmary of Edinburgh.* Edinburgh: Balfour and Smellie, 1778.

Stewart, Miller. *Moving the Wounded: Litters, Carolets and Ambulance Wagons.* Ft. Collins, Colo.: Old Army Press, 1979.

"Street Cabs and Contagious Diseases." *The Lancet,* April 12, 1856.

Strouse, Richard. "Riding Bus with a Hospital Interne." *New York Times,* January 2, 1949.

Stuart, Roger. "Ambulance Score." *Pittsburgh Press,* January 11, 1970.

———. "Ex-Jobless Rushing to Rescue." *Pittsburgh Press,* November 11, 1968.

———. "Ex-Jobless to the Rescue." *Pittsburgh Press,* November 17, 1968.

Surgeon General, United States Army. *Medical and Surgical History of the War of the Rebellion.* Part 3, Vol. 2. Washington, D.C.: U.S. Government Printing Office, 1883.

———. *Reports on the Extent and Nature of the Materials Available for the Preparation of a Medical and Surgical History of the Rebellion.* Philadelphia: Lippincott, 1865.

"Survey of Ambulance Service Shows ... It's Awful." *The Modern Hospital* 85, no.2 (1955).

"Survey Shows Decrease in Private Ambulances." *The Modern Hospital* 109, no. 4 (October 1967).

Taylor, Blaine. "Close Encounters of the Cowley Kind." *Maryland State Medical Journal* 27, no. 6 (1978).

"Telephones in Mine Rescue Work." *The Modern Hospital* 4, no. 6 (1915).

"Texas Ambulance Crisis Growing." *The Modern Hospital* 113, no. 5 (November 1969).

"Texas Cities Take Over Ambulance Services as Undertakers Quit." *The Modern Hospital* 109, no. 1 (July 1967).

Thomas, M.W. *Police Communications.* Springfield, Ill.: C.C. Thomas, 1974.

Thompson, Judy. Email to author, January 27, 2004.

Timmermans, Stefan. "Hearts Too Good to Die." *Journal of Historical Sociology* 14, no. 1 (March 2001).

"To the Editor." *Times,* October 23, 1854.

Travell, Janet. *Office Hours: Day and Night.* New York: New American Library, 1968.

Truby, Albert. "History of the Airplane Ambulance." Typescript, Office of the Chief of Air Service, 1922.

"A true Report of the great Costs and Charges of the five Hospitals in the city of London under the Care of the Lord Mayor, Commonalty and Citizens of London, in the maintaining of a very great Number of poore the yeare last past [dated] 11th day of Aprill, 1653." London: n.p., 1653.

"A true report of the great costs and charges of the foure hospitals, in the city of London: in the maintenance of their great number of poore, this present yeare, 1644, as followeth." London: n.p., 1644.

"Turkey." *Times,* October 13, 1854.

"Twelve Can Ride." *The Modern Hospital* 79, no. 4 (1952).

United States Bureau of the Census. *Census of the Population: 1960.* Washington, D.C.: U.S. GPO, 1963.

United States Census Bureau. *Decennial Census Abstract 1940.* Washington, D.C.: U.S. GPO, 1941.

———. *Decennial Census Abstract 1950.* Washington, D.C.: U.S. GPO, 1951.

United States Department of Health and Human Services. Office of the Inspector General. "Medicare Payments for Ambulance Transports." OEI-05-02-00590. January 2006.

United States Department of Health, Education and

Welfare. *Ambulance Services and Hospital Emergency Departments.* DHEW Publication No. (HSM) 72-2022. Washington: U.S. Printing Office, 1972.

United States Department of Health, Education and Welfare. Division of Emergency Health Services. *Compendium of State Statutes on the Regulation of Ambulance Services, Operation of Emergency Vehicles and Good Samaritan Laws.* Washington, D.C.: U.S. GPO, June 1969.

United States House of Representatives. *House Journal,* February 8, 1859.

United States Surgeon General's Office. "Ambulance Corps." In *Medical and Surgical History of the War of the Rebellion.* Part 3, Vol. 2. Washington, D.C.: U.S. GPO, 1883.

University of Cincinnati. "Hospital History 1850–1880." University of Cincinnati College of Medicine, 2001–2008. www.med.uc.edu/about/history/htmlversion/page14.cfm.

Van Zandt, Raymond. "What 316 Patients Paid in Five Rochester Hospitals." *The Modern Hospital* 38, no. 6 (1932).

Vogt, Fred. "Open Memorandum: Standards." *Emergency Medical Services* 4, no. 1 (Jan./Feb. 1975).

Waller, Julian. "Reflections on Half a Century of Injury Control." *American Journal of Public Health* 84, no. 4 (April 1994).

Warren, Michael. "A Chronology of State Medicine, Public Health, Welfare and Related Services in Britain: 1066–1999." www.chronology.ndo.co.uk/1500-1699.htm.

Waters, John. "Am I My Brother's Keeper?" *Journal of Emergency Services* 6, no. 6 (1973).

Weaver, Jay. "History of the Boston Emergency Medical Services, 1891–1900." City of Boston, Oct. 16, 2007. http://www.bostonems.com/execoffice/history.html.

Weed, Guy. Correspondence from the Portland Accident Prevention Committee to the Officers and Members of the Townsend Old Age Pension Clubs. July 20, 1936. Multnomah County Central Library, Portland, Oregon.

Weingroff, Richard. "President Dwight D. Eisenhower and the Federal Role in Highway Safety, Chapter One." Federal Highway Administration. www.fhwa.dot.gov/infrastructure/safety01.htm.

Welles, Gideon. *Diary of Gideon Welles.* Vol. 1. Boston: Houghton, Mifflin, 1911.

West, Irma, et al. *Study of Emergency Ambulance Operations — A Preliminary Report.* Typescript, California State Department of Health/State Highway Patrol, 1964.

White, John. "Bellevue." *Fourth Annual Report of the Commissioners of Public Charities and Corrections.* New York: Frank McElroy, 1864.

White, Roger. "Shocking History." *Journal of Emergency Medical Services,* October 1995.

"White Car to the Rescue." *The Modern Hospital* 83, no. 5 (November 1954).

Wiegenstein, J. "The Need for Training Physicians in Emergency Medicine." *Journal of Trauma* 12, no. 5 (1972).

Wilbur, R.K. *Revolutionary Medicine.* N.p., 1976.

Willard, DeForest. *Ambulance Service in Philadelphia.* Philadelphia, 1883.

Williamson, Jeffrey. "The Structure of Pay in Britain: 1710–1911." *Research in Economic History* 7 (1982).

Wilson, Blake. *Music and Merchants: The Laudesi Companies of Republican Florence.* New York: Oxford University Press, 1992.

"Winged Ambulance of the United States Army." *Scientific American,* December 7, 1918.

Withington, E.T. *Medical History from the Earliest Times.* London: Scientific Press, 1894.

Woodward, Arthur. *Lances at San Pascual.* San Francisco: California Historical Society, 1948.

Woolf, S.J. "A New Hand Guides the Police Force." *New York Times,* January 29, 1929.

Young, Charles. *Clara Barton, A Centenary Tribute.* Boston: Gorham Press, 1922.

Young, Peter. "City Ambulance Associations." *Edinburgh Medical Journal* 30, no. 4 (1884).

Zoll, Paul, et al. "Termination of Ventricular Fibrillation in Man by Externally Applied Electric Counter Shock." *New England Journal of Medicine* 254, no. 16 (1956).

Index

Abbot, Downing Company 60, 173
Accidental Death and Disability 246, 249–250, 298
Adamson, Robert 194
Aherns, Henry 87
air ambulances 122; fixed wing 158–166 (*see also* Ardmore, Oklahoma; Colonial Air; Royal Flying Doctor Service; Scully-Walton; U.S. Army Air Service); helicopter 166–173 (*see also* Arizona Highway Patrol; Bell Aircraft; Maryland Police Aviation Command; MAST; Santa Monica Hospital)
Alberta, Canada 228
Allegheny County Medical Society 262
Amalfi, Italy 126, 129
ambulance crashes 182–189
ambulance design standards 244, 298–300, 319–322
ambulance operating costs 62, 233, 235, 239, 268, 335; automobiles 150–151, 153; horse drawn 150; offsets 295; wages 247–248
ambulance traffic regulations 177–183
ambulancias 11
American Ambulance Association 326, 336
American College of Surgeons 240, 252; Ambulance Report (1959) 228–229; equipment recommendations 244–245
American Legion ambulance 199
American Medical Response 225, 327
American Red Cross 135–136
American Revolution 30
American Women's Voluntary Services 122–123
Ardmore, Oklahoma 161
Arena, Ernest 109
Arizona Highway Patrol 169
Asclepius 3
attendants *see* interns; training

Baltimore Fire Department 220–221, 351
Baltimore Shock Trauma Center 169–171
Banks, Sam 252
barber-surgeons 14, 334
bariatric ambulance 225
Barr, Joseph 261, 271
Barringer, Emily *see* Dunning, Emily
Barton, Clara 135
Beck, C.S. 350
Beekman, James 57
Belfast Royal Victoria Hospital 254
Bell Aircraft Corporation 166–168
Bellevue Ambulance Service 58–65, 84, 107, 109
Bellevue Hospital 53–55, 61
Belmar Rescue and First Aid Squad 194–196, 199
Bernecker, Edward 110
best practices 338
Bigallo Hospital 9, 10, 13, 342
Bischoffsheim, H.L. 90
Blackwell, Elizabeth 114
Bliss, George 305
block grants 324
Boder, Mrs. Bartlett 123
Bonaparte, Napoleon 21
Borneo 132
Borsi, Pietro 7
Boston emergency ambulances 144
Boston Police Department 96
Bowditch, Henry 35, 37, 40
Boyd, David 315
Brandwell, Stephen 13
Bridgeport, Connecticut 146
Bringing Out the Dead 328
British Columbia 322–324
British National Aid Society 129
Brookes, Walter 282
Brooklyn, New York 74, 177, 181, 235
Brooklyn Health Service 67
Brooklyn Homeopathic Hospital 67
Brooklyn Hospital 67
Brooklyn infectious disease ambulances 68
Brooklyn Jewish Hospital 185, 235
Brooklyn Methodist-Episcopal Hospital 67
Brothers of Mercy 5–10, 12; *see also* Misericordia

Brown, Mitchell 272, 275
Buck Ambulance Company 155, 218, 294
Buffalo, New York 94, 166
Bull Run, Battle of 35, 37, 91
Bush, George W. 334

Cagle, Frances 282
call boxes 102–103
Canadian ambulance services *see* Alberta; British Columbia
Caroline, Nancy 276, 295, 296–297
Carter, Mary 122
Centre Street Hospital 65, 138
Chadwick, Walter 214
Chambers Street Hospital 67
Channing, W.F. 102
Chicago Fire Department 168, 231, 233, 252, 304
Chicago Police Department 231, 307
Chicago, private ambulances 72, 231, 305–310
cholera 24, 54, 55
Cholera Interdiction Squad 54, 55
Cincinnati Commercial Hospital 50
Cincinnati Police Department 96
Cinader, Robert 311
Citizens' Ambulance Service 266, 272
Civil Defense 238–239
Cleary, Joseph 91
Cleveland, Ohio 71, 94
Cloncurry, Queensland 164
Cobb, Leonard 292
Cody, Samuel 159
Cold War 236
Coleman, Morton 261
Colonial Air 155
Columbus, Ohio 290
communications 332; *see also* call boxes; telegraph
Confederate ambulances 41
Corcoran, Eugene 214
Cortese, James 269
Cowley, R Adams 169
Crane, Mary 157
Crane Oxygen and Ambulance Company 157
Cranston, Alan 316
Criley, Michael 290

379

Crimea 22, 23
Crossman, James 46, 89, 90
Crouse-Irving Hospital 256
Cummings, Patrick 93, 95

Dalton, Edward B. 54, 57, 79, 347
Daugherty, John 185
Davis, Arthur 268
Dean, Man Mountain 140
defibrillator 96, 254, 281, 349
design standards *see* ambulance design standards
Detroit, Michigan 94
dispatch 99; *see also* communications; telegraph
dreckapotheke 12
Dumas, Alexander 10
Duncan, Francis 129, 131
Dunning, Emily 113–121
du Puy, Raymond 126
Dusseldorf, O.L. 74

Edinburgh, Scotland 14
Edward, Prince of Wales 132
electric ambulances 146–147, 150, 152
Electromobile Company 91
Elm Park Riot 64–65
Emergency! 311, 316
emergency hospitals 137–145
emergency rooms 15, 143, 145
EMS Act (1973) 316
EMT training 215, 253, 271, 295–297; *see also* paramedic training
equipment standards 202, 224, 231, 240; *see also* American College of Surgeons
Esposito, Gerald 260, 263, 266
Etheridge, Anna 113

Farmer, Moses 102
Farrington, Joseph "Deke" 251, 295, 298
FDNY *see* New York City Fire Department
federal funding *see* block grants; Medicaid; Medicare
Feichter, Ralph 279
Fici, Lorenzo 6
fire surgeons 194, 199
Flaherty, Peter 269, 271, 275
Florence, Italy 5, 13,
Flushing Hospital 123
flying squads 301
Flynn, John 163
Foley, Mary 113, 122
fourgon 12
Frank, Aaron 189, 203
Frederick, Dolores 273
Frederick Wood and Son 146
Freedom House Ambulance Service 255–261, 296
Freedom House Enterprises Corporation 260
Fuller, Robert 312
Furley, John 129, 132

Gallagher, Bill 167
gasoline ambulances 146–154
Genesee Hospital 79, 123

George Baker Emergency Car 200–203
Georgia Street Receiving Hospital 140, 142
Gerard, Tonque (The Blessed) 126
German Samaritan Association 135
Gernster Field, Louisiana 159
Ghislieri, Francesco 6
Goler, George 185
Goodwin, E.B. 279, 281
Gouverneur Hospital 113
Grace, William 288, 290
Graf, Walter 290
Grant, Ulysses 32, 54
Grenfell, William 182
Grosman, George 158

Hadden, Adam 75
Hahnemann Hospital (Rochester, New York) 100, 108, 122
Halleck, Henry 32, 37
Hallen, Phil 255, 257, 277
Hammond, William 37
Harbor General Hospital (Los Angeles, California) 290
Harborview Hospital (Seattle, Washington) 292
Harlem Hospital (New York City) 112
Hasan, Sayyid 161
Hasbrouck, Stephen 83
Haywood County, North Carolina 278
Haywood County Volunteer Rescue Squad 278
Heart Mobiles 254, 290–294
helicopter ambulance 166–173; *see also* air ambulance
Henderson, Sir Edmund 90
Hess and Eisenhardt 176, 218
Heydecker, Mary 157
highway traffic safety planning 239–240, 244, 246; *see also* U.S. Department of Transportation
Hill District (Pittsburgh, Pennsylvania) 258
Hirschmann, Jim 285
Homeland Security, Department of 333–334
hospital ambulances 229, 233, 248; *see also* individual infirmaries
hospital wagons 31
Hospitallers of St. John 126–128
hospitals, pre-modern 4
Howard, Benjamin 28, 44–45, 54, 67, 89
Howell, Charlene 278, 279
Howell, Gene 278, 282
Hunt, William 270, 273

industrial emergency hospitals 144
infectious disease 27–30; *see also* cholera
interns 104–112
Isabella I, Queen 11, 12

Jackson City Hospital (Michigan) 150

Jackson Memorial Hospital (Mississippi) 285
James Cunningham and Son, and Company 15, 151, 218, 219
Jerusalem Ophthalmic Hospital 132
Johnson, Lyndon 245, 335
Jones, William 305
J.W. Stevens Disaster Car 181–183, 189, 203

Katz, David 262
Kenmore Hospital (Buffalo, New York) 167–168
Kenney, Lawrence 285
Kings County Hospital (New York City) 147
KKK-A-1822 Ambulance Standards 321, 337
Klotzback, Walter 209
Knights Hospitaller *see* Hospitallers of St. John
Knights of Malta *see* Sovereign Order of Malta
Koenigstein, Saxony 21
Korean War 166, 168
Kouwenhoven, William 349

LaGuardia, Fiorello 109
Laird, Melvin 171
Landini, Placido 6, 341
Larrey, Dominique 18–22
Laudesi Brotherhood of Or San Michele 341
Lawrence, David 256, 271
Lee, Duncan 58
Leipzig, Saxony 14
Letterman, Jonathan 32
Lieb, John 349
Life Care Ambulance 188
Limbourg, Belgium 18
London 24, 25, 91; charity hospitals 13, 47; plague (1665) 13; workhouses 25
London, Julie 312
London Boards of Guardians 24, 25
London Hospital Carriage Society 26, 27, 46, 132
London Metropolitan Police 87, 90
Long Island, New York 304
Los Angeles County Fire Department 141, 287, 291–292
Los Angeles Police Department 140–141
Low, Seth 114
Ludlow Massacre 191
Lynchburg Volunteer Life Saving and First Aid Crew 197

Magliabechi, Antonio 6
Malaga, Spain 11
Manchester Board of Health (England) 16, 25
Margerum, Mike 220–222
Marmon Company 153
Marvingt, Marie 121, 122
Maryland State Police Aviation Command 97, 170

Massachusetts General Hospital 68, 173
Massachusetts Homeopathic Hospital 151
MAST Program 97, 171–172
Mauricius 3, 5
McClean, Alice 122
McClellan, George 23, 32
McCoy, James 260
McElligott, John 194
McGann, Thomas 151
McGuire, Daniel 61
McMahon, Martin 220
Measure, Charles 194
medevac *see* air ambulance; MAST
Medicaid, reimbursement 334–336
Medicare, reimbursement 334–336
Medici, Coismo 9
Metropolitan Asylums Board (London) 28
Miami-Dade County Fire and Rescue 286
Miami Fire and Rescue 284–289
Michael Reese Hospital (Chicago, Illinois) 146
Middlesex Hospital (London, England) 15, 24
Milhon, Frank 196
Miller-Meteor 175, 247
Mine Safety Appliance Company 351
Misericordia 6, 10, 341–343
Mississippi Hospital Association 238
Moon, John 275
Moore, Margaret 150
mortuary ambulances 70, 72, 230, 246–249, 314
Moses, Israel 31
Mother, Jugs and Speed 328
Mount Sinai Hospital (New York City) 150
Muckle, Dave 109
Mulrooney, Edward 211
Murray, Tim 119

Nachtel, Henri 74
Nader, Ralph 245
Nagel, Eugene 284, 287
Nassau County Police Department 96
National Safety Bureau (United States) 96
New Orleans Charity Hospital 177
New York City 233
New York City Board of Ambulance Service 179
New York City Fire Department 193, 332
New York City Police Department 60; Emergency Services 207–216, 332
New York City Police Surgeons 61–65, 180
New York Hospital (New York City) 56–57, 67, 152, 181

Newark, New Jersey 87, 112
Night Medical Service: Europe 73; United States 74–75
99th Street Hospital (New York City) 67
Nixon, Richard 313, 316
non-emergency transfer service 157
Northern Hospital (Liverpool, England) 47, 70

occupational injury 337
Order of St. John 128
Otrera, Spain 11

Page, James 312
Pancoast, William 70
Pantridge, Frank 254, 279; *see also* Heart Mobiles
paramedic training 254–255, 264–267, 280–282, 289, 294, 295
Paris, France 74
Park Street Hospital *see* Centre Street Hospital
Peel, Sir Robert 81
Pennsylvania Hospital (Philadelphia) 69
Pennsylvania State Police 168
Percy, Baron 21
Peter of Verona 342
pharmacies 52, 139
Philadelphia, Pennsylvania 77
Philadelphia Alms House Hospital 70
Philadelphia Board of Health 69
Philadelphia Fire Companies 42, 69
Philadelphia Police Department 87
Pittsburgh, Pennsylvania 256
Pittsburgh Police Ambulances 257, 270, 274
Platt, Melville 295
police patrol ambulances 89, 138, 140–142, 227; *see also* individual police departments
police surgeons 81–87, 136; New York 81–86, 137; Philadelphia 87; San Francisco 86, 140
Polyclinic Hospital (New York City) 150
Poor Law Act (United Kingdom, 1881) 24
Poplar Accident Hospital (London, England) 138
popular culture, the ambulance in 328–330, 333; *see also* "Emergency!"
Port Authority Police (New York and New Jersey) 332
"Port of Broken Heads" 139; *see also* pharmacies
Portland, Oregon 138, 181, 188
Portland Emergency Hospital (Oregon) 143
Portland Fire Bureau (Oregon) 200
Portland Police Department (Oregon) 188

Presbyterian-University Hospital (Pittsburgh, Pennsylvania) 261

railroad accidents 77
Rayzer, Dave 268
Reagan, Ronald 324
Recktenwald, William 305
regionalized EMS 304, 317–319
Rescue 911 328
Rescue Squad 1 (FDNY) 193–194; *see also* New York City Fire Department
Rexall Drug Company 167
Reynolds, Kevin 215
Rhoades, A.L. 158
Richmond Ambulance Committee 41
Roanoke Life Saving and First Aid Crew 196
Roberts, Fred 200
Rochester, New York 72, 100, 185, 238
Rochester City Hospital (New York) 42, 100, 157, 174
Rochester Fire Department (New York) 201, 238
Rochester General Hospital *see* Rochester City Hospital
Rochester Homeopathic Hospital (New York) 69, 73, 100
Rochester Police Department (New York) 82, 91–95
Rochester Town Watch (New York) 80
Roosevelt Hospital (New York City) 67, 146, 179
Rose, Leonard 294
Royal Flying Doctor Service (Australia) 163–165

Safar, Peter 260, 262, 265, 270, 272, 298
St. Andrew's Ambulance Association 132
St. Bartholomew's Hospital (London, England) 91
St. Catherine's Hospital (Brooklyn) 67
St. John Ambulance Association 28, 129–134; *see also* hospitallers
St. John Ambulance Society 87, 126, 132–134
St. John Invalid Transportation Corps 132
Saint Louis, Missouri 52, 218
St. Tobit (Tobias) 343
St. Vincent's Hospital (New York City) 146, 288
Sampson, Grover 79
San Francisco, California 139
San Francisco Emergency Hospitals 140, 141
Sanitary Act (United Kingdom, 1860) 27
Sanitary Commission (United States) 36, 41, 217
Santa Monica Hospital (Los Angeles, California) 168

Seattle, Washington 95, 155, 231, 292
Seattle Fire Department 292
Second Alarmers Rescue Squad 234
Schultz, Jackson 56
Scully-Walton Ambulance Service 155
sedan chairs 13, 14, 17
Shephard Ambulance Service 155, 292
siren regulations 183–186
Smyrna, Delaware 199
Sovereign Order of Malta 128
Soviet Union ambulance services 314
speed limits 186–187
Stamey, Marty 279, 282
Stanton, Edwin 32, 37
Starrs, Ernest 228
Starzenski, Gene 277
steam powered ambulances 147, 150, 152
Stone, James 61
Stout, Samuel 41
streetcar ambulances 218, 219
Superior Ambulance Corporation 176
Swab Wagon Company 220–226
Swedish railroads 126

Taylor, Robert 58
telegraph dispatch 42, 51, 55, 57, 69, 99–102
Theresa, Sister Marie 113
Thomas, David 268
Tighe, Kevin 312
training 131–132, 240, 250–254, 264; *See also* EMT training; interns; paramedic training
trauma hospitals 326
Travell, Janet 152, 181
Traverso, Daniel 194
240-Robert 328; *see also* popular culture

Unfallstationen (Germany) 135
U.S. Army Air Service 161
U.S. Army motor ambulances 146–147
U.S. Bureau of Mines emergency services 190
U.S. Department of Emergency Medical Services 243, 295, 315
U.S. Department of Health, Education, and Welfare *see* U.S. Department of Emergency Medical Services
U.S. Department of Transportation 169, 246, 250, 253, 295, 298
U.S. Public Health Service 243
University of Maryland Shock Trauma Center 169

Vehicle Safety Act (United States, 1966) 319
Vickery, Gordon 292
Viet Nam War 171; *see also* MAST
Vogt, Fred 319
volunteer rescue squads 194, 227, 279; *see also* individual squads by name
von Esmarch, Johannes 134
Voorhis, James 85

wages 247; *see also* ambulance operating costs; Medicaid; Medicare
Walker, Jimmy 209
Walters, John 331
Waterloo 21
Webb, Jack 311, 316; *see also* "Emergency!"
Welles, Gideon 37
Wellington, Duke of 21, 22
Wenzel, F.G. 281
Whalen, Grover 209
White, Tom 119
White Motor Truck Company 208
Wise, Julian 196, 198, 246
women's contributions 122–125; *see also* named individuals
Women's Voluntary Service 122–123
Wood, Barbara 123
Wood, Fernando 81, 93
World War I 122, 198
World War II 122–123
wurst wagons 21

Y.M.C.A. 136; *see also* training

Zaharias, George 140
Zoll, Paul 350